THE YEAR IN
HEART FAILURE
VOLUME I

THE YEAR IN HEART FAILURE

VOLUME 1

Edited by

**ILEANA PIÑA, SIDNEY GOLDSTEIN,
MARK E DUNLAP**

CLINICAL PUBLISHING

OXFORD

Distributed worldwide by
CRC Press

Boca Raton   London   New York   Washington, DC

Clinical Publishing

an imprint of Atlas Medical Publishing Ltd

Oxford Centre for Innovation
Mill Street, Oxford OX2 0JX, UK

Tel: +44 1865 811116
Fax: +44 1865 251550
Web: www.clinicalpublishing.co.uk

Distributed by:

CRC Press LLC
2000 NW Corporate Blvd
Boca Raton, FL 33431, USA
E-mail: orders@crcpress.com

CRC Press UK
23–25 Blades Court
Deodar Road
London SW15 2NU, UK
E-mail: crcpress@itps.co.uk

A catalogue record for this book is available from the British Library

ISBN 1 904392 38 5
ISSN 1742-3074

**The publisher makes no representation, express or implied, that the dosages in this book are correct.
Readers must therefore always check the product information and clinical procedures with the
most up-to-date published product information and data sheets provided by the manufacturers and
the most recent codes of conduct and safety regulations. The authors and the publisher do not accept
any liability for any errors in the text or for the misuse or misapplication of material in this work**

Project manager: Rosemary Osmond
Typeset by Footnote Graphics Ltd, Warminster, Wiltshire, UK
Printed in Spain by T. G. Hostench, Barcelona

Contents

Part III

Innovative therapies, special populations

Part IV

The future

Editors

ILEANA L PIÑA, MD, Professor of Medicine, Case Western Reserve University; Division of Cardiology, University Hospitals of Cleveland, Cleveland, Ohio, USA

SIDNEY GOLDSTEIN, MD, Division Head Emeritus, Division of Cardiovascular Medicine, Henry Ford Hospital, Detroit, Michigan, USA

MARK E DUNLAP, MD, Associate Professor of Medicine, Physiology and Biophysics, Louis B Stokes VA Medical Center, Case Western Reserve University, Cleveland, Ohio, USA

Contributors

KIRKWOOD F ADAMS, MD, Associate Professor, Departments of Medicine and Radiology, School of Medicine, University of North Carolina, Chapel Hill, North Carolina, USA

INDER S ANAND, MD, FRCP, DPhil(Oxon), FACC, Professor of Medicine, Division of Cardiology, University of Minnesota Medical School; Director, Heart Failure Clinic, Veterans Administration Medical Center, Minneapolis, Minnesota, USA

EMILY L BURKETT, MS, Research Associate and Genetic Counsellor, Division of Cardiology, Oregon Health and Science University, Portland, Oregon, USA

MARK E DUNLAP, MD, Associate Professor of Medicine, Physiology and Biophysics, Louis B Stokes VA Medical Center, Case Western Reserve University, Cleveland, Ohio, USA

SIDNEY GOLDSTEIN, MD, Division Head Emeritus, Division of Cardiovascular Medicine, Henry Ford Hospital, Detroit, Michigan, USA

RAY E HERSHBERGER, MD, Associate Professor, Division of Cardiology, Oregon Health and Science University, Portland, Oregon, USA

STEVEN J KETEYIAN, PhD, Program Director, Preventive Cardiology, Division of Cardiovascular Medicine, Henry Ford Heart and Vascular Institute, Detroit, Michigan, USA

MIKHAIL KOSIBOROD, MD, Fellow, Section of Cardiovascular Medicine, and Clinical Scholar, Robert Wood Johnson Clinical Scholars Program, Yale University School of Medicine, New Haven, Connecticut, USA

HARLAN M KRUMHOLZ, MD, MSc, Professor of Medicine (Cardiology) and Epidemiology and Public Health, Yale University School of Medicine, New Haven, Connecticut, USA

PATRICK M McCARTHY, MD, Chief, Cardiothoracic Surgery, Co-Director, Northwestern Cardiovascular Institute, Galter; Professor of Surgery, Northwestern Medical School, Chicago, Illinois, USA

MANDEEP R MEHRA, MD, MBBS, Director, Ochsner Heart Failure and Cardiac Transplantation Program, Oschsner Clinic Foundation, New Orleans, Louisiana, USA

MARIA EUGENIA NATALE, MD, Clinical Cardiologist, Hospital Italiano, Buenos Aires, Argentina

CARLOS EDUARDO NEGRÃO, PhD, Professor of Medicine, Heart Institute (InCor), University of São Paulo Medical School, São Paulo, Brazil

JAMES O O'NEILL, MRCPI, Fulbright Scholar, Department of Cardiovascular Medicine, George M and Linda H Kaufman Center for Heart Failure, Cleveland Clinic Foundation, Cleveland, Ohio, USA

J HERBERT PATTERSON, PharmD, Associate Professor of Pharmacy, School of Pharmacy, and Research Associate Professor, School of Medicine, University of North Carolina, Chapel Hill, North Carolina, USA

ILEANA L PIÑA, MD, Professor of Medicine, Case Western Reserve University; Division of Cardiology, University Hospitals of Cleveland, Cleveland, Ohio, USA

MARGARET M REDFIELD, MD, Director, Mayo Heart Failure Program and Mayo Cardiorenal Research Laboratory, Mayo Clinic College of Medicine, Rochester, Minnesota, USA

MATT SAVAL, MS, Research Coordinator, Henry Ford Heart and Vascular Institute, Division of Cardiovascular Medicine, Detroit, Michigan, USA

RICARDO SERRA-GRIMA, MD, Professor of Cardiology and Sports Medicine, University of Barcelona; Director of Exercise Testing and Cardiac Rehabilitation, Holy Cross and St. Paul Hospital, Barcelona, Spain

JAMES B YOUNG, MD, FACC, Chairman, Division of Medicine, Professor and Academic Chair, Department of Medicine, Lerner College of Medicine of Case Western Reserve University; Medical Director, Kaufman Center for Heart Failure, Cleveland Clinic Foundation, Cleveland, Ohio, USA

Foreword

I would argue that there is no more important problem in cardiology than heart failure—for both the patient and society. Heart failure also presents an immense management challenge to physicians, surgeons, nurses and other members of the healthcare team. Fortunately, we are meeting this challenge and heart failure is one of the most vibrant and fruitful areas for clinical science and clinical trials in cardiology. Important developments occur almost monthly, creating a new challenge which is keeping up to date with all of these exciting reports. Help is at hand! *The Year in Heart Failure* provides a superb summary of the key recent publications in every important area of heart failure. A valuable commentary, placing these new reports in context, is also provided by a team of recognized experts. Epidemiology, pathophysiology, pharmacology, devices and surgical treatment are all covered. I particularly like the inclusion of a section on comorbidities, special populations and innovative therapies. I also like the inclusion of European and South American authors and perspectives on what is a global problem.

Drs Piña, Goldstein and Dunlap are to be congratulated on their selection of topics and authors and for their skilful editing. Each of the contributing authors, all distinguished investigators, must also be thanked for their elegant contributions. Everyone with an interest in heart failure will gain from having this fine book and, hopefully, so will more patients with that condition.

John McMurray
Professor of Medical Cardiology and
Honorary Consultant Cardiologist
Division of Cardiovascular Medicine
Gardiner Institute, Western Infirmary
Glasgow, Scotland

Part I

Epidemiology and pathophysiology

1

General trends in epidemiology

HARLAN KRUMHOLZ, MIKHAIL KOSIBOROD

Introduction

Recent studies have emphasized several important themes in the field of heart failure epidemiology. With the ageing of the US population, elderly patients with many coexisting medical conditions represent a growing majority of heart failure patients |**1**|. Moreover, a large proportion of older heart failure patients have preserved systolic left ventricular function (see Masoudi *et al.* below). These patients have been excluded from randomized clinical trials of heart failure therapies. As a result, little is known about effective therapies for these patients. Finally, even when effective therapies are known, studies suggest that many heart failure patients still do not receive guideline-recommended treatments such as angiotensin-converting enzyme inhibitors and β blockers |**2**|.

Given the magnitude of the problem, understanding the reasons behind the heart failure epidemic and the development of strategies to reverse it should be top public health priorities. Research contributions reviewed in this chapter have been selected from a large body of excellent work published in the preceding 12–18 months. They offer valuable insights into the latest trends in heart failure epidemiology and highlight potential approaches to improving care for patients with heart failure. These studies are grouped into four major categories: general trends in heart failure epidemiology, heart failure with preserved systolic function, predictors of prognosis in heart failure patients, and quality of care in heart failure patients.

Long-term trends in the incidence of and survival with heart failure
Levy D, Kenchaiah S, Larson MG, *et al. N Engl J Med* 2002; **347**(18): 1397–402

B A C K G R O U N D . **Long-term trends in the incidence of heart failure and survival after the diagnosis of heart failure in the community have not been well characterized. The Framingham Heart Study provides an excellent opportunity to track these trends over time.**

INTERPRETATION. Investigators examined temporal trends in the incidence of and survival with heart failure among patients in the Framingham Heart Study during a 50-year interval from the 1950s through the 1990s. The Framingham Heart Study used uniform criteria and methods of ascertainment for the diagnosis of heart failure. Cases of heart failure were classified according to the date of onset: 1950–1969, 1970–1979, 1980–1989, and 1990–1999. Age-adjusted mortality rates for 30 days, 1 year and 5 years were calculated. Heart failure occurred in 1075 subjects (51% women). As compared with the rate for the period between 1950 and 1969, the incidence of heart failure remained unchanged in men in three subsequent periods, but declined by 31% in women (rate ratio for the period from 1990 to 1999, 0.69; 95% confidence interval [CI] 0.51–0.93). The 30-day, 1-year and 5-year age-adjusted mortality rates among men declined from 12, 30 and 70%, respectively, in the period from 1950 to 1969, to 11, 28 and 59%, respectively, in the period from 1990 to 1999. The corresponding rates in women were 18, 28, and 57% for the period from 1950 to 1969, and 10, 24, and 45% for the period between 1990 and 1999. After multivariable adjustment, long-term mortality was significantly lower in both men and women for the period from 1990 to 1999 as compared with the period from 1950 to 1969, but not for other time periods (Table 1.1).

Comment

This was one of the largest community-based studies of trends in heart failure incidence and mortality. Some of the major attributes of this Framingham investigation included prospective collection of data from an unselected cohort of patients in the community, with over 50 years of follow-up, and using uniform criteria for the diagnosis of heart failure. The study demonstrated a significant reduction in heart failure mortality in both men and women in the period 1990–1999, as compared with the period 1950–1969. Whether this was due to better management of risk factors such as hypertension, valve disease and coronary disease, increasing use of pharmacological

Table 1.1 Long-term trends in the adjusted risk of death after the onset of heart failure, 1950–1999 (hazard ratio [95% confidence interval])

Period	Men		Women	
	Age-adjusted*	Adjusted for multiple variables†	Age-adjusted*	Adjusted for multiple variables†
1950–1969‡	1.00	1.00	1.00	1.00
1970–1979	1.06 [0.79–1.41]	1.02 [0.76–1.37]	0.96 [0.68–1.33]	0.93 [0.67–1.30]
1980–1989	0.85 [0.63–1.13]	0.82 [0.61–1.10]	0.80 [0.58–1.11]	0.77 [0.55–1.07]
1990–1999	0.74 [0.54–1.01]	0.69 [0.50–0.95]	0.71 [0.50–1.00]	0.68 [0.48–0.98]
Overall trend	0.90 [0.82–0.99]	0.88 [0.80–0.97]	0.89 [0.80–0.99]	0.88 [0.78–0.98]
P value for trend	0.03	0.01	0.03	0.02

*All values were adjusted for age (<55, 55–64, 65–74, 75–84, and ≥85 years).
†All values were adjusted for age (<55, 55–64, 65–74, 75–84, and ≥85 years) and the presence or absence of hypertension, electrocardiographic evidence of left ventricular hypertrophy, diabetes mellitus, valve disease, and a history of myocardial infarction.
‡This period served as the reference category.
Source: Levy *et al.* (2002).

agents that improve survival in heart failure such as angiotensin-converting enzyme inhibitors and β blockers, or changes in the pathophysiology of heart failure such as the increasing proportion of patients with preserved left ventricular systolic function, is unclear.

However, several words of caution in the interpretation of the study are in order. First, the mortality rates for the period between 1990 and 1999 were only directly compared with the mortality rates for the period 1950–1969—the era when the treatment of risk factors for heart failure, as well as heart failure itself, was minimal. As no direct comparison was performed for the period of 1990–1999 with the decade of 1980–1989, it is unclear whether any significant improvement in mortality has occurred in the past 20 years. Secondly, the data on the baseline characteristics of patients enrolled into the study (including the aetiology of heart failure, the degree of left ventricular systolic dysfunction and comorbidities) were not provided. Therefore, the study did not account for the changing cause of heart failure over time, and it is also unclear whether the patients in this study were representative of the typical heart failure patient population. Finally, the patients enrolled in the Framingham cohort could have had better access to preventive care and more rigorous follow-up than other patients with heart failure—a limitation the authors have acknowledged in the article.

Mortality trends for 23 505 Medicare patients hospitalized with heart failure in Northeast Ohio, 1991 to 1997

Baker DW, Einstadter D, Thomas C, Cebul RD. *Am Heart J* 2003; **146**(2): 258–64

BACKGROUND. Mortality trends in patients with heart failure during the 1990s have not been well described.

INTERPRETATION. Investigators analysed mortality trends from 1991 to 1997 for 23 505 Medicare patients hospitalized with a first admission for heart failure at 29 northeast Ohio hospitals. The data were abstracted from the Cleveland Health Quality Choice Program and Medicare administrative databases. Logistic regression was used to analyse trends in risk-adjusted in-hospital, 30-day and 1-year mortality. Between 1991 and 1997, the mean length of stay declined steeply from 9.2 to 6.6 days (*P* <0.001 for trend). Risk-adjusted in-hospital mortality also decreased significantly (absolute decline 3.7%; 95% CI 3.0–4.3%), which corresponded to 52.8% relative decline. However, this was accompanied by a significant rise in post-discharge mortality (Fig. 1.1). As a result, the decline in 30-day mortality was less impressive (absolute decline 1.4%; relative decline 15.3%). There was also a modest decline in 1-year mortality (absolute decline 5.3%; relative decline 14.6%).

Comment

This was the largest population-based study to examine recent trends in heart failure mortality. Although the investigators found modest declines in short- and long-term

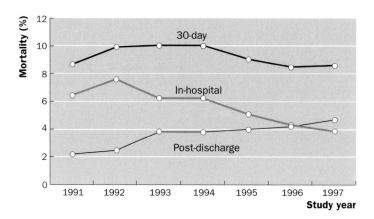

Fig. 1.1 Trends in unadjusted in-hospital, post-discharge (between discharge and 30 days after admission, and 30-day mortality rates from 1991 to 1997 for Medicare patients discharged with a principal diagnosis of heart failure from 29 hospitals participating in the Cleveland Health Quality Choice Program. All trends were significant at $P < 0.001$. Source: Baker *et al.* (2003).

mortality between 1991 and 1997, mortality rates remain extremely high for patients with heart failure. The study revealed another troubling trend. As the length of hospital stay declined sharply during the study period, there was a corresponding fall in in-hospital mortality. However, most of this decline was negated by a sharp rise in post-discharge mortality. Studies that focus on in-hospital mortality would miss this rise in early post-discharge mortality. The main limitation of this study was that the diagnosis of heart failure was determined from the administrative databases, and not confirmed with clinical chart review.

Heart failure and the aging population: an increasing burden in the 21st century?

Stewart S, MacIntyre K, Capewell S, McMurray JJV. *Heart* 2003; **89**(1): 49–53

BACKGROUND. Despite an overall decline in the age-adjusted mortality from coronary disease, there is evidence to suggest that the number of patients with heart failure is rising. This may result from the ageing of the population, with an increasing proportion of patients with major risk factors for heart failure, such as hypertension and coronary artery disease, as well as the longer survival of patients with coronary artery disease and acute myocardial infarction. There is, therefore, a need to project a future burden of heart failure in the community.

INTERPRETATION. Current estimates of prevalence, general practice consultation rates and hospital admission rates related to heart failure were applied to the entire population of Scotland. These estimates were then projected over the period 2000–2020 on an age- and sex-specific basis, using expected changes in the age structure of the Scottish population. The aim was to calculate the current (year 2000), short-term (2005), medium-term (2010) and long-term (2020) burden of heart failure in Scotland. The investigators estimated that there will be 105 000 (33%) more men and 122 000 (28%) more women aged ≥65 years in Scotland in the year 2020, as compared with 2000. The number of men with chronic heart failure was estimated to rise by 2300 (6%), 4900 (12%) and 12 300 (31%) in the years 2005, 2010 and 2020, respectively. The corresponding numbers in women were estimated to rise by 1500 (3%), 3100 (7%) and 7800 (17%) in the years 2005, 2010 and 2020, respectively. The number of hospital admissions for heart failure is expected to rise by 52% in men and 16% in women in the year 2020, as compared with the year 2000.

Comment

This study projected a substantial increase in the burden of heart failure over the next 20 years. Even though the investigators made a number of assumptions to arrive at their projections (such as assuming no change in heart failure prevalence over the next 20 years and no change in outcomes, such as the rate of hospital admissions for heart failure), they clearly pointed out that the ageing of the population will most likely lead to a marked increase in the number of patients with heart failure and in the utilization of healthcare resources due to heart failure. This information highlights the importance of the heart failure 'epidemic' as one of the top public health priorities, and is invaluable for future healthcare planning.

Natural history of asymptomatic left ventricular systolic dysfunction in the community

Wang TJ, Evans JC, Benjamin EJ, Levy D, LeRoy EC, Vasan RS. *Circulation* 2003; **108**(8): 977–82

BACKGROUND. The natural history of asymptomatic left ventricular systolic dysfunction (ALVD) in the community is not well described. Specifically, information regarding the rates of progression to overt heart failure and mortality in these patients is limited.

INTERPRETATION. The authors studied an unselected group of 4257 patients who participated in the Framingham Heart Study and underwent routine echocardiography as part of the study protocol. The patients were subsequently followed for up to 12 years, and carefully monitored for the development of cardiovascular disease events. The overall prevalence of ALVD was 3% (95% CI 2.5–3.5%), and increased with age. The majority of ALVD patients (61%) had mild ALVD (ejection fraction [EF] 40–50%), 33% of patients had moderate ALVD, and 6% had severe ALVD. About one-third of patients with ALVD did not have either a prior history of myocardial infarction or significant valve disease. During the

12 years of follow-up, overt heart failure developed in 26% of patients with ALVD. Patients with ALVD were at higher risk of developing heart failure than patients without ALVD, and the risk increased with greater severity of ALVD (Fig. 1.2). After multivariable adjustment there was a gradient of rising heart failure risk with increasing degrees of ALVD (hazard ratio [HR] 3.3; 95% CI 1.65–6.64 for mild ALVD; HR 7.77; 95% CI 3.86–15.63 for moderate to severe ALVD, no ALVD—referent). The risk of heart failure was also markedly increased even in those ALVD patients without a history of myocardial infarction or significant valve disease, in whom baseline echocardiography would not be typically indicated (HR 6.50; 95% CI 3.13–13.50). ALVD was also associated with increased risk of mortality (HR 1.6; 95% CI 1.1–2.4).

Comment

This study is the best description of the natural history of ALVD in the community. It has clearly documented that ALVD is not infrequent in the community, and is associated with a markedly increased risk of developing overt heart failure, as well as a higher risk of mortality. However, data on the appropriate treatment of patients with mild ALVD (the most prevalent form of ALVD in the study) were lacking, and the majority of patients with ALVD had a history of myocardial infarction or valve disease—which would typically necessitate echocardiographic evaluation. Therefore, whether community-wide screening with echocardiography will reduce the incidence of overt heart failure or improve outcomes is unclear.

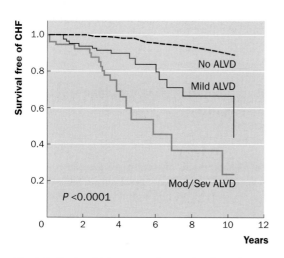

Fig. 1.2 Kaplan–Meier curves for survival free of congestive heart failure (CHF). The referent group consisted of subjects with normal left ventricular systolic function (EF >50%); those with mild asymptomatic left ventricular systolic dysfunction (ALVD) had an EF of 40–50%; those with moderate to severe (Mod/Sev) ALVD had an EF <40%. Source: Wang et al. (2003).

Most hospitalized older persons do not meet the enrolment criteria for clinical trials in heart failure

Masoudi FA, Havranek EP, Wolfe P, *et al. Am Heart J* 2003; **146**(2): 250–7

BACKGROUND. The magnitude of the discrepancy between patient populations in clinical trials and in the community is not well documented. The authors determined the proportion of older persons meeting enrolment criteria of randomized clinical trials of agents proven to prolong life in heart failure.

INTERPRETATION. The investigators evaluated the medical records of a representative group of 20 388 Medicare beneficiaries aged ≥65 years, hospitalized in acute care facilities in the US with the principal diagnosis of heart failure, who had an assessment of left ventricular systolic function. The enrolment criteria of the Studies of Left Ventricular Dysfunction (SOLVD), Metoprolol CR/LX Randomized Intervention Trial in Congestive Heart Failure (MERIT-HF) and Randomized Aldactone Evaluation Study (RALES) trials were applied to the population. The mean age of the population was 78 years, most of the patients were women (57%), and non-cardiac comorbidities were common (chronic obstructive pulmonary disease 32%, diabetes 38%, dementia, cancer or hepatic failure 10%). Only a small minority of patients would have qualified for randomized trials (25% for RALES, 17% for SOLVD and 13% for MERIT-HF; see Table 1.2). Of the total cohort, 67% of the patients did not fit the enrolment criteria of any of the three randomized trials, and the proportion of ineligible patients increased with age and was higher in women (75%) than in men (59%). The proportion of patients not included because of preserved left ventricular systolic function was at least twice as large as the proportion of patients who fit the enrolment criteria.

Table 1.2 Proportions of the total National Heart Failure cohort and the subgroup with impaired left ventricular systolic function meeting all the enrolment criteria for selected clinical trials of heart failure pharmacotherapy

	SOLVD			RALES			MERIT-HF		
	Total	Male	Female	Total	Male	Female	Total	Male	Female
Number meeting enrolment criteria	3579	2002	1557	5158	2787	2371	2726	1495	1231
Percentage of total cohort	17	23	13*	5	32	21*	13	17	11*
Percentage of cohort with impared LVSF	38	40	35*	55	55	54†	25	26	23†

SOLVD, Studies of Left Ventricular Dysfunction; RALES, Randomized Aldactone Evaluation Study; MERIT-HF, Metoprolol CR/LX Randomized Intervention Trial in Congestive Heart Failure.
*P <0.0001 compared with men.
†P <0.01 compared with men.
Source: Masoudi *et al.* (2003).

Comment

In this large, nationally representative cohort, more than two-thirds of the patients would not have met the enrolment criteria for any of the three major randomized clinical trials that evaluated life-saving therapies in patients with heart failure. This investigation highlighted a striking disparity between the patient populations evaluated in the randomized trials and those seen in 'real-world' clinical practice. Most of this disparity stems from the exclusion of older patients, women, and those with preserved systolic function from clinical trials. As these patients represent the majority of patients with heart failure – a trend which is likely to continue with the ageing of the population – this study has highlighted the importance of trials that address the needs of this specific group.

Heart failure with preserved left ventricular systolic function

Burden of systolic and diastolic ventricular dysfunction in the community: appreciating the scope of the heart failure epidemic
Redfield MM, Jacobson SJ, Burnett JC, Mahoney DW, Bailey KR, Rodeheffer RJ. *JAMA* 2003; **289**(2): 194–202

BACKGROUND. It is estimated that nearly half of all patients with overt congestive heart failure have diastolic dysfunction without a reduction in systolic left ventricular function. However, the prevalence of diastolic dysfunction and its relation to systolic dysfunction and symptomatic heart failure in the community is unknown.

INTERPRETATION. Investigators performed a cross-sectional survey of 2042 randomly identified residents of Olmsted County, Minnesota, aged ≥45 years. All participants underwent a complete physical examination and Doppler echocardiography, which included detailed measurements of systolic and diastolic left ventricular function, and were then followed for 3 years. Trained personnel abstracted the medical records of the participants for diagnosis of heart failure (using Framingham criteria), coronary artery disease, hypertension, other medical history and selected comorbidities. The prevalence of confirmed heart failure was 2.2% (95% CI 1.6–2.8%), and 44% of patients with heart failure had preserved left ventricular ejection fraction (LVEF). The prevalence of validated heart failure increased with age, and was higher in men (2.7%) than in women (1.7%).

Overall, 20.8% of participants had mild, 6.6% moderate, and 0.7% severe diastolic dysfunction. Of patients with preserved left ventricular function, 5.6% had moderate or severe diastolic dysfunction. The prevalence of diastolic dysfunction increased with age, was equally common in men and women, and was more common in patients with coronary artery disease, diabetes, and in those with systolic dysfunction. The prevalence of systolic dysfunction (LVEF ≤50%) was 6.5%. Less than half of the patients with either systolic dysfunction or moderate/severe diastolic dysfunction had a confirmed diagnosis of heart failure. Both mild and moderate/severe diastolic dysfunction parameters were powerful predictors of all-cause mortality, both in unadjusted analysis (Fig. 1.3) and after multivariable adjustment (HR 8.31; 95% CI 3.00–23.1 for mild, and HR 10.17; 95% CI 3.28–31.0 for moderate/severe diastolic dysfunction).

Comment

This study clearly demonstrated that diastolic dysfunction is common in the community. Both systolic as well as diastolic dysfunction parameters were frequently present in patients without a confirmed diagnosis of heart failure. Any degree of diastolic dysfunction was strongly predictive of higher all-cause mortality. The average age in this study was considerably younger than that seen in a typical representative sample of patients with heart failure. Because the prevalence of heart failure increases with age and older patients with heart failure are more likely to have preserved systolic function, the ageing of the population is likely to result in higher numbers of patients with both symptomatic and asymptomatic diastolic dysfunction. Whether screening patients in the community for pre-clinical systolic and diastolic dysfunction will result in the prevention of clinical heart failure and improvement in patient outcomes is unknown.

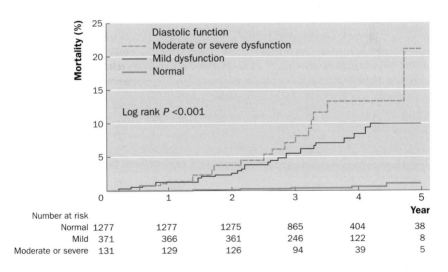

Fig. 1.3 Kaplan–Meier mortality curves for participants with normal diastolic function versus subjects with mild or moderate or severe diastolic dysfunction.
Source: Redfield *et al.* (2003).

Outcomes in heart failure patients with preserved ejection fraction: mortality, re-admission and functional decline

Smith GL, Masoudi FA, Vaccarino V, Radford MJ, Krumholz HM. *J Am Coll Cardiol* 2003; **41**(9): 1510–18

BACKGROUND. The trajectory of illness in patients hospitalized for heart failure with preserved LVEF is not well established. The authors assessed the risks of mortality, all-cause and heart failure re-admissions, and decline in functional status in patients with preserved LVEF hospitalized for heart failure.

INTERPRETATION. The investigators evaluated 413 consecutive patients admitted to a single medical centre between 1996 and 1998 with the clinically confirmed diagnosis of heart failure. Of 413 patients, 200 (48%) had preserved EF (defined as EF ≥40%), and these patients tended to be older, female, and more likely to have a history of hypertension. The patients with preserved EF had lower 6-month mortality as compared with patients who had depressed EF (13 vs 21%; $P = 0.02$). In multivariable analysis, preserved EF continued to be associated with better survival, as compared with depressed EF (HR 0.51; 95% CI 0.27–0.96). There was no difference in all-cause or heart failure re-admissions between patients with preserved versus depressed EF (HR 1.01; 95% CI 0.72–1.43, and HR 0.77; 95% CI 0.38–1.56, respectively). Although more patients with preserved EF had declined in activities of daily living at 6 months, as compared with patients who had depressed EF, this difference was not statistically significant (30 vs 23%; $P = 0.14$).

Comment

Even though this study was limited by the relatively small numbers and the single centre experience, it has illuminated the substantial morbidity and mortality experienced by patients hospitalized with heart failure who have preserved EF. Even though the mortality was lower in this group, patients with preserved EF and heart failure were at as high a risk of re-admissions and functional decline as patients with depressed EF.

Gender, age, and heart failure with preserved left ventricular systolic function

Masoudi FA, Havranek EP, Smith GL, *et al. J Am Coll Cardiol* 2003; **41**(2): 217–23

BACKGROUND. Whether women are more likely to have heart failure with preserved LVEF has not been well established. The authors examined the data from the Centers for Medicare and Medicaid Services' National Heart Failure Project to determine the relative contributions of gender, age and comorbidity to the prevalence of heart failure with preserved left ventricular systolic function.

INTERPRETATION. The investigators evaluated a cohort of 19 710 patients hospitalized with clinically confirmed heart failure, aged ≥65 years, who had an assessment of left ventricular systolic function. Of these patients, 6754 (34%) had normal left ventricular systolic function. In women, preserved left ventricular systolic function was present in 43%, whereas in men it was present in 23% of patients. After adjustment for demographic and clinical variables, female gender (relative risk [RR] 1.71; 95% CI 1.63–1.78) was significantly associated with preserved left ventricular systolic function. The association between increasing age and preserved left ventricular systolic function was also present, although it was not as striking (for age group 70–74 years, RR 1.09; 95% CI 1.01–1.17). Comorbidities associated with preserved left ventricular systolic function included hypertension, chronic obstructive pulmonary disease, atrial fibrillation and aortic stenosis.

Comment

This large, nationally representative study demonstrated that heart failure with preserved left ventricular systolic function is a condition that much more commonly affects women. This association was observed across a wide spectrum of patient characteristics, and was not affected by multivariable adjustments. As major randomized clinical trials include only patients with depressed left ventricular systolic function, therapeutic strategies for a large proportion of women with heart failure have not been adequately evaluated.

Predictors of prognosis in patients with heart failure

Predicting mortality among patients hospitalized for heart failure. Derivation and validation of a clinical model

Lee DS, Austin PC, Rouleus JL, Liu PP, Naimark D, Tu JV. *JAMA* 2003; **290**(19): 2581–7

BACKGROUND. A predictive model of mortality in heart failure could be useful for clinicians to improve risk stratification, counselling and management of hospitalized patients. Such well-developed models are not currently available for patients with heart failure.

INTERPRETATION. The authors studied 4031 community-based patients hospitalized with heart failure in Ontario, Canada (2624 patients in the derivation cohort from 1999 to 2001, and 1407 patients in the validation cohort from 1997 to 1999). Multivariable predictors of mortality at 30 days and 1 year included older age, lower systolic blood pressure, higher respiratory rate, higher blood urea nitrogen level, hyponatraemia, and comorbidities (such as cerebrovascular disease, chronic obstructive pulmonary disease, cirrhosis, dementia, and cancer). A risk index was subsequently developed, which stratified patients into low-, intermediate- and high-risk individuals. Patients with very high risk scores (>150) had a mortality rate of 59% at 30 days and 78.8% at 1 year, whereas patients with very low risk scores had corresponding rates of 0.8 and 9.0%. The risk index remained highly predictive of mortality in the validation cohort.

Comment

This study developed a community-based risk assessment tool that allows for both short- and long-term assessment of prognosis in patients with heart failure. It is relatively simple, and could be easily used by clinicians to improve counselling and management of patients with heart failure. As this risk index was developed for patients hospitalized with heart failure, whether it will be applicable to outpatients with heart failure is unclear.

Temporal relations of atrial fibrillation and congestive heart failure and their joint influence on mortality: the Framingham Heart Study

Wang TJ, Larson MG, Levy D, *et al. Circulation* 2003; **107**(23): 2920–5

BACKGROUND. Heart failure and atrial fibrillation frequently coexist, and both disproportionately affect the elderly. Although several studies have addressed the joint prognosis of heart failure and atrial fibrillation, they had multiple limitations and offered conflicting results. The authors' objective was to characterize the joint epidemiology of heart failure and atrial fibrillation in a large, well-monitored community-based cohort.

INTERPRETATION. The investigators evaluated 1470 patients from the Framingham Heart Study, aged ≥50 years, who developed new-onset atrial fibrillation or heart failure between 1948 and 1995. They examined whether survival after the onset of atrial fibrillation was affected by the subsequent development of heart failure, and vice versa. In addition, they tested whether survival after the onset of atrial fibrillation was affected by the pre-existing diagnosis of heart failure, and vice versa. The time period (1948–1969, 1970–1979, 1980–1989, 1990 or later) was included to account for secular trends in mortality.

Overall, 382 patients (26%) developed both atrial fibrillation and heart failure, of which 38% had atrial fibrillation first, 41% had heart failure first, and 21% had both diagnosed the same day. Among those patients with new-onset atrial fibrillation who were initially free of heart failure (*n* = 144), the subsequent development of heart failure was associated with considerably higher mortality (HR 2.7; 95% CI 1.9–3.7 for men, and HR 3.1; 95% CI 2.2–4.2 in women). The subsequent development of atrial fibrillation in patients with new-onset heart failure (*n* = 159) was also associated with increased mortality during follow-up (HR 1.6; 95% CI 1.2–2.1 for men, HR 2.7; CI 2.0–3.6 in women). Whereas the prior diagnosis of heart failure adversely influenced survival in patients with new-onset atrial fibrillation, prior diagnosis of atrial fibrillation did not have an effect on mortality in patients with new-onset heart failure (Table 1.3).

Comment

This investigation had several distinct strengths, including the predominant use of incident cases for both conditions, the evaluation of a relatively unselected community-based cohort over several decades of observation, and the use of uniform criteria for the diagnosis of heart failure. It provides support for the common clinical perception that the combination of atrial fibrillation and heart failure is associated with worse prognosis than either condition alone. Even though aggressive maintenance of sinus rhythm has not been shown to affect outcomes in all patients with atrial fibrillation, these findings raise the question of whether rhythm maintenance therapy should be considered in patients with heart failure.

However, several important limitations deserve attention. Left ventricular systolic function was not determined in these patients. Therefore, it is unclear whether the prognostic effects of atrial fibrillation and heart failure may be different in patients with preserved versus impaired left ventricular systolic function. In addition, the study period spanned several decades, during which the management of both atrial fibrillation and heart failure changed dramatically. As the results were not stratified by time period, the trends in the prognostic implications of atrial fibrillation and heart failure were not specified. Finally, because most patients in this study were evaluated prior to 1990, it is unclear whether these results can be accurately extrapolated to the patients currently diagnosed with atrial fibrillation and heart failure.

Table 1.3 Cox multivariable proportional hazards models examining the impact of the cormorbid condition on mortality

Models	Men, adjusted HR (95% CI)	Women, adjusted HR (95% CI)
Comorbid condition as a time-dependent variable		
(a) Mortality after AF		
Impact of incident CHF	2.7 (1.9 to 3.7)*	3.1 (2.2 to 4.2)*
(b) Mortality after CHF		
Impact of incident AF	1.6 (1.2 to 2.1)†	2.7 (2.0 to 3.6)*
Comorbid condition as a categorical variable		
(c) Mortality after AF		
Impact of prior CHF	2.2 (1.6 to 3.0)*	1.8 (1.3 to 2.3)*
Impact of concurrent CHF‡	2.4 (1.6 to 3.5)*	1.4 (1.0 to 1.9)
(d) Mortality after CHF		
Impact of prior AF	0.8 (0.6 to 1.0)	1.2 (0.9 to 1.6)
Impact of concurrent AF‡	1.0 (0.7 to 1.4)	1.1 (0.8 to 1.5)

*$P \leq 0.0001$, †$P < 0.01$.
‡Diagnosed on same day. Each letter (a through d) denotes a separate model. Models with the comorbid condition as a time-dependent variable (a and b) are restricted to those without the comorbid condition at the index event. Hazard ratios (HR) are adjusted for age, time period, myocardial infarction, stroke/transient ischaemic attack, diabetes, valvular disease, ECG left ventricular hypertrophy, systolic blood pressure, antihypertensive therapy, and smoking.
Source: Wang *et al.* (2003).

Inflammatory markers and risk of heart failure in the elderly subjects without prior myocardial infarction: the Framingham Heart Study

Vasan RS, Sullivan LM, Roubenoff R, *et al. Circulation* 2003; **107**(11): 1486–91

BACKGROUND. Studies have suggested that the serum levels of pro-inflammatory cytokines, such as tumour necrosis factor-α, interleukin-6 and C-reactive protein, are elevated in patients with established heart failure, and associated with adverse outcomes. However, whether the levels of cytokines can predict the development of heart failure in asymptomatic individuals is unknown.

INTERPRETATION. The authors evaluated 732 elderly (mean age 78 years) participants in the Framingham Heart Study, who had measurements of pro-inflammatory cytokines and no evidence of heart failure at baseline, and followed them closely for a mean of 5.2 years. All patients were under continuous surveillance for the development of cardiovascular disease events. On follow-up, 56 patients (7.6%) developed heart failure. The cumulative incidence of heart failure increased with higher levels of inflammatory cytokines (Fig. 1.4). In multivariable analysis, the RR of developing heart failure increased by 68% per tertile increase in concentration of interleukin-6, and 60% per tertile increase in concentration of tumour necrosis factor-α. Patients with elevated C-reactive protein levels (≥5 mg/dl) were also at increased risk of heart failure (HR 2.81; 95% CI 1.22–6.50). Patients with elevation of all three pro-inflammatory cytokines had a markedly increased risk of heart failure (HR 4.07; 95% CI 1.34–12.37). Stepwise backward elimination analysis identified the interleukin-6 level as the best predictor of heart failure among the three inflammatory markers.

Comment

This was the first study to prospectively identify inflammatory cytokines as risk factors for the development of heart failure in asymptomatic community-based patients. Whether elevated cytokine levels are markers of an inflammatory state that antedates the development of heart failure or mediators of adverse outcomes is unclear. To date, therapies aimed at the inhibition of inflammation have not proven effective in patients with heart failure. It is also unclear whether cytokine levels will substantially improve the ability of clinicians to identify patients at high risk for *de novo* heart failure. Most of these patients are likely to have other cardiovascular risk factors, and may be identified with careful clinical follow-up and echocardiography alone (patients in this investigation did not undergo echocardiography, and it is unclear what proportion of patients with elevated cytokine levels could have had asymptomatic systolic and/or diastolic dysfunction).

(a) Serum IL-6 and CHF risk

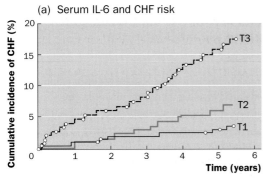

(b) Spontaneous production of TNF-α by
    PBMC and CHF risk

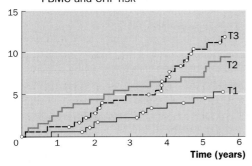

(c) Serum C-reactive protein and CHF risk

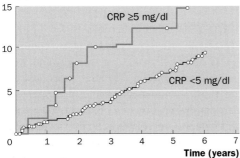

Fig. 1.4 (a) Kaplan–Meier plots showing the crude cumulative incidence of CHF in subjects according to tertiles of serum interleukin-6 (IL-6), (b) the spontaneous production of tumour necrosis factor-α (TNF-α) by peripheral blood mononuclear cells (PBMC), and (c) for individuals with serum C-reactive protein (CRP) values above and below 5 mg/dl. T1, T2 and T3 represent the tertiles of the marker (T3 being the top tertile). Number of CHF cases/number at risk for each tertile: serum IL-6 (pg/ml); T1, 7/220 (3.2%); T2, 11/167 (6.6%); T3, 24/165 (14.5%). PBMC spontaneous production of TNF-α (ng/ml): T1, 9/217 (4.1%); T2, 18/220 (8.2%); T3, 19/199 (9.5%). For serum CRP: <5 mg/dl, 48/657 (7.3%); ≥5 mg/dl, 8.66 (12.1%). Source: Vasan et al. (2003).

Plasma homocysteine and risk for congestive heart failure in adults without prior myocardial infarction

Vasan RS, Beiser A, D'Agostino RB, et al. JAMA 2003; **289**(10): 1251–7

BACKGROUND. Elevated homocysteine levels have been associated with greater risk of coronary artery disease, stroke and cardiovascular mortality. However, the relationship between homocysteine levels and the risk of heart failure is unknown.

INTERPRETATION. The authors evaluated 2491 patients with no prior history of heart failure or myocardial infarction, who participated in the Framingham Heart Study during the 1979–1982 and 1986–1990 examinations. The patients were monitored for the first episode of heart failure during an 8-year follow-up. Overall, 23% of men and 28% of women had elevated homocysteine levels. During a follow-up period, 156 patients (6.3%) developed heart failure. In addition, 6% of women and 12% of men experienced myocardial infarction. The crude cumulative incidence of heart failure was considerably higher in women and men in the top two quartiles, as compared with the patients in the lower two quartiles, and of the incident cases of heart failure, about a third had myocardial infarction. After multivariable adjustment for other heart failure risk factors, interim development of myocardial infarction and prevalent coronary artery disease, women in quartiles with the higher homocysteine levels were at greater risk than those in the quartile with the lowest homocysteine level (HR 1.47 per quartile; 95% CI 1.19–1.82; *P* for trend 0.008). In men, there was no statistically significant difference between quartiles of homocysteine.

Comment

This study was the first to demonstrate an association between elevated homocysteine levels and the risk of *de novo* heart failure in a prospective cohort of community-based patients. This elevated risk was observed mainly in women, and was not pronounced (and not statistically significant) in men. The reason for this gender difference is unclear. Whether an elevated homocysteine level is a marker of sub-clinical systolic or diastolic left ventricular dysfunction or a mediator of adverse outcomes is also unknown (echocardiography was not routinely performed in the study patients). As such, whether screening of high-risk individuals with homocysteine levels will have any additional value to clinical follow-up and echocardiography, and whether treatment of hyperhomocysteinaemia will improve outcomes remain to be determined.

Systolic blood pressure, diastolic blood pressure, and pulse pressure as predictors of risk for congestive heart failure in the Framingham Heart Study

Haider AW, Larson MG, Franklin SS, Levy D. *Ann Intern Med* 2003; **138**(1): 10–16

BACKGROUND. Even though hypertension is a well-recognized risk factor for the development of heart failure, the specific relationship of systolic, diastolic, and pulse pressure with the risk for heart failure is incompletely defined.

INTERPRETATION. The authors prospectively followed 2040 community-based patients enrolled in the Framingham Heart Study between 1968 and 1973, who had no antecedent history of heart failure or coronary artery disease, and were not receiving any antihypertensive therapy at baseline. The patients were monitored for the onset of congestive heart failure through mid-1994. Overall, heart failure developed in 234 (11.8%) patients. Myocardial infarction preceded heart failure in 59 (25%) of these patients. After multivariable adjustment, increments of one standard deviation were associated with a 56% increase in the RR of heart failure for systolic pressure (HR 1.56; 95% CI 1.37–1.77), 55% for pulse pressure (HR 1.56; 95% CI 1.37–1.75) and 24% for diastolic pressure (HR 1.24; 95% CI 1.08–1.42). A similar effect was seen when systolic, diastolic and pulse pressure were analysed as continuous variables, and this effect was consistent across age and secular time subgroups.

Comment

This study confirmed that systolic blood pressure and pulse pressure are strong predictors of *de novo* heart failure in a prospective, community-based cohort with over 20 years of follow-up. Pulse pressure, which can be easily calculated, was the strongest risk factor of the three blood pressure measurements, and should probably be routinely used in clinical practice along with other predictors of risk. The study highlighted the importance of tight blood pressure control as a means of primary prevention of heart failure. The implications for treatment of elevated blood pressure that results in the lowering of diastolic in greater proportion to systolic, increasing the pulse pressure, are not clear. Also, as echocardiography was not routinely performed in the study patients, the differential contribution of systolic, diastolic and pulse pressure to systolic versus diastolic left ventricular dysfunction is unclear.

Non-cardiac comorbidity increases preventable hospitalizations and mortality among Medicare beneficiaries with chronic heart failure

Braunstein JB, Anderson GF, Gerstenblith G, *et al. J Am Coll Cardiol* 2003; **42**(7): 1226–33

BACKGROUND. Chronic heart failure disproportionately affects elderly patients, who typically have extensive comorbidity. However, how non-cardiac comorbidity affects outcomes and complicates care in these patients is incompletely defined.

INTERPRETATION. The authors evaluated data from the Medicare administrative database, using a 5% (*n* = 122 630) nationally representative random sample of Medicare beneficiaries with a diagnosis of heart failure in 1999. The main outcomes were potentially preventable heart failure hospitalizations, potentially preventable all-cause hospitalizations, and all-cause mortality occurring at any time in 1999. The mean age was 79.6 years, and most patients were women (60%). Non-cardiac comorbidities were highly prevalent, and 39% of the patients had five or more non-cardiac comorbidities. The most common non-cardiac comorbidities were hypertension (55%), diabetes (31%) and chronic obstructive pulmonary disease (26%). The probability of heart failure and all-cause preventable hospitalizations increased incrementally with the rising number of comorbidities (Fig. 1.5). Patients with five or more comorbidities accounted for 81% of the total hospital days. After multivariable adjustments, secondary or complicated hypertension (RR 1.51; 95% CI 1.45–1.56), chronic renal failure (RR 1.43; 95% CI 1.36–1.50) and chronic obstructive pulmonary disease (RR 1.40; 95% CI 1.36–1.44) were the strongest predictors of preventable heart failure hospitalizations. Lower respiratory disease (RR 2.34; 95% CI 2.27–2.41), renal failure (RR 1.65; 95% CI 1.58–1.73), dementia (RR 1.24; 95% CI 1.20–1.29), cerebrovascular disease (RR 1.23; 95% CI 1.15–1.31) and chronic obstructive pulmonary disease (RR 1.12; 95% CI 1.09–1.16) were the strongest predictors of mortality.

Comment

Despite the limitations (such as the use of administrative databases and the risk of residual confounding), this study clearly demonstrated the profound adverse impact of non-cardiac comorbidity burden on survival and quality of life of elderly patients with heart failure. It also highlighted a striking gap between the overwhelming majority of heart failure patients in 'real-world' practice and the typical randomized clinical trial patient population, and suggests that non-cardiac comorbidity should be strongly considered in risk stratification of patients with heart failure. Some of the potential reasons for poor outcomes in older heart failure patients with extensive comorbidity may include underutilization of effective heart failure therapies (due to absolute or relative contraindications), polypharmacy, poor adherence to medications secondary to complex regimens, and poor coordination of care. Reducing fragmentation of care, introducing disease management programmes, and focusing

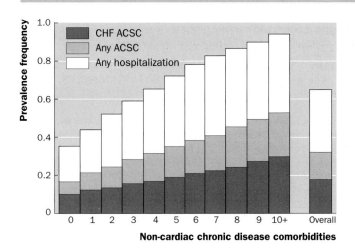

Fig. 1.5 Impact of non-cardiac comorbidity burden on the annual probability of a Medicare beneficiary with chronic heart failure (*n* = 122 630) experiencing a hospitalization due to any cause, a preventable hospitalization or a preventable hospitalization due to chronic heart failure (CHF). Data are represented as mean probabilities. *P* <0.0001 for linear trend for all outcomes. ACSC, ambulatory care sensitive conditions.
Source: Braunstein *et al.* (2003).

on patient-centred care are some of the strategies that may improve outcomes in this increasingly growing majority of patients with heart failure.

The association of left ventricular ejection fraction, mortality, and cause of death in stable outpatients with heart failure
Curtis JP, Sokol SI, Wang Y, *et al. J Am Coll Cardiol* 2003; **42**(4): 736–42

BACKGROUND. Although LVEF is a well-recognized indicator of prognosis in patients with heart failure, the relationship between LVEF and mortality across the full spectrum of LVEF is incompletely defined.

INTERPRETATION. The authors examined the association between LVEF and mortality among 7788 stable outpatients with heart failure enrolled in the Digitalis Investigation Group trial. The mean follow-up was 37 months. The patients were divided into six groups according to LVEF: ≤15, 16–25, 26–35, 36–45, 46–55, and >55%. Overall, mortality increased with successively lower LVEF values, but was substantial in all LVEF groups (range, LVEF ≤15%, 51.7%, LVEF >55%, 23.5%). When LVEF was analysed as a continuous variable, among patients with LVEF <45% mortality rates increased in near linear manner with successively lower LVEF, whereas mortality rates were similar for all patients with LVEF >45% (Fig. 1.6). After multivariable adjustment, lower LVEF values were still independently associated with higher mortality in patients with LVEF ≤45%, but the mortality in groups of patients with LVEF >45% remained comparable (Table 1.4). Worsening heart failure and arrhythmias were the leading causes of death in all LVEF groups.

Comment

The study demonstrated that the relationship between LVEF and mortality changed across the spectrum of LVEF. There was an essentially linear increase in mortality with successively lower LVEF values for patients with LVEF ≤45%, with no clear plateau effect even in those patients with severely depressed LVEF. In contrast, in those patients with LVEF >45%, higher LVEF did not appear to confer any survival advantage. The causes of death did not differ among patients across the LVEF groups. These findings may aid in more effective risk stratification of patients with heart failure. Even though the investigators did not adjust the results for functional status, and evaluated patients who were younger and had less extensive comorbidity than a typical heart failure population, this study has highlighted a very poor prognosis associated with the diagnosis of heart failure across the spectrum of LVEF— even in this, relatively 'healthy' patient population.

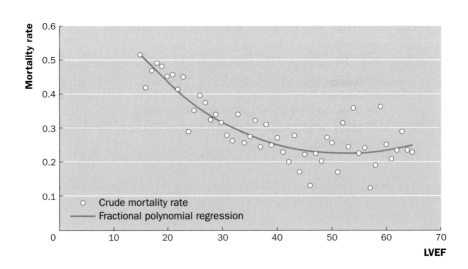

Fig. 1.6 Linear trend for LVEF as a continuous variable and unadjusted all-cause mortality. Each point represents the mortality rate associated with each LVEF point. Source: Curtis *et al.* (2003).

Table 1.4 LVEF and mortality: multivariable analysis

	LVEF ≤ 15%	LVEF 16% to 25%	LVEF 26% to 35%	LVEF 36% to 45%	LVEF 46% to 55%	LVEF > 55%
Unadjusted	2.66 (2.26, 3.14)	1.85 (1.66, 2.07)	1.28 (1.14, 1.43)	1.00	0.88 (0.73, 1.05)	0.88 (0.71, 1.08)
Adjusted: [1]	2.66 (2.25, 3.14)	1.82 (1.63, 2.04)	1.26 (1.12, 1.41)	1.00	0.85 (0.71, 1.02)	0.82 (0.66, 1.02)
Adjusted: [2]	2.03 (1.71, 2.41)	1.56 (1.39, 1.75)	1.15 (1.02, 1.29)	1.00	0.87 (0.73, 1.05)	0.83 (0.67, 1.04)
Adjusted: [3]	1.84 (1.54, 2.18)	1.47 (1.30, 1.65)	1.13 (1.01, 1.26)	1.00	0.91 (0.76, 1.09)	0.89 (0.71, 1.10)
Adjusted: [4]	1.77 (1.49, 2.11)	1.44 (1.28, 1.61)	1.10 (0.98, 1.28)	1.00	0.92 (0.97, 1.10)	0.88 (0.71, 1.09)

*Reference group left ventricular ejection fraction (LVEF) 36% to 45%. [1] Demographics + History. [2] Demographics + History + Admission. [3] Demographics + History + Admission + Laboratory. [4] Demographics + History + Admission + Laboratory + Previous medications + Study drug assignment. Source: Curtis *et al.* (2003).

Quality of care in heart failure patients

Race, quality of care, and outcomes of elderly patients hospitalized with heart failure

Rathore SS, Foody JM, Wang Y, *et al. JAMA* 2003; **289**(19): 2517–24

BACKGROUND. Even though it has been previously reported that black patients hospitalized with heart failure receive poorer quality of care and have worse outcomes than white patients, these studies were limited by selected patient populations. Therefore, it is unclear if racial differences in quality of care and outcomes of heart failure patients currently exist in the USA.

INTERPRETATION. The authors evaluated the medical records from the national sample of 29 732 Medicare beneficiaries hospitalized with heart failure between 1998 and 1999. The measures of quality of care included rates of LVEF assessment, use of angiotensin-converting enzyme inhibitors and angiotensin receptor blockers. The outcomes were 1-year all-cause re-admission and 30-day and 1-year all-cause mortality.

Overall, black and white patients had similar rates of LVEF assessment (67.8 vs 66.7%, respectively; *P* = 0.29), and angiotensin-converting enzyme inhibitor or angiotensin receptor blocker use (85.7 vs 82.5%, respectively; *P* = 0.08). These results were not altered after multivariable adjustment (LVEF assessment RR 0.99; 95% CI 0.95–1.03; angiotensin-converting enzyme inhibitor or angiotensin receptor blocker use RR 1.03; 95% CI 0.97–1.07). Black patients had higher rates of re-admission than white patients (68.2 vs 63.0%; *P* <0.001), but lower 30-day (6.3 vs 10.7%; *P* <0.001) and 1-year

(31.5 vs 40.1%; $P < 0.001$) mortality rates. After multivariable adjustment, black patients remained at slightly higher risk of re-admission at 1 year (RR 1.09; 95% CI 1.06–1.13), but lower risk of 30-day (RR 0.78; 95% CI 0.68–0.91) and 1-year mortality (RR 0.93; 95% CI 0.88–0.98).

Comment

Using the data from the largest contemporary sample of elderly patients hospitalized with heart failure, this study demonstrated that black and white Medicare patients received comparable quality of care and had similar outcomes. The absence of racial differences in this study could be due to the fact that all patients had medical insurance (Medicare), at least for inpatient care, and demonstrated an ability to access the healthcare system by virtue of their hospitalization. It should be noted that the current quality indicators for heart failure are quite limited and treatment of these groups may differ in other ways. Also, the study was not able to assess differences in functional status.

Metformin and thiazolidinedione use in Medicare patients with heart failure

Masoudi FA, Wang Y, Inzucchi SE, *et al*. *JAMA* 2003; **290**(1): 81–5

BACKGROUND. According to the Food and Drug Administration prescribing information, metformin is contraindicated in patients receiving drug therapy for heart failure, and thiazolidinediones are not recommended in patients with moderate–severe heart failure. However, the patterns of use of these antihyperglycaemic agents in diabetic patients with heart failure are not well described.

INTERPRETATION. The authors evaluated the medical records of 25 663 patients with diabetes from the National Heart Care Project, a nationally representative sample of Medicare beneficiaries hospitalized with heart failure in the USA between 1998 and 1999 or 2000 and 2001. Patients prescribed insulin-sensitizing medications at discharge were divided into groups according to the agent prescribed (metformin, thiazolidinediones, or both).

In 1998–1999, 7.1% of patients were prescribed metformin, and 7.2% were prescribed thiazolidinediones at hospital discharge. By 2000–2001, the proportion of patients prescribed these medications increased to 11.2% for metformin (relative increase 61%) and 16.1% for thiazolidinediones (relative increase 124%). The proportion of patients prescribed either agent increased from 13.5% in 1998–1999 to 24.4% in 2000–2001. In addition, 4.4% of patients with renal insufficiency were treated with metformin in 1998–1999, which increased to 6.7% in 2000–2001. Over 98% of patients who were prescribed metformin were receiving active drug therapy for heart failure.

Comment

The study demonstrated that the use of metformin and thiazolidinediones in diabetic patients with heart failure is widespread, contrary to explicit recommendations by the Food and Drug Administration. In addition, there was a marked increase in the use of these medications between 1998–1999 and 2000–2001, even in patients considered at high risk for side effects (such as patients with heart failure and renal insufficiency who were prescribed metformin).

The question remains whether this pattern of care is causing harm. These drugs are beneficial in treating diabetes and it is unclear whether the increasing use of these medications is causing adverse outcomes. This study has clearly highlighted the urgent need for further data to clarify the safety and effectiveness of these medications in diabetic patients with heart failure.

References

1. Vasan RS, Larson MG, Benjamin EJ, Evans JC, Reiss CK, Levy D. Congestive heart failure in subjects with normal versus reduced left ventricular ejection fraction: prevalence and mortality in a population-based cohort. *J Am Coll Cardiol* 1999; **33**(7): 1948–55.
2. McCullough PA, Philbin EF, Spertus JA, Sandberg KR, Sullivan RA, Kaatz S. Opportunities for improvement in the diagnosis and treatment of heart failure. *Clin Cardiol* 2003; **26**(5): 231–7.

2

Cardiac physiology

SIDNEY GOLDSTEIN, ILEANA PIÑA

Introduction

Major advances in our understanding of the treatment and progression of heart fail-ure related to cell function, survival and transplantation have occurred in the last year. The papers included in this review are examples of some of these advances. The importance of the effect of the differentiation of transplanted cells is crucial to the ability to successfully restore function in the recipient myocardium with undifferen-tiated cell implantation. In addition to being able to transplant cells, the maintenance of the integrity of cells and the prevention of apoptosis is a major goal in therapy with a variety of pharmacological agents. Caspase activation is one of the mechan-isms that can initiate and accelerate apoptosis. The ability to inhibit caspase activity has important implications in the development of future therapy for heart failure and the progression of ventricular remodelling characteristic of the failing myocardium. The initiation of the remodelling process that leads to activation of the sympathetic and renin angiotensin systems and the increase in expression of caspases is thought to result from an increase in stretch. The studies included in this review discuss observations in this regard. In addition, the ability to measure non-invasively the change in gene transfer will allow investigators to understand the dynamics of gene determinants in heart function in disease.

Differentiation of human embryonic stem cells to cardiomyocytes; role of coculture with visceral endoderm-like cells

Mummery C, Ward-van Oostwaard D, Doevendans P, *et al. Circulation* 2003; **107**: 2733–40

BACKGROUND. Cardiomyocytes derived from human embryonic stem cells could be useful in restoring heart function after myocardial infarction or in heart failure. Cardiomyocyte differentiation of human embryonic stem cells was induced using a novel method. The electrophysiological properties and coupling of the cells were then compared with those of primary human fetal cardiomyocytes. Human embryonic stem cells were cocultured with visceral endoderm-like cells from mice, which initiated differentiation in the beating muscle. Sarcomeric marker proteins, chronotropic responses, and ion channel expression and function were typical of cardiomyocytes. Electrophysiology demonstrated that most cells resembled human fetal ventricular cells. Real time intracellular calcium measurements, Lucifer Yellow injection, and connexin 43 expression demonstrated that fetal and human embryonic stem cell-derived cardiomyocytes were coupled by gap junctions in culture. Inhibition of electrical responses by verapamil demonstrated the presence of functional α_{ic} calcium ion channels.

INTERPRETATION. This was the first demonstration of the induction of cardiomyocyte differentiation in human embryonic stem cells that did not undergo spontaneous cardiogenesis. It provides a model for the study of human cardiomyocytes in culture and could be a step forward in the development of cardiomyocyte transplantation therapies.

Comment

The identification of the visceral endoderm as a cellular source of signals that result in human embryonic stem cells differentiating to cardiomyocytes is an important step forward in the identification of the markers of cell function.

Inhibition of cardiac myocyte apoptosis improves cardiac function and abolishes mortality in the peripartum cardiomyopathy of Gαq transgenic mice

Hayakawa Y, Chandra M, Miao W, *et al. Circulation* 2003; **108**: 3036–41

BACKGROUND. Although the occurrence of cardiac myocyte apoptosis during heart failure has been documented, its importance in pathogenesis is unknown. Transgenic mice with cardiac-restricted over-expression of Gαq exhibit a lethal, peripartum cardiomyopathy accompanied by apoptosis. In order to test whether apoptosis is causally linked to heart failure, the effect of the inhibition of cell death would improve left ventricular function and survival in the Gαq peripartum cardiomyopathy model. The potent polycaspase inhibitor IDN-1965 or vehicle was administered subcutaneously to Gαq mice by osmotic minipump, beginning on day 12 of pregnancy and continuing through to euthanasia at day 14 post-partum. As expected, IDN-1965 markedly suppressed cardiac caspase-3-like activity (86.5%; P <0.01), accompanied by a reduction in the frequency of cardiac myocyte apoptosis from 1.9 ± 0.3 to 0.2 ± 0.1% (P <0.01). Animals receiving IDN-1965 exhibited significant improvement in left ventricular end-diastolic dimension (vehicle, 4.7 ± 0.1 mm; IDN-1965, 4.2 ± 0.1 mm; P <0.01), fractional shortening (vehicle; 30.7 ± 1.2%; IDN-1965, 38.9 ± 1.0%; P <0.01), positive (vehicle, 3972 ± 412; IDN-1965, 5870 ± 295; P <0.01), and negative (vehicle, 2365 ± 213; IDN-1965, 3413 ± 201; P <0.01) dP/dt, and complete suppression of mortality (vehicle, 6/20 died; IDN-1965, 0/14 died; P <0.05) (Fig. 2.1).

INTERPRETATION. The reduction in cardiac myocyte apoptosis by caspase inhibition improved left ventricular function and survival in pregnant Gαq mice. These data indicate that cardiac myocyte apoptosis plays a causal role in the pathogenesis of cardiomyopathy in this model. Caspase inhibition may provide a novel therapeutic target for heart failure.

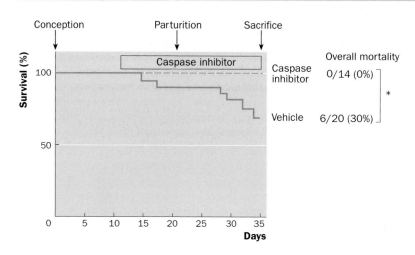

Fig. 2.1 Kaplan–Meier survival analysis. All-cause mortality of vehicle-treated ($n = 20$) versus IDN-1965-treated ($n = 14$) pregnant Gαq transgenic mice over the course of the experiment, starting on day 12 after conception and ending on day 14 post-partum before euthanasia. All animals that entered the study were included in the analysis. *$P < 0.05$. Source: Hayakawa *et al.* (2003).

Comment

Reports are emerging that demonstrate that troponin 'leaks' are occurring in patients with heart failure who are admitted for decompensation. These observations may represent ongoing cell necrosis and apoptosis with each decompensation. This study demonstrated that inhibition of caspase reduces the development of apoptosis, improves cardiac function and limits mortality in a peripartum cardiomyopathy model. Future studies could be directed to determine whether the prognosis of patients with 'leaks' is different from those patients who decompensate but have no abnormal troponin levels.

Noninvasive imaging of transgene expression by use of positron emission tomography in a pig model of myocardial gene transfer

Bengel FM, Anton M, Richter T, *et al*. *Circulation* 2003; **108**: 2127–33

B A C K G R O U N D . Radionuclide imaging of reporter gene expression may be useful for non-invasive monitoring of clinical cardiac gene therapy. Experience until now, however, has been limited to small animals. To evaluate feasibility in a clinically applicable setting, pigs were studied by conventional positron emission tomography 2 days after regional intramyocardial injection of control adenovirus or adenovirus carrying herpesviral thymidine kinase reporter gene (*HSV1-tk*). Myocardial blood flow was quantified by use of [^{13}N]ammonia. Subsequently, kinetics of the reporter substrate [^{124}I]-2'-fluoro-2'-deoxy-5-iodo-1-β-ᴅ-arabino-furanosyluracil (FIAU) were assessed over a period of 2 h. Areas infected with adenovirus expressing *HSV1-tk* showed significantly elevated FIAU retention during the first 30 min after injection. At later times, washout was observed, and retention was not different from that in areas infected with control virus or remote myocardium. Early *in vivo* FIAU uptake correlated with *ex vivo* images, autoradiography and immunohistochemistry for reporter gene product after euthanasia. After intramyocardial injection of both adenoviruses, myocardial blood flow was mildly elevated compared with that in remote areas, consistent with histological signs of regional inflammation.

INTERPRETATION. *In vivo* quantification of regional myocardial transgene expression is feasible with clinical positron emission tomography methodology, the radio-iodinated reporter probe FIAU, and the *HSV1-tk* reporter gene. Radioactivity efflux after specific initial uptake has not been observed previously in tumour studies, suggesting that tissue-specific differences in nucleoside metabolism influence reporter probe kinetics. By coregistering reporter gene expression with additional biological parameters such as myocardial blood flow, positron emission tomography allows for non-invasive characterization of the success of cardiac gene transfer along with its functional correlates.

Comment

On the basis of these data, it is clear that positron emission tomography provides the possibility that cardiac gene therapy can be monitored externally. Not only the location, but also the magnitude, of gene expression can be determined with this methodology.

Reversal of chronic molecular and cellular abnormalities due to heart failure by passive mechanical ventricular containment

Sabbah HN, Sharov VG, Gupta RC, *et al*. *Circ Res* 2003; **93**: 1095–101

BACKGROUND. Passive mechanical containment of a failing left ventricle with the Acorn cardiac support device (CSD) was shown to prevent progressive left ventricular dilation in dogs with heart failure and increase ejection fraction (EF). To examine possible mechanisms for improved left ventricle function with the CSD, the effect of CSD therapy on the expression of cardiac stretch response proteins, myocyte hypertrophy, sarcoplasmic reticulum Ca^{2+}ATPase (SERCA) activity and uptake, and mRNA gene expression for myosin heavy chain isoforms was examined. Heart failure was produced in twelve dogs by intracoronary microembolization. Six dogs were implanted with the CSD and six served as concurrent controls. Left ventricle tissue from six normal dogs was used for comparison. Compared with normal dogs, untreated heart failure dogs showed reduced cardiomyocyte contraction and relaxation, up-regulation of stretch response proteins (p21ras, c-fos and p38 α/β mitogen-activated protein kinase), increased myocyte hypertrophy, reduced SERCA activity with unchanged affinity for calcium, reduced proportion of mRNA gene expression for α-myosin heavy chain, and increased proportion of β-myosin heavy chain. Therapy with the CSD was associated with improved cardiomyocyte contraction and relaxation, down-regulation of stretch response proteins, attenuation of cardiomyocyte hypertrophy, increased affinity of the pump for calcium, and restoration of the α- and β-myosin heavy chain isoform ratio.

INTERPRETATION. These observations suggest that preventing left ventricular dilation and stretch with the CSD promotes down-regulation of stretch response proteins, attenuates myocyte hypertrophy and improves sarcoplasmic reticulum calcium cycling. These data offer possible mechanisms for improvement of left ventricular function after CSD therapy.

Comment

This study demonstrated that a broad spectrum of stretch-initiated proteins can be modified by limiting the mechanical stretch that occurs in the failing myocardium. These observations clearly establish that diastolic stretch initiates much of what we currently understand as neurohumoral activation that leads to myocardial remodelling in heart failure.

Changes in myocardial gene expression associated with β-blocker therapy in patients with chronic heart failure
Yasumura Y, Takemura K, Sakamoto A, Kitakaze M, Miyatake K. *J Card Fail* 2003; **9**: 469–74

BACKGROUND. The improvement in ventricular function by β blocker therapy in dilated cardiomyopathy is attributed to changes in the biology of the myocytes. These investigators examined the effects of β blockers on an array of contractility-regulating gene expressions in patients with dilated cardiomyopathy. Patients were selected who had an absence of any significant coronary artery disease or serious comorbidities. Gene expressions were assessed by myocardial biopsy. At baseline, brain natriuretic peptide (BNP) levels were obtained with the myocardial biopsy. Patients were then administered β blocker therapy (bisoprolol or carvedilol) with up-titration for a total of 4 months. Biopsy samples were again obtained after therapy. EF improved from 22 ± 3 to $35 \pm 12\%$; $P <0.01$. BNP levels tended to drop; $P <0.072$. Levels of β-myosin heavy chain mRNA decreased significantly. In addition, levels of SERCA mRNA increased significantly ($P <0.01$) and correlated significantly with the degree of changes in left ventricular ejection fraction (LVEF) ($r = 0.679$; $P <0.05$) (Fig. 2.2). Although the levels of $Na^+ Ca^{2+}$ exchanger mRNA did not change, the ratio of SERCA/$Na^+ Ca^{2+}$ exchanger increased significantly. None of the gene changes correlated with BNP levels.

INTERPRETATION. This study confirmed other reports that have shown that SERCA gene expression improves with chronic β blockade. Of added importance is the relationship between SERCA expression and the improvement in EF. The restoration of calcium handling is another valuable finding from this trial.

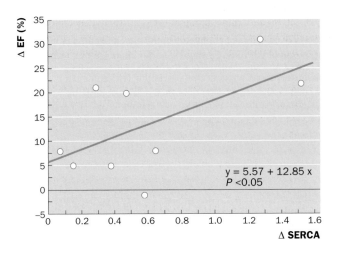

y = 5.57 + 12.85 x
P <0.05

Fig. 2.2 Relation between increases in LVEF and increases in SERCA mRNA expression. LVEF, left ventricular ejection fraction; SERCA, sarcoplasmic-reticulum calcium ATPase; mRNA, messenger RNA. Source: Yasumura *et al.* (2003).

Comment

Beta blockers have become part of the armamentarium of medical therapy in patients with chronic heart failure. The effects on EF can be striking. Mechanisms of improvement have been somewhat elusive. This report relates specific changes in various mRNAs with changes in EF.

Relation between pulse pressure and survival in patients with decompensated heart failure

Aronson E, Burger AJ. *Am J Cardiol* 2004; **93**: 785–8

B A C K G R O U N D . Pulse pressure widening has been attributed to stiff arteries, but in fact it is a complex interaction between arterial wall composition and pulse wave velocity, among others. The relationship between pulse pressure and mortality in heart failure is important clinically. Pulse pressure is easily measured at the patient's bedside and hence may be useful to the clinician. The Vasodilation in the Management of Acute Congestive Heart Failure study compared nesiritide with nitroglycerin in patients with decompensated heart failure. In order to analyse the association of mean arterial and pulse pressure with mortality, tertiles of measurements were used and relative risks calculated. The population was 489 patients and the mean arterial and pulse pressure measurements at baseline and prior to randomization were used. Tertiles of pulse pressure were: <43, 44–58 and >59 mmHg. Higher tertiles were associated with advanced age, female gender, the presence of diabetes and higher serum creatinine. Of interest, higher pulse pressure was also associated with higher EFs. During 6 months of follow-up, 110 patients died; 52, 30 and 28 occurring in the first, second and third tertiles, respectively. After adjusting for covariates, pulse pressure remained a strong predictor of mortality, whereas mean arterial pressure became non-significant. Other risk variables that still predicted mortality were diabetes and serum creatinine.

INTERPRETATION. This study is in contradistinction to other studies of heart failure that have shown a direct relationship between elevated pulse pressure and subsequent cardiac events. Pulse pressure has been seen as a surrogate of arterial stiffness, which is harmful to the heart by increasing afterload and myocardial oxygen demand. In this study, however, the higher pulse pressure was associated with more preserved left ventricular function and, therefore, some element of ventricular function is needed to maintain a higher pulse pressure. As contractility is also necessary to maintain a higher pulse pressure, patients with decompensation and an inherently decreased contractility may explain the findings of this study. Therefore, in the patient with more advanced disease, the pulse pressure relationship may be different and represent poor ventricular reserve.

Comment

A simple blood pressure measurement with derivation of pulse pressure may help the clinician to predict outcome in those patients with advanced disease who are admitted with decompensation. Each clinical setting is different.

Gender differences in advanced heart failure: insights from the BEST study

Ghali JK, Krause-Steinrauf HJ, Adams Jr KF, *et al. J Am Coll Cardiol* 2003; **42**: 2128–34

BACKGROUND. The goal of this study was to determine the influence of gender on baseline characteristic responses to treatment and prognosis in patients with heart failure secondary to impaired systolic function. Women have been underrepresented in heart failure trials. The Beta-blocker Evaluation of Survival Trial (BEST) randomized 2708 patients with New York Heart Association class III–IV heart failure to either bucindolol or placebo. Although the trial did not show overall mortality benefits from bucindolol, the trial is replete with important data. There were 593 women in the study. The women were younger, more likely to be black and had a higher number of dilated cardiomyopathies. Ischaemic aetiology and measures of heart failure severity were prognostic predictors in both men and women. Coronary artery disease and LVEF appeared to be stronger predictors of prognosis in women (Fig. 2.3).

INTERPRETATION. Historically, the number of women in heart failure trials has been approximately 20%. The general opinion has been that women have an overall better prognosis than men with equal EFs. The investigators in BEST took the time to look further into mortality in women by aetiology. However, data are emerging that women with

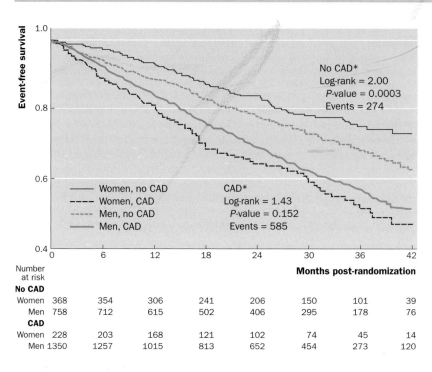

Fig. 2.3 Multivariate predictors of mortality in women. The hazard ratio for coronary artery disease (CAD) in women was 2.47 compared to 1.47 in the men.
Source: Ghali *et al.* (2003).

coronary disease and heart failure have a worse prognosis than their male counterparts. These observations were made in BEST, although the women had lower norepinephrine levels. Elevations of norepinephrine are associated with a worse prognosis among patients with heart failure.

Comment

Women with heart failure should not be assumed to have non-ischaemic or dilated cardiomyopathy. A thorough diagnostic investigation should be carried out to evaluate women for coronary disease. Rather than being influenced by reports of a better survival in women with heart failure, this study tells us differently.

Left ventricular wall stress as a direct correlate of cardiomyocyte apoptosis in patients with severe dilated cardiomyopathy

Di Napoli P, Al Taccardi A, Grilli A, *et al*. *Am Heart J* 2003; **146**: 1105–11

BACKGROUND. Apoptosis, programmed cell death, is implicated as one of the mechanisms of 'cell dropout' in patients with heart failure, leading to more abnormal remodelling. Although early after an insult, myocardial growth occurs as a compensatory mechanism, stimulated by various cytokines such as tumour necrosis factor and the renin–angiotensin system, among others. These factors are thought to 'turn on' genes that are pro-apoptotic, such as *Bax*, and some that are antipro-apoptotic, such as *Bcl-2*. The mechanisms involved with apoptosis have not been completely elucidated. Inflammatory cytokines have been implicated, as have mechanical stretch and wall stresses. This study examined 90 myocardial tissue samples from eight patients who were undergoing ventricular reduction surgery. The specimens included subendocardial, midmyocardial and epicardial thickness. The investigators analysed the samples to determine the placement on the ventricular wall of *Bax* and *Bcl-2*. *Bax* intensity (apoptotic) was highest in the subendocardial regions in all patients, while *Bcl-2* was weakly and uniformly concentrated and distributed evenly throughout the wall thickness. Apoptosis was detected using terminal deoxynucleotidyl transferase-mediated deoxyuridine triphosphate nick end labelling (TUNEL). The percentage of TUNEL-positive cells is defined as the apoptotic index and was directly related to systolic and end-diastolic wall stress, which were calculated by echocardiography (Fig. 2.4).

INTERPRETATION. In patients with dilated cardiomyopathy in whom programmed cell death or apoptosis is occurring, left ventricular wall stress may be at the root of the subendocardial concentration of apoptotic indices.

Comment

Pharmacological therapy that is directly impacting on left ventricular wall stress includes angiotensin-converting enzyme inhibitors, angiotensin II receptor blockers, diuretics, nitrates and β blockers, among others. One could extrapolate that one of the mechanisms of improvement in the progression of remodelling is a drop in wall stress with the currently indicated pharmacotherapy in heart failure. The relationship of drug therapy to the drop in apoptosis rate is a new field of study and more data are needed.

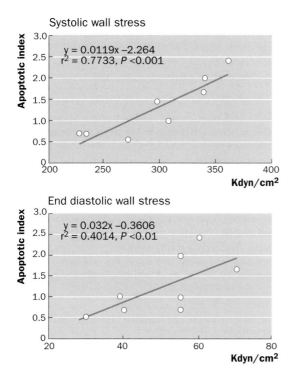

Fig. 2.4 Linear regression and correlation coefficients between systolic (top) or end diastolic (bottom) wall stresses and the apoptotic index. Source: Di Napoli *et al.* (2003).

Partial reversal of cachexia by β-adrenergic receptor blocker therapy in patients with chronic heart failure

Hryniewicz K, Androne AS, Hudaihed A, Katz SD. *J Card Fail* 2003; **9**: 464–8

BACKGROUND. Cachexia, often accompanied by loss of appetite, is a predictor of poor outcome in heart failure patients with advanced chronic disease. Cachexia has been attributed to inflammatory cytokines such as tumour necrosis factor-α. The investigators hypothesized that the neuroendocrine abnormalities associated with heart failure that could be attenuated with β blocker therapy would have beneficial effects on the catabolic and anabolic hormones in cachectic and non-cachectic patients with heart failure. Twenty-seven subjects were studied: 13 were cachectic and 14 non-cachectic. Both carvedilol 25 mg bid and long-acting metoprolol with a target dose of 200 mg daily were chosen as beta blockers of choice and uptitrated over an 8-week period. Cachectic patients had signs of more advanced disease with higher New York Heart Association

class, lower EFs and more frequent use of diuretics and digoxin. The cachectic group also had higher plasma catecholamine levels. After 6 months of β blocker therapy, subjects with baseline cachexia had greater increases in weight gain, a greater increase in leptin levels and a greater decrease in norepinephrine levels when compared with non-cachectic patients. There were no differences in any of these parameters if the patients were treated with carvedilol or long-acting metroprolol.

INTERPRETATION. In patients with cachexia and advanced heart failure, sympathetic activation may be associated with a loss of weight by promotion of pro-inflammatory cytokines and with a decrease in leptin. These patients may be the most difficult to administer β blockers to. However, evidence is accumulating to justify the use of β blockers in this group of more advanced patients, even if it is difficult to initiate.

Comment

The use of a placebo would not have been ethical in this population due to the known mortality benefits of β blockers in patients with heart failure. Larger patient groups are needed to confirm these preliminary findings. Cytokine inhibitors to date, such as etanercept, have not proven to be beneficial in larger studies of heart failure patients.

Conclusion

This chapter illustrates the complexity of ventricular remodelling and some of the mechanisms that may be at play. The resolution of 'remodelling' or reverse remodelling has been noted and attributed to β blocker therapy. The mechanism involved, however, has not been fully explained. Yasumura and colleagues offer one mechanism which may be in part responsible. In addition, we have illustrated a group of publications that touch on various aspects of heart failure, such as cachexia and narrow pulse pressure, that can directly impact clinical care. Future research will continue to elucidate mechanisms of the heart's response to insult and the manifestations of its consequences on clinical presentation of patients with HF.

Further reading

1. Mummery C, Ward-van Oostwaard D, Doevendans P, Spijker R, van den Brink S, Hassink R, van der Heyden M, Opthof T, Pera M, de la Riviere AB, Passier R, Tertoolen L. Differentiation of human embryonic stem cells to cardiomyocytes: role of coculture with visceral endoderm-like cells. *Circulation* 2003; **107**: 2733–40.

2. Hayakawa Y, Chandra M, Miao W, Shirani J, Brown JH, Dorn GW 2nd, Armstrong RC, Kitsis RN. Inhibition of cardiac myocyte apoptosis improves cardiac function and abolishes mortality in the peripartum cardiomyopathy of Gαq transgenic mice. *Circulation* 2003; **108**: 3036–41.

3. Bengel FM, Anton M, Richter T, Simoes MV, Haubner R, Henke J, Erhardt W, Reder S, Lehner T, Brandau W, Boekstegers P, Nekolla SG, Gansbacher B, Schwaiger M. Non-invasive imaging of transgene expression by use of positron emission tomography in a pig model of myocardial gene transfer. *Circulation* 2003; **108**: 2127–33.

4. Sabbah HN, Sharov VG, Gupta RC, Mishra S, Rastogi S, Undrovinas AI, Chaudhry PA, Todor A, Mishima T, Tanhehco EJ, Suzuki G. Reversal of chronic molecular and cellular abnormalities due to heart failure by passive mechanical ventricular containment. *Circ Res* 2003; **93**: 1095–101.

5. Yasumura Y, Takemura K, Sakamoto A, Kitakaze M, Miyatake K. Changes in myocardial gene expression associated with beta-blocker therapy in patients with chronic heart failure. *J Card Fail* 2003; **9**: 469–74.

6. Aronson E, Burger AJ. Relation between pulse pressure and survival in patients with decompensated heart failure. *Am J Cardiol* 2004; **93**: 785–8.

7. Ghali JK, Krause-Steinrauf HJ, Adams KF, Khan SS, Rosenberg YD, Yancy CW, Young JB, Goldman S, Peberdy MA, Lindenfeld J. Gender differences in advanced heart failure: insights from the BEST study. *J Am Coll Cardiol.* 2003; **42**: 2128–34.

8. Hryniewicz K, Androne AS, Hudaihed A, Katz S. Partial reversal of cachexia by b-adrenergic receptor blocker therapy in patients with chronic heart failure. *J Card Fail* 2003; **9**: 464–8.

3

Heart failure with preserved ejection fraction: is it really 'diastolic' heart failure?

MARGARET REDFIELD

Introduction

Heart failure is an extremely common and costly condition which primarily afflicts the elderly. The age- and sex-specific incidence of heart failure has not changed in recent decades |1|. Thus, heart failure does not meet the strict definition of an 'epidemic'. Nonetheless, as persons over the age of 65 years have the highest incidence of heart failure and as this segment of the population is growing rapidly, the number of persons developing heart failure will increase dramatically in coming decades |2| contributing to the perception of a heart failure epidemic. Thus, heart failure will have a growing impact on public health and the limited healthcare resources available to attend to it.

Clinical and epidemiology studies published over the last 30 years have established that 40–50% of patients with heart failure have a normal (≥50%) ejection fraction (EF) |3–8|, a clinical syndrome which has come to be referred to as 'diastolic' heart failure (DHF). These studies have consistently reported a few basic features of the clinical syndrome of DHF. As compared with patients with heart failure and reduced EF (systolic heart failure, SHF), patients with DHF are older, more often female and hypertensive and less likely to have recognized coronary artery disease. Most studies have shown comparable rates of diabetes, atrial fibrillation, and renal disease among those with SHF and DHF. Acute episodes of DHF are often associated with hypertensive episodes or the onset of atrial fibrillation |9|, while the nature and severity of symptoms in chronic or less severe DHF are poorly characterized. While still controversial, many studies have shown that mortality rates subsequent to a diagnosis of DHF are nearly equivalent to those observed in patients given a diagnosis of SHF |4,10|. Beyond these basic clinical features, and in contrast to the wealth of information concerning SHF |11–13|, we know relatively little concerning the natural history, diagnosis, pathophysiology, myocardial histological features and therapeutic approach to DHF. Although few would now question the importance of this syndrome as a major healthcare problem, our incomplete understanding of the syndrome continues to engender controversy.

Articles published within the last 15 months have provided some answers and stimulated some questions regarding DHF. Three studies and a major editorial addressed the pathophysiology of DHF. Two studies have expanded our understanding of the epidemiology of DHF, providing data on the prevalence of what some consider to be 'pre-clinical' DHF, that is Doppler echocardiographic evidence of diastolic dysfunction in the absence of clinical heart failure. Two novel studies have provided new insights into the natural history of DHF. An important study reported multicentre experience with the use of plasma brain natriuretic peptide (BNP) levels for the diagnosis of DHF. Facilitating the diagnosis of DHF is an important clinical issue, as many clinicians find it difficult to confidently establish the diagnosis. Finally, the second major placebo-controlled, randomized multicentre trial of a pharmacological agent in DHF was published in 2003.

Pathophysiology of DHF

Given the complexity of heart failure, the paucity of studies in actual patients with DHF, and the potential for heterogeneity in this condition, caution in making assumptions regarding the pathophysiology of DHF has been advised. Whether patients with DHF share most pathogenic mechanisms with SHF remains to be established.

Pathophysiological characterization of isolated diastolic heart failure in comparison to systolic heart failure
Kitzman DW, Little WC, Brubaker PH, et al. JAMA 2002; **288**: 2144–50

BACKGROUND. Many older patients with symptoms of congestive heart failure (CHF) have a preserved left ventricular EF (LVEF). However, the pathophysiology of this disorder, presumptively termed DHF, is not well characterized and it is unknown whether it represents true heart failure. This study sought to assess the four key pathophysiological domains that characterize classic heart failure by systematically performing measurements in older patients with presumed DHF and comparing these results with those from age-matched healthy volunteers and patients with classic SHF. In total, 147 subjects aged at least 60 years were studied. Fifty-nine had isolated DHF defined as clinically presumed heart failure, LVEF of at least 50%, and no evidence of significant coronary, valvular, or pulmonary disease. Sixty had typical SHF (LVEF ≤35%). Twenty-eight were age-matched healthy volunteer controls. Left ventricular structure and function, exercise capacity, neuroendocrine function and quality of life were assessed.

INTERPRETATION. By echocardiography, mean (standard error) LVEF was 60% (2%) in patients with DHF versus 31% (2%) in those with SHF and 54% (2%) in controls. The mean (standard error) left ventricular mass–volume ratio was markedly increased in patients with DHF (2.12 [0.14] g/ml) versus those with SHF (1.22 [0.14] g/ml) (P <0.001) and versus controls (1.49 [0.17] g/ml) (P = 0.002). Peak oxygen consumption by expired gas analysis during cycle ergometry was similar in the DHF and SHF groups (14.2 [0.5] and 13.1 [0.5] ml/kg/min, respectively; P = 0.40) and in both was markedly reduced compared with healthy controls (19.9 [0.7] ml/kg/min) (P = 0.001 for both). Norepinephrine levels were similar in the DHF (306 [64] pg/ml) and SHF (287 [62] pg/ml) groups (P = 0.56) and in both were markedly increased versus healthy controls (169 [80] pg/ml) (P = 0.007 and 0.03, respectively). BNP was substantially increased in both the DHF (56 [30] pg/ml) and SHF (154 [28] pg/ml) groups compared with healthy controls (3 [38] pg/ml) (P = 0.02 and 0.001, respectively). The quality of life decrement score as assessed by the Minnesota Living with Heart Failure Questionnaire was substantially increased from the benchmark score of 10 in both groups (SHF: 43.8 [3.9]; DHF: 24.8 [4.4]). Patients with isolated DHF had similar, although not as severe, pathophysiological characteristics compared with patients with typical SHF, including severely reduced exercise capacity, neuroendocrine activation, and impaired quality of life.

Comment

This landmark study characterized left ventricular structure, neurohumoral activation, exercise capacity and quality of life in stable outpatients with DHF and established the validity of the term 'heart failure' in such patients by demonstrating perturbations in these key components of the heart failure syndrome. It must be noted that this study was performed in stable outpatients and quality of life, exercise parameters and neurohumoral function may be more severely perturbed in more symptomatic patients studied in a hospital setting. This was one of the first studies to demonstrate activation of the sympathetic nervous system and the naturietic peptide system in DHF. Unfortunately, characterization of the renin–angiotensin–aldosterone system, endothelin and cytokines in DHF was not provided and remains an important area for future studies. It should also be noted that this study is pertinent to those patients with DHF but without coronary disease. This is a strength as it provides a homogenous and well-defined population, but more studies are needed to better define the prevalence of coronary disease in patients with DHF, as many patients with DHF are very elderly and do not undergo definitive evaluation of their coronary status. Whether patients with DHF and coronary disease have a different prognosis and whether revascularization is an effective therapeutic strategy for DHF with coronary disease remain to be established. The issues have been recently reviewed [14].

Crucial to the understanding of the pathogenesis of DHF is an appreciation of the fundamental abnormality in ventricular function that causes or at least accompanies the clinical syndrome. Young patients with hypertrophic, infiltrative or primary restrictive cardiomyopathy may present with heart failure despite normal EF. In these rare conditions, a discrete and well-characterized abnormality in the myocardium (hypertrophy with myofibre disarray, amyloid infiltration or extensive fibrosis) results in impairment in both the rate of active left ventricular relaxation and the compliance of the ventricle without reduced EF or left ventricular cavity dilatation. These abnormalities in diastolic function mandate increased dependence on filling with atrial contraction and higher atrial pressures to maintain filling and cardiac output. It was assumed that elderly patients presenting with heart failure and a normal EF had primary diastolic dysfunction similar to that observed in these rarer conditions.

However, the assumption that primary abnormalities in diastolic function are the fundamental perturbation leading to DHF has now been challenged.

Combined ventricular systolic and arterial stiffening in patients with heart failure and preserved ejection fraction: implications for systolic and diastolic reserve limitations

Kawaguchi M, Hay I, Fetics B, Kass DA. *Circulation* 2003; **107**: 714–20

BACKGROUND. Heart failure with preserved EF is common in aged individuals with systolic hypertension and is frequently ascribed to diastolic dysfunction. It was hypothesized that such patients also display combined ventricular systolic and arterial stiffening that can exacerbate blood pressure lability and diastolic dysfunction under stress.

INTERPRETATION. Left ventricular pressure–volume relationships were measured in patients with heart failure with preserved EF ($n = 10$) and contrasted with asymptomatic age-matched ($n = 9$) and young ($n = 14$) normotensives and age- and blood pressure-matched controls ($n = 25$). End-systolic elastance (stiffness) was higher in patients with heart failure and preserved EF (4.7 ± 1.5 mmHg/ml) than in controls (2.1 ± 0.9 mm Hg/ml for normotensives and 3.3 ± 1.0 mmHg/ml for hypertensives; $P <0.001$). Effective arterial elastance was also higher (2.6 ± 0.5 vs 1.9 ± 0.5 mmHg/ml) due to reduced total arterial compliance; the latter inversely correlated with end-systolic elastance ($P = 0.0001$) (Fig. 3.1). Body size and stroke volumes were similar and could not explain differences in ventricular arterial stiffening. Patients with HF with preserved EF also displayed diastolic abnormalities, including higher left ventricular end-diastolic pressures (EDPs) (24.3 ± 4.6 vs 12.9 ± 5.5 mmHg), caused by an upward-shifted diastolic pressure–volume curve. However, isovolumic relaxation and the early/late filling ratio were similar in age- and blood pressure-matched controls (Fig. 3.2). Ventricular arterial stiffening amplified stress-induced hypertension, which worsened diastolic function, and predicted higher cardiac energy costs to provide reserve output (Fig. 3.3). Patients with HF with preserved EF have systolic ventricular and arterial stiffening beyond that associated with ageing and/or hypertension. This may play an important pathophysiological role by exacerbating systemic load interaction with diastolic function, augmenting blood pressure lability, and elevating cardiac metabolic demand under stress.

Comment

This was a very important study which has expanded our understanding of the pathophysiology of DHF. While few patients were studied, the methods included pressure–volume analysis using high-fidelity pressure transducers and a conductance catheter to measure pressure and volume instantaneously during changes in pre-load produced by inferior vena cava occlusion. These methods have been considered to be the 'gold standard' for the assessment of diastolic function. Several studies have suggested that ageing is associated with decreases in aortic compliance, a phenomenon which may be independent of atherosclerosis. Here, the authors demonstrated that ventricular systolic stiffening is also observed in elderly hypertensives and in

(a)

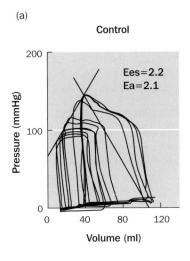
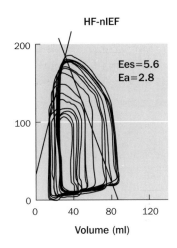

(b)

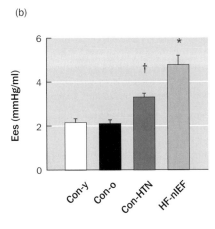
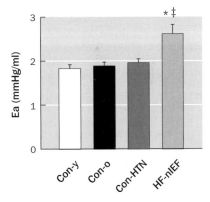

Fig. 3.1 Increased arterial elastance (Ea) and end-systolic elastance (Ees) in patients with heart failure and preserved ejection fraction (HF-nIEF). (a) An example of pressure–volume data in a control (Con) (age 65 years) and a patient with HF-nIEF (age 66 years). There is near matching of Ees and Ea in the control patient, but both are increased with a disproportionate rise in Ees in the HF-nIEF patient. (b) Group data for Ees and Ea. *$P <0.005$; †$P <0.03$ versus young (Con-y) and age-matched (Con-o) normotensive controls; ‡$P <0.005$ versus Con-HTN (patients with hypertension but without heart failure). Source: Kawaguchi et al. (2003).

(a)

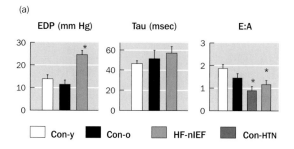

(b)

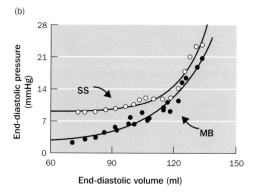

(c)

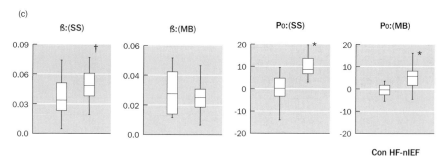

Fig. 3.2 Diastolic relaxation and stiffness in patients with heart failure and preserved EF. (a) Mean group data for end-diastolic pressure (EDP), relaxation time constant (tau), and early/late filling ratio (E:A). *P <0.001 versus young (Con-y) and age-matched (Con-o) normotensive controls. (b) An example of diastolic pressure–volume data and fits from resting steady-state (SS) beat and multibeat (MB) analyses after internal vena cava obstruction. SS data were typically shifted upwards and were more abruptly non-linear due to pressure elevation in the early filling phase. (c) Summary data for end-diastolic volume pressure–volume relationship exponential fits from SS and MB analyses. Data for all normotensive controls were very similar and were therefore combined (Con). *P <0.001; †P <0.02. Source: Kawaguchi et al. (2003).

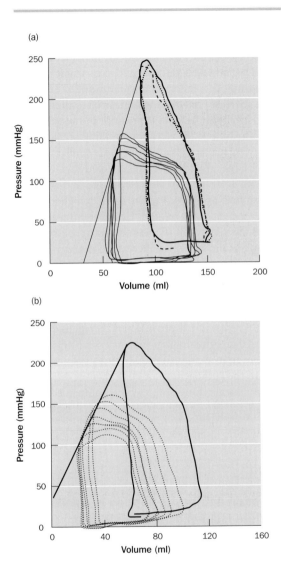

(a)

(b)

Fig. 3.3 Exaggerated increase in left ventricular systolic and diastolic pressures with exercise in patients with heart failure and preserved EF (HF-nlEF). Pressure–volume relationships before (dashed line) and after (dark solid line) sustained isometric handgrip in two patients with HF-nlEF. Baseline loops display elevated end-systolic elastance (E_{es}) and arterial elastance (E_a), predicting the marked hypertensive response with loading. This was accompanied by increased end-diastolic pressure and prolonged relaxation, supporting a mechanism whereby ventricular arterial stiffening could couple to diastolic dysfunction. Source: Kawaguchi *et al.* (2003).

patients with DHF. Increased systolic left ventricular stiffness can be due to enhanced contractility whereby the thickness of the myocardium is increased at end-systole due to enhanced fibre shortening making the myocardium stiffer. However, hypertrophy and fibrosis may also increase systolic stiffness without an increase, or even despite a decrease, in contractility. The increased vascular and ventricular systolic stiffness may impair the ability to accommodate increases in volume due to excessive salt intake (or due to exercise where increases in stroke volume are required), thus exacerbating increases in aortic and left ventricular systolic pressure and systolic load which impairs relaxation and may contribute to the elevation in filling pressures. In this study, at baseline, the speed of ventricular relaxation (τ) was similar to that observed in controls. However, other larger studies have documented impaired left ventricular relaxation in patients with DHF |15|. In this study, the end-diastolic pressure–volume relationship was shifted upwards, indicating that higher filling pressures were present for any given end-diastolic volume. However, a measure of the slope of that relationship, the stiffness coefficient (β) was similar in controls and in patients with DHF. The significance of the lack of an increase in β and τ despite marked increases in filling pressures in this small number of patients is unclear, but the findings concerning arterial and ventricular systolic stiffness are important and indicate that factors other than intrinsic diastolic dysfunction may contribute to the propensity for the development of DHF, at least in the sizeable subgroup of patients who present with labile hypertension. These findings provide new therapeutic targets for DHF as agents which modify vascular stiffening are under clinical testing |16|. While the value of this study lies more in its demonstration of potential additional mechanisms which may contribute to the pathogenesis of DHF than in disproving the role of primary abnormalities in diastolic function, it was accompanied by an editorial that raised the question of whether we should refer to HF with preserved EF as DHF until more data are available to document the presence of diastolic dysfunction in most patients |17|.

Elevation of plasma brain natriuretic peptide is a hallmark of diastolic heart failure independent of ventricular hypertrophy

Yamaguchi H, Yoshida J, Yamamoto K, *et al. J Am Coll Cardiol* 2004; **43**: 55–60

BACKGROUND. The clinical characteristics of DHF are not well acknowledged, although DHF has become a great social burden. Such a lack of clinical information leads to inaccuracy in the diagnosis of DHF. Enhancement of the ventricular production of BNP has been demonstrated with the progression of maladaptive ventricular hypertrophy, but not with the development of compensatory hypertrophy in an animal DHF model. The hypothesis that elevation of the plasma level of BNP is one of the characteristics of patients with DHF independent of left ventricular hypertrophy was tested. Of 372 patients who presented to the emergency department because of acute pulmonary congestion without acute coronary syndrome between January 1996 and May 2002, those with EF ≥45% upon admission, who were stably controlled for at least 1 year in the outpatient clinics, comprised the DHF group (*n* = 19). A control group consisted of 22 hypertensive patients with a left ventricular mass index greater than or equal to its minimum value of the DHF group and EF ≥45%, in whom cardiac symptoms had not occurred.

INTERPRETATION. Despite a similar distribution of left ventricular mass index, the BNP level was higher in the DHF group than in the control group (149 ± 38 vs 31 ± 5 pg/ml, *P* <0.01). There was no difference in left ventricular cavity size or parameters derived from pulsed Doppler transmitral flow velocity curves. An elevation in BNP may be a hallmark of patients with or at risk of DHF among subjects with preserved systolic function independent of left ventricular hypertrophy.

Comment

This was a small but important study demonstrating that the natriuretic peptides are activated in patients with DHF as compared with a clinically relevant control group. Of note, norepinephrine, plasma renin activity and aldosterone were not activated in the DHF patients. As neurohumoral activation is a hallmark of HF with reduced EF and as the degree of neurohumoral activation varies with the clinical status of the patient, further studies are needed to clearly define whether the same neurohumoral and cytokine activation present in heart failure with reduced EF is present in those with DHF. As the observation of neurohumoral activation served as the seminal observation leading to the use of angiotensin-converting enzymes, β blockers and aldosterone antagonists in heart failure with reduced EF, documentation of neuro-humoral activation would seem key to efforts directed at testing these therapies in DHF.

Epidemiology of DHF

Epidemiology studies have been crucial to the appreciation of DHF as a major public health problem. Because much of the heart failure literature focuses on clinical trials and studies carried out at referral centres focused on the care of patients referred for consideration of cardiac transplantation, in the past cardiologists often did not see the type of patients who develop DHF. Investigators from the Framingham Heart Study generated an exhaustive review of the clinical literature regarding DHF in the mid-1990s |7|. In this article they critically reviewed the clinical literature and empha-sized the need for epidemiological studies defining the relative prevalence of SHF and DHF in the populations. A number of excellent epidemiology studies followed and established that 40–50% of patients with clinical heart failure have preserved systolic function |4–6,8|. At the same time, our perception of the natural history of heart failure was changing with a greater focus on the progressive nature of the syndrome from cardiovascular disease (stage A heart failure) to asymptomatic or 'pre-clinical' ventricular remodelling and dysfunction (stage B heart failure) to overt or 'clinical' heart failure (stage C heart failure) and finally to pre-terminal HF (stage D heart failure) and death |**11**|. A number of epidemiology studies defined the prevalence of pre-clinical systolic dysfunction in the population by performing echocardiographic assessment of EF in large cross-sectional samples of the population. The prevalence and prognostic significance of pre-clinical diastolic dysfunction remained unclear. However, data from two epidemiological studies suggested that even simple Doppler parameters suggestive of diastolic dysfunction predicted future heart failure and death in the general population |**18,19**|. A limitation of these studies, however, was the relatively rudimentary assessment of diastolic function performed. While pressure–volume analysis remains the gold standard for assessment of diastolic function, Doppler echocardiography can provide insight into diastolic function and filling pressures. While limitations exist, if a comprehensive examination is performed and appropriately interpreted, Doppler echocardiography can detect the presence of impaired relaxation (grade I diastolic dysfunction) and impaired relaxation with moderate (grade II diastolic dysfunction) or severe (grade III diastolic dysfunction) elevation of filling pressures. Furthermore, patients with restrictive physiology indicating advanced diastolic dysfunction (grade IV diastolic dysfunction) can be identified |**20,21**|. Population-based studies using these methods have now defined the prevalence of clinical and pre-clinical diastolic dysfunction in the population.

Burden of systolic and diastolic ventricular dysfunction in the community: appreciating the scope of the heart failure epidemic

Redfield M, Jacobsen SJ, Burnett JC Jr, *et al. JAMA* 2003; **289**: 194–202

BACKGROUND. Approximately half of patients with overt CHF have diastolic dysfunction without reduced EF. Yet, the prevalence of diastolic dysfunction and its relationship to systolic dysfunction and CHF in the community remain undefined. The objective of this study was to determine the prevalence of CHF and pre-clinical diastolic dysfunction and systolic dysfunction in the community and to determine if diastolic dysfunction is predictive of all-cause mortality. This was a cross-sectional survey of 2042 randomly selected residents of Olmsted County, Minnesota, aged 45 years or older from June 1997 to September 2000. Doppler echocardiographic assessment of systolic and diastolic function was performed and the presence of CHF diagnosis was established by the review of medical records with designation as validated CHF if Framingham criteria were satisfied. Subjects without a CHF diagnosis but with diastolic or systolic dysfunction were considered as having pre-clinical diastolic or systolic dysfunction.

INTERPRETATION. The prevalence of validated CHF was 2.2% (95% confidence interval [CI] 1.6–2.8%) with 44% having an EF higher than 50%. Overall, 20.8% (95% CI 19.0–22.7%) of the population had mild diastolic dysfunction, 6.6% (95% CI 5.5–7.8%) had moderate diastolic dysfunction, and 0.7% (95% CI 0.3–1.1%) had severe diastolic dysfunction with 5.6% (95% CI 4.5–6.7%) of the population having moderate or severe diastolic dysfunction with normal EF. The prevalence of any systolic dysfunction (EF ≤50%) was 6.0% (95% CI 5.0–7.1%) with moderate or severe systolic dysfunction (EF ≤40%) being present in 2.0% (95% CI 1.4–2.5%). CHF was much more common among those with systolic or diastolic dysfunction than in those with normal ventricular function. However, even among those with moderate or severe diastolic or systolic dysfunction, less than half had recognized CHF (Table 3.1). In multivariate analysis, controlling for age, sex, and EF, mild diastolic dysfunction (hazard ratio [HR] 8.31; 95% CI 3.00–23.1; P <0.001) and moderate or severe diastolic dysfunction (HR 10.17; 95% CI 3.28–31.0; P <0.001) were predictive of all-cause mortality (Fig. 3.4; Table 3.2). In the community, systolic dysfunction is frequently present in individuals without recognized CHF. Furthermore, diastolic dysfunction as rigorously defined by comprehensive Doppler techniques is common, often not accompanied by recognized CHF, and associated with marked increases in all-cause mortality.

Table 3.1 Prevalence (95% confidence interval) of pre-clinical systolic and diastolic dysfunction in the community*

Variable	No. of participants	Ejection fraction (%)		Diastolic dysfunction	
		≤40	≤50	Mild	Moderate to severe
General adult population					
All	1991	1.1 (0.7–1.7)	4.9 (4.0–6.0)	20.6 (18.7–22.6)	6.8 (5.6–8.0)
Men	952	2.0 (1.2–3.1)	7.9 (6.3–9.8)	22.3 (19.5–25.3)	6.2 (4.7–8.1)
Women	1039	0.3 (0.1–0.8)	2.2 (1.4–3.3)	19.1 (16.7–21.8)	7.3 (5.7–9.1)
High-risk population (age ≥65 years and hypertension or coronary artery disease)					
All	396	2.8 (1.4–4.9)	10.9 (8.0–14.4)	47.6 (42.1–53.1)	16.5 (12.6–20.9)
Men	196	5.1 (2.5–9.2)	16.8 (11.9–22.8)	48.7 (40.7–56.8)	14.6 (9.5–21.0)
Women	200	0.5 (0.0–2.8)	5.0 (2.4–9.0)	46.5 (38.8–54.3)	18.2 (12.7–24.9)

*Pre-clinical denotes no previous validated CHF diagnosis. EF was assessed by a two-dimensional visual method.
Source: Redfield *et al.* (2003).

Table 3.2 Diastolic dysfunction is an independent predictor of all-cause mortality in the population

Variable	Hazard ratio (95% confidence interval)	P value
Age per year	1.06 (1.03–1.10)	0.004
Male sex	1.40 (0.74–2.68)	0.30
Ejection fraction, per 5 ejection fraction percentage points	0.81 (0.71–0.92)	0.02
Mild diastolic dysfunction versus normal diastolic function	8.31 (3.00–23.10)	<0.001
Moderate to severe diastolic dysfunction versus normal diastolic function	10.17 (3.28–31.00)	<0.001

Source: Redfield *et al.* (2003).

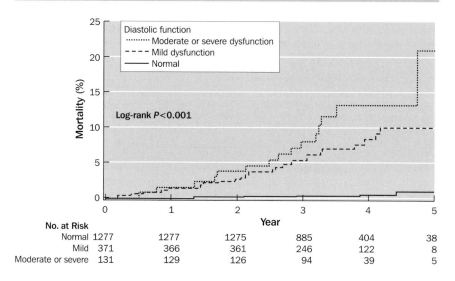

Fig. 3.4 Diastolic dysfunction predicts mortality in the population. Kaplan–Meier mortality curves for participants with normal diastolic function versus subjects with mild or moderate or severe diastolic dysfunction. Source: Redfield *et al.* (2003).

Comment

This study viewed the heart failure epidemic as a spectrum, from pre-clinical systolic and diastolic dysfunction (stage B heart failure) to clinically overt heart failure (stages C and D heart failure). The prevalence of pre-clinical systolic and diastolic dysfunction far exceeds that of clinically overt heart failure. Previous studies have demonstrated the risk associated with pre-clinical systolic dysfunction |22|. This study established the prevalence of and risk associated with pre-clinical diastolic dysfunction. Future studies are needed to establish methods to identify those with pre-clinical ventricular dysfunction and clinical trials are needed to establish the efficacy and cost effectiveness of strategies focused on the early identification and treatment of pre-clinical heart failure.

 Prevalence of left ventricular diastolic dysfunction in the community: results from a Doppler echocardiographic-based survey of a population sample
Fischer M, Baessler A, Hense HW, *et al. Eur Heart J* 2003; **24**(4): 320–8

B A C K G R O U N D . The prevalence of left ventricular diastolic abnormalities in the general population is largely unclear. Thus, the aims of this study were, first, to identify

abnormal diastolic function by echocardiography in an age-stratified population-based European sample (MONICA [Monitoring Trends and determinants in Cardiovascular Disease] Augsburg, $n = 1274$, 25–75 years, mean 51 ± 14) and, secondly, to analyse clinical and anthropometric parameters associated with diastolic abnormalities.

INTERPRETATION. The overall prevalence of diastolic abnormalities, as defined by the European Study Group on Diastolic Heart Failure (i.e. age-dependent isovolumic relaxation time [92–105 ms] and early [E-wave] and late [A-wave] left ventricular filling [E/A ratio 1–0.5]) was 11.1%. When only subjects treated with diuretics or with left atrial enlargement were considered (suggesting diastolic dysfunction) the prevalence was 3.1%. The prevalence of diastolic abnormalities varied according to age: from 2.8% in individuals aged 25–35 years to 15.8% among those older than 65 years (P <0.01). Significantly higher rates of diastolic abnormalities were observed in men as compared with women (13.8 vs 8.6%; P <0.01). Independent predictors of diastolic abnormalities were arterial hypertension, evidence of left ventricular hypertrophy, and coronary artery disease. Interestingly, in the absence of these predisposing conditions, diastolic abnormalities (4.3%) or diastolic dysfunction (1.1%) were rare, even in subjects older than 50 years of age (4.6 and 1.2%, respectively). In addition to these factors, diastolic dysfunction was related to high body mass index, high body fat mass, and diabetes mellitus. The prevalence of diastolic abnormalities and diastolic dysfunction is higher than that of systolic dysfunction and is increased (despite age-dependent diagnostic criteria) in the elderly. However, in the absence of risk factors for diastolic abnormalities or diastolic dysfunction, namely left ventricular hypertrophy, arterial hypertension, coronary artery disease, obesity and diabetes, the condition is rare even in elderly subjects. These data allow speculation on whether DHF may be prevented by improved implementation of measures directed against predisposing conditions.

Comment

This was another study defining the prevalence of diastolic dysfunction in the population and establishing the association between diastolic dysfunction and cardiovascular risk factors and disease. While the Doppler echocardiographic methods were relatively rudimentary, the findings confirmed the association between cardiovascular disease and diastolic dysfunction. Until studies establish whether treating the diastolic dysfunction specifically modifies prognosis or symptoms, studies such as this reaffirm the need to control risk factors and established cardiovascular disease.

Natural history of DHF

While basic clinical characteristics of patients with DHF have been established, there is still much to learn regarding the clinical heterogeneity and natural history of this syndrome. Two excellent studies published in 2003 provide greater insight into the natural history of DHF.

The association of left ventricular ejection fraction, mortality, and cause of death in stable outpatients with heart failure

Curtis JP, Sokol SI, Yongfei Wang, *et al. J Am Coll Cardiol* 2003; **42**(4): 736–42

BACKGROUND. Although LVEF is an accepted prognostic indicator in heart failure patients, the relationship of LVEF and mortality across the full spectrum of LVEF is incompletely understood. The aim of this study was to assess the prognostic importance of LVEF in stable outpatients with heart failure. The association of LVEF and outcomes was examined among 7788 stable heart failure patients enrolled in the Digitalis Investigation Group trial.

INTERPRETATION. During a mean follow-up of 37 months, mortality was substantial in all LVEF groups (range, LVEF ≤15%, 51.7%; LVEF >55%, 23.5%). Among patients with LVEF ≤45%, mortality decreased in a near linear manner across successively higher LVEF groups (LVEF <15%, 51.7%; LVEF 36–45%, 25.6%; P <0.0001). This association was present after multivariable adjustment, although the magnitude of this associated risk was reduced (LVEF ≤15%: HR 1.77; 95% CI 1.48–2.11; LVEF 16–25%: HR 1.44; 95% CI 1.28–1.61; LVEF 26–35%: HR 1.10; 95% CI 0.98–1.28; LVEF 36–45%: referent). In contrast, mortality rates were comparable among patients with LVEF >45% both before (LVEF 46–55%: 23.3%; LVEF >55%: 23.5%; P = 0.25) and after multivariable adjustment (LVEF 46–55%: HR 0.92; 95% CI 0.77–1.10; LVEF >55%: HR 0.88; 95% CI 0.71–1.09; LVEF 36–45%: referent). Patients with lower LVEF were at increased absolute risk of death due to arrhythmia and worsening HF, but these were leading causes of death in all LVEF groups. Among HF patients in sinus rhythm, higher LVEFs were associated with a linear decrease in mortality up to an LVEF of 45%. However, increases above 45% were not associated with further reductions in mortality.

Comment

This analysis has provided some of the best data to date on the cause of death in patients with DHF. The Digitalis Investigation Group Trial included a small subgroup of patients with heart failure and preserved EF. In this post-hoc analysis from that study, the investigators reported that the relationship between heart failure mortality and EF was not linear. While mortality was highest with the lowest EF, the relationship was lost once the EF approached 40% and greater. More importantly, while the number of DHF patients was much smaller than those with reduced EF and the clinical data available on their characteristics relatively limited, this study suggested that the causes of death are somewhat different in patients with DHF (Fig. 3.5). While worsening heart failure and arrhythmias were the leading causes of death in all heart failure patients regardless of EF, deaths due to non-cardiovascular causes were more frequent in DHF patients, consistent with the older age of these patients. As with most clinical trials, the mean age of even the DHF patients (68 ± 10 years) was

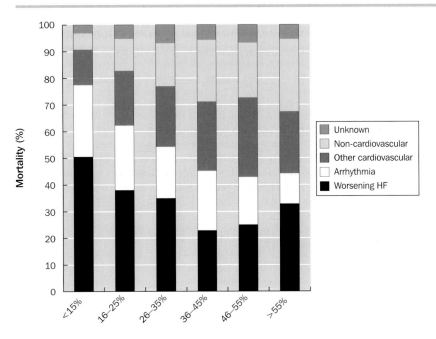

Fig. 3.5 Cause of mortality according to EF in stable outpatients with heart failure. Proportion of death attributed to specific causes of death across left ventricular EF groups. HF, heart failure. Source: Curtis *et al.* (2003).

below the average age of patients with DHF in the community. One might speculate that, in the community, patients with DHF may have even higher rates of non-cardiovascular deaths. Furthermore, this study dealt with stable outpatients with DHF and cardiovascular mortality may be higher in studies including more DHF patients with more severe HF symptoms and including hospitalized patients. These data need to be confirmed in more contemporary and better characterized cohorts, but suggest that treatment strategies for DHF and clinical trials testing such strategies will need to account for the considerable non-cardiovascular morbidity and mortality in DHF patients.

Outcomes in heart failure patients with preserved ejection fraction: mortality, re-admission, and functional decline
Smith GL, Masoudi FA, Vaccarino V, Radford MJ, Krumholz HM. *J Am Coll Cardiol* 2003; **41**(9): 1510–18

BACKGROUND. Although the poor prognosis of heart failure with depressed EF has been extensively documented, there are only limited and conflicting data concerning clinical outcomes for patients with preserved EF. The 6-month clinical trajectory of patients hospitalized for heart failure with preserved EF was evaluated, as the natural history of this condition has not been well established. Mortality, hospital re-admission, and changes in functional status were examined in patients with preserved versus depressed EF. In total, 413 patients hospitalized for heart failure were prospectively evaluated to determine whether EF ≥40% was an independent predictor of mortality, re-admission, and the combined outcome of functional decline or death.

INTERPRETATION. After 6 months, 13% of patients with preserved EF died, compared with 21% of patients with depressed EF ($P = 0.02$). However, the rates of functional decline were similar among those with preserved and depressed EF (30 vs 23%; $P = 0.14$). After adjusting for demographic and clinical covariates, preserved EF was associated with a lower risk of death (HR 0.49; 95% CI 0.26–0.90; $P = 0.02$), but there was no difference in the risk of re-admission (HR 1.01; 95% CI 0.72–1.43; $P = 0.96$) or the odds of functional decline or death (odds ratio 1.01; 95% CI 0.59–1.72; $P = 0.97$). Heart failure with preserved EF confers a considerable burden on patients, with the risk of re-admission, disability, and symptoms subsequent to hospital discharge, comparable with that of HF patients with depressed EF.

Comment

This study has provided a prospective and comprehensive follow-up of patients with heart failure and preserved as compared with reduced systolic function. Mortality was only slightly lower in DHF than in heart failure associated with reduced EF and morbidity (heart failure re-admissions and function decline) was considerable and equivalent to that observed with heart failure and reduced EF. This was an extremely important and well carried out study and has provided extensive characterization of patients.

Diagnosis of DHF

A confident diagnosis of DHF remains challenging for clinicians. When patients who present with fulminate pulmonary oedema have a normal EF, the diagnosis is clear. However, less dramatic presentations in elderly patients with comorbidities, including other potential causes of dyspnoea, are common. Advanced Doppler echocardiographic characterization of diastolic function and filling pressures is often not available. There has been great interest in the use of the measurement of plasma BNP to aid in the diagnosis of DHF.

Bedside B-type natriuretic peptide in the emergency diagnosis of heart failure with reduced or preserved ejection fraction: results from the Breathing Not Properly Multinational Study

Maisel AS, McCord J, Nowak RM, *et al.* and Breathing Not Properly Multinational Study Investigators. *J Am Coll Cardiol* 2003; **41**(11): 2010–17

BACKGROUND. Preserved systolic function is increasingly common in patients presenting with symptoms of CHF, but is still difficult to diagnose. This study examined BNP levels in patients with systolic versus non-systolic dysfunction presenting with shortness of breath. The Breathing Not Properly Multinational Study was a seven-centre, prospective study of 1586 patients who presented with acute dyspnoea and had BNP measured upon arrival. A subset of 452 patients with a final adjudicated diagnosis of CHF who underwent echocardiography within 30 days of their visit to the emergency department was evaluated. An EF >45% was defined as non-systolic CHF.

INTERPRETATION. Of the 452 patients with a final diagnosis of CHF, 165 (36.5%) had preserved left ventricular function on echocardiography, whereas 287 (63.5%) had systolic dysfunction. Patients with non-systolic CHF had significantly lower BNP levels than those with systolic CHF (413 vs 821 pg/ml; P <0.001). As the severity of HF worsened by New York Heart Association class, the percentage of systolic CHF increased, whereas the percentage of non-systolic CHF decreased. When patients with non-systolic CHF were compared with patients without CHF ($n = 770$), a BNP value of 100 pg/ml had a sensitivity of 86%, a negative predictive value of 96%, and an accuracy of 75% for detecting abnormal diastolic dysfunction. Using logistic regression to differentiate systolic CHF from non-systolic CHF, BNP entered first as the strongest predictor followed by oxygen saturation, history of myocardial infarction, and heart rate. It was concluded that non-systolic CHF is common in the setting of the emergency department and that differentiating non-systolic from systolic CHF is difficult in this setting using traditional parameters. Whereas BNP adds modest discriminatory value in differentiating non-systolic from systolic CHF, its major role is still the separation of patients with CHF from those without CHF.

Comment

This study suggested that BNP is helpful but less accurate for diagnosing DHF than for diagnosing heart failure with reduced EF. The data suggested that BNP levels may be lower in patients with DHF than in those with heart failure and reduced EF. However, the heart failure was less severe in those with DHF. Further studies are needed in patients with equivalent severity of heart failure.

Therapy of DHF

To date, only two randomized placebo-controlled multicentre drug trials in patients with DHF have been completed and published. The first was the Digitalis Investigation Group trial where the study included a small subgroup who had heart failure and normal EF. In that trial, digoxin did not alter mortality but did reduce heart failure hospitalizations. The second trial was the CHARM-Preserved Trial published in 2003.

Effects of candesartan in patients with chronic heart failure and preserved left-ventricular ejection fraction: the CHARM-Preserved Trial

Yusuf S, Pfeffer MA, Swedberg K, *et al.* and CHARM Investigators and Committees. *Lancet* 2003; **362**(9386): 777–81

BACKGROUND. Half of patients with chronic heart failure have preserved LVEF, but few treatments have specifically been assessed in such patients. In previous studies of patients with chronic heart failure and low LVEF or vascular disease and preserved LVEF, inhibition of the renin–angiotensin system is beneficial. The effect of the addition of an angiotensin receptor blocker to current treatments was investigated. Between March 1999 and July 2000, 3023 patients were randomly assigned candesartan (*n* = 1514, target dose 32 mg once daily) or matching placebo (*n* = 1509). Patients had New York Heart Association functional class II–IV chronic heart failure and LVEF higher than 40%. The primary outcome was cardiovascular death or admission to hospital for chronic heart failure. The analysis was carried out by intention to treat.

INTERPRETATION. The median follow-up was 36.6 months. In total, 333 (22%) patients in the candesartan and 366 (24%) in the placebo group experienced the primary outcome (unadjusted HR 0.89; 95% CI 0.77–1.03; *P* = 0.118; covariate adjusted 0.86; 0.74–1.0; *P* = 0.051). Cardiovascular death did not differ between groups (170 vs 170), but fewer patients in the candesartan group than in the placebo group were admitted to hospital for chronic heart failure once (230 vs 279; *P* = 0.017) or multiple times. Composite outcomes that included non-fatal myocardial infarction and non-fatal stroke showed similar results to the primary composite (388 vs 429; unadjusted 0.88 [0.77–1.01]; *P* = 0.078; covariate adjusted 0.86 [0.75–0.99]; *P* = 0.037). Candesartan had a moderate impact in preventing admissions for chronic heart failure among patients who had heart failure and LVEF higher than 40%.

Comment

This study was predicated on the assumption that patients with DHF share similar pathogenetic mechanisms with patients who have heart failure and reduced EF, i.e. that the renin–angiotensin–aldosterone system is activated in patients with DHF and contributes to the progression of heart failure. While many feel that initial therapeutic trials in DHF should test those strategies proven useful in heart failure with reduced EF, there are few data to establish the neurohumoral hypothesis in DHF. The modest beneficial effect observed with angiotensin receptor antagonism in DHF might support the need for more studies evaluating the pathophysiology of DHF and the role of neurohumoral activation prior to further trials of this nature. Furthermore, this study defined preserved EF as 40% or greater, whereas 50% is the more common discriminatory value. No subgroup analysis, i.e. hazard ratios, in those with different EF, age, blood pressure, etc. was performed to provide insight into the mechanism of observed effects. This was an important study and really the first foray into drug trials in DHF in the contemporary era. Another trial with a different angiotensin receptor antagonist and one with spironolactone are reportedly planned. One might speculate that trials are not using angiotensin-converting enzyme inhibitors due to pharmaceutical company considerations given that most angiotensin-converting enzyme inhibitors are off patent. Trials in patients with DHF will be more difficult for a number of reasons. Cardiologists in heart failure clinics are most likely to participate in clinical trials, but many, if not most, patients with DHF are cared for by non-cardiologists. Patients with DHF are more elderly and only a few clinical trials have had a good track record in enrolling large numbers of elderly patients. Patients with DHF have multiple comorbidities and as illustrated by the study by Curtis *et al.* discussed above, may have higher non-cardiovascular event rates which will complicate study end-points and may mandate larger trials |23|. Finally, many patients with DHF may already be treated with multiple cardioactive medications (angiotensin-converting enzyme inhibitors, angiotensin receptor antagonists, β blockers, aldosterone antagonists and calcium channel antagonists) for control of their hypertension and/or coronary artery disease. This will make it difficult to design trials evaluating any one of these agents. This is in contrast to trials in heart failure with reduced EF where few patients were treated with angiotensin-converting enzyme inhibitors, angiotensin receptor antagonists or β blockers prior to the onset of the clinical trials which established their role in the treatment of heart failure.

Conclusion

The studies reviewed here indicate that the scientific community is, at last, fully engaged in addressing the important public health problem posed by DHF. While much remains to be accomplished, these studies and those that preceded them have done much to define the clinical syndrome and have begun to address the pathophysiology, natural history, epidemiology, and clinical approach to the diagnosis and management of DHF. Currently, formal heart failure management guidelines can offer little beyond a 'common sense' approach to the management of DHF and focus on controlling underlying cardiovascular disease (hypertension and coronary disease) and managing fluid overload with diuretics |11|. It is likely to be some time before clinical trials validating a treatment approach are completed. In the mean time, clinicians need to expand their understanding of DHF and its pathophysiology and natural history and remain open to the possibility that the therapeutic approach to DHF may well evolve into one quite different from that of heart failure with reduced EF.

Since this article was submitted, Zile *et al.* |**24**| reported that left ventricular diastolic stiffness assessed with Doppler echocardiographic assessment of ventricular volume coupled with invasive assessment of diastolic pressures was increased in patients with DHF as compared to age matched controls. This important paper provides support for the presence of intrinsic diastolic dysfunction in DHF.

References

1. Levy D, Kenchaiah S, Larson MG, Benjamin EJ, Kupka MJ, Ho KKL, Murabito JM, Vasan RS. Long-term trends in the incidence of and survival with heart failure. *N Engl J Med* 2002; **347**(18): 1397–402.

2. Redfield MM. Heart failure—an epidemic of uncertain proportions. *N Engl J Med* 2002; **347**(18): 1442–4.

3. Senni M, Redfield MM, Ling LH, Danielson GK, Tajik AJ, Oh JK. Left ventricular systolic and diastolic function after pericardiectomy in patients with constrictive pericarditis: Doppler echocardiographic findings and correlation with clinical status. *J Am Coll Cardiol* 1999; **33**(5): 1182–8.

4. Senni M, Tribouilloy CM, Rodeheffer RJ, Jacobsen SJ, Evans JM, Bailey KR, Redfield MM. Congestive heart failure in the community: a study of all incident cases in Olmsted County, Minnesota, in 1991. *Circulation* 1998; **98**(21): 2282–9.

5. Devereux RB, Roman MJ, Liu JE, Welty TK, Lee ET, Rodeheffer R, Fabsitz RR, Howard BV. Congestive heart failure despite normal left ventricular systolic function in a population-based sample: the Strong Heart Study. *Am J Cardiol* 2000; **86**(10): 1090–6.

6. Kitzman DW, Gardin JM, Gottdiener JS, Arnold A, Boineau R, Aurigemma G, Marino EK, Lyles M, Cushman M, Enright PL; Cardiovascular Health Study Research Group. Importance of heart failure with preserved systolic function in patients ≥65 years of age; Cardiovascular Health Study. *Am J Cardiol* 2001; **87**(4): 413–19.

7. Vasan RS, Benjamin EJ, Levy D. Prevalence, clinical features and prognosis of diastolic heart failure: an epidemiologic perspective. *J Am Coll Cardiol* 1995; **26**: 1565–73.

8. Vasan RS, Larson MG, Benjamin EJ, Evans JC, Reiss CK, Levy D. Congestive heart failure in subjects with normal versus reduced left ventricular ejection fraction. *J Am Coll Cardiol* 1999; **33**: 1948–55.

9. Chen HH, Lainchbury JG, Senni M, Bailey KR, Redfield MM. Diastolic heart failure in the community: clinical profile, natural history, therapy, and impact of proposed diagnostic criteria. *J Card Fail* 2002; **8**(5): 279–87.

10. Senni M. Heart failure with preserved systolic function. A different natural history? *J Am Coll Cardiol* 2001; **38**(5): 1277–82.

11. Hunt SA, Baker DW, Chin MH, Cinquegrani MP, Feldman AM, Francis GS, Ganiats TG, Goldstein S, Gregoratos G, Jessup ML, Noble RJ, Packer M, Silver MA, Stevenson LW, Gibbons RJ, Antman EM, Alpert JS, Faxon DP, Fuster V, Jacobs AK, Hiratzka LF, Russell RO, Smith SC Jr. ACC/AHA guidelines for the evaluation and management of chronic heart failure in the adult: a report of the American College of Cardiology/American Heart Association Task Force on Practice Guidelines (Committee to Revise the 1995 Guidelines for the Evaluation and Management of Heart Failure). (http://www.acc.org/clinical/guidelines/failure/hf_index.htm).

12. Eichhorn EJ, Bristow MR. Medical therapy can improve the biological properties of the chronically failing heart: a new era in the treatment of heart failure. *Circulation* 1996; **94**: 2285–96.

13. Jessup M, Brozena S. Heart failure. *N Engl J Med* 2003; **348**(20): 2007–18.

14. Choudhury L, Gheorghiade M, Bonow RO. Coronary artery disease in patients with heart failure and preserved systolic function. *Am J Cardiol* 2002; **89**(6): 719–22.

15. Zile MR, Gaasch WH, Carroll JD, Feldman MD, Aurigemma GP, Schaer GL, Ghali JK, Liebson PR. Heart failure with normal ejection fraction: is measurement of diastolic function necessary to make the diagnosis of diastolic heart failure. *Circulation* 2001; **104**: 779–82.

16. Vasan S, Foiles PG, Founds HW. Therapeutic potential of AGE-inhibitors and breakers of AGE-protein crosslinks. *Expert Opin Investig Drugs* 2001; **10**(11): 1–11.

17. Burkhoff D, Maurer M, Packer M. Heart failure with a normal ejection fraction: is it really a disorder of diastolic function? *Circulation* 2003; **107**(5): 656–8.

18. Aurigemma GP, Gottdiener JS, Shemanski L, Gardin J, Kitzman D. Predictive value of systolic and diastolic function for incident congestive heart failure in the elderly: the cardiovascular health study. *J Am Coll Cardiol* 2001; **37**(4): 1042–8.

19. Bella JN, Palmieri V, Roman MJ, Liu JE, Welty TK, Lee ET, Fabsitz RR, Howard BV, Devereux RB. Mitral ratio of peak early to late diastolic filling velocity as a predictor of mortality in middle-aged and elderly adults: the Strong Heart Study. *Circulation* 2002; **105**(16): 1928–33.

20. Nishimura RA, Tajik AJ. Evaluation of diastolic filling of left ventricle in health and disease: Doppler echocardiography in the clinician's Rosetta stone. *J Am Coll Cardiol* 1997; **30**: 8–18.

21. Ommen SR, Nishimura RA, Appleton CP, Miller FA, Oh JK, Redfield MM, Tajik AJ. Clinical utility of Doppler echocardiography and tissue Doppler imaging in estimation of left ventricular filling pressures: a comparative simultaneous Doppler–catheterization study. *Circulation* 2000; **102**: 1788–94.

22. Wang TJ, Evans JC, Benjamin EJ, Levy D, LeRoy EC, Vasan RS. Natural history of asymptomatic left ventricular systolic dysfunction in the community. *Circulation* 2003; **108**: 977–82.

23. Curtis JP, Sokol SI, Wang Y, Rathore SS, Ko DT, Jadbabaie F, Portnay EL, Marshalko SJ, Radford MJ, Krumholz HM. The association of left ventricular ejection fraction, mortality, and cause of death in stable outpatients with heart failure. *J Am Coll Cardiol* 2003; **42**(4): 736–42.

24. Zile MR, Baicu CF, Gaasch WH. Diastolic heart failure—abnormalities in active relaxation and passive stiffness of the left ventricle. *N Engl J Med* 2004; **350**(19): 1953–9.

4

Epidemiology and aetiology of heart failure in South America

CARLOS EDUARDO NEGRÃO

Countries to the south of the North American continent continue to experience significant changes in demography, economics and epidemiological aspects. Modernization of countries often brings diseases of the cardiovascular system in parallel. Hence, it is not surprising that cardiovascular disease has risen from 20 to 27% over the last 20 years in Central and South America, with 31 of 35 countries reporting the single most frequent cause of death to be cardiovascular |1–3|. Although the countries are diverse and populations may be different, most of the data published on heart failure epidemiology in South and Central America come from Brazil and Argentina.

Brazil is the largest country of South America, with an area of 8 547 403.05 km^2 and 169 799 170 inhabitants. According to the DATASUS statistics, cardiovascular diseases accounted for 1 834 903 of Brazil's Sistema Unificado de Saúde (SUS; government medical care) hospitalizations in 2001 |4|. This number represents the second greatest cause of this type of hospitalization in the country. In addition, these statistics do not include people with private health insurance or those with private medical care. Heart failure due to cardiovascular disease is the most common cause of hospitalization in Brazil. In 1996, Freitas |5| reported that dilated cardiomyopathy was the principal diagnosis in 45% of a group of patients with heart failure followed in a tertiary hospital in Sao Paulo. Chagas' disease accounted for 20% of the group but had the worst prognosis. Ischaemic heart disease accounted for only 19%. By 1998, in the same hospital, ischaemic disease accounted for 33% of cases, with Chagas' disease dropping to 6% |6|. There are reports, however, that these numbers underestimate the prevalence of Chagas'-induced heart failure and that it may account for as many as one third of all cases throughout Brazil |7|. In 2001, 385 758 heart failure patients were hospitalized, of which 49.64% were male and 50.36% female. The age distribution was: 6294 (1.63%) below 20 years of age, 117 625 (30.49%) between 20 and 60 years, 261 839 (67.88%) older than 60 years |4|. With regard to the aetiology data from the Heart Institute (InCor), Medical School, University of São Paulo, which is a tertiary public hospital, heart failure represents 9.38% of all hospitalizations due to cardiovascular diseases |6|. This statistic includes 75% of SUS hospitalizations and 25% of private hospitalizations.

According to the DATASUS from the Brazilian Health Ministry, 25 511 people died in 2001 due to heart failure |4|. As expected, the mortality rate was higher in those older than 60 years of age. The Brazilian statistics also show that the rate of mortality for heart failure increases during the wintertime, especially in the south-eastern and southern regions of Brazil, in which the temperature during the winter-time is lower than other parts of the country. During 2001, the expenditure by the Brazilian Ministry of Health for cardiovascular disease reached R$ 898 122 874.99 (~US$ 310 million), R$ 201 939 410.42 (~US$ 70 million) of this value due to heart failure.

Argentina, another large country of the South American continent, is varied in geography, cultures and social economic status. In 1992, heart failure accounted for 20% of all hospital admissions to coronary care units. Dilated cardiomyopathy and hypertension accounted for 60 and 37% of all aetiologies, with Chagas' disease at 6% |8|. In a more recent survey of 31 hospitals in Argentina, ischaemic aetiology accounted for 30% of heart failure and Chagas' disease only 3%. This survey may be a better representation of Argentina's heart failure burden |9|.

In summary, although the continents of Central and South America are large, they are not homogenous for the epidemiology and aetiology of heart failure, similar to their differences in social structure, political and economic status.

References

1. Nicholls ES, Peruga A, Restrepo HE. Cardiovascular disease mortality in the Americas. *World Health Stat Q* 1993; **46**(2): 134–50.

2. Secretaria de Salud M. Main results of mortality statistics in Mexico 1998. *Salud Publica Mex* 2000; **42**: 155–61.

3. Mendez GF, Cowie MR. The epidemiological features of heart failure in developing countries: a review of the literature. *Int J Cardiol* 2001; **80**(2–3): 213–19.

4. DATASUS. Ministério da Saúde. 1 January 2001.

5. Freitas HFG. Chagas' disease as an etiology of severe heart failure with worse prognosis. *Circulation* 1996; **94**: 138.

6. Barretto ACP, Nobre MR, Wajngarten M, Canesin MF, Ballas D, Serro-Azul JB. Insufi-ciência cardíaca em grande hospital terciário de São Paulo [Heart failure at a large tertiary hospital of Sao Paulo]. *Arq Bras Cardiol* 1998; **71**: 15–20.

7. Mady C, Nacruth R. Natural history of chronic Chagas' heart disease: prognosis factors. *Rev Paul Med* 1995; **113**(2): 791–6.

8. Bazzino O. Encuesta Nacional de Unidades Coronarias: insuficiencia cardiaca. *Rev Argent Cardiol* 1993; **63**: 9–16.

9. Amarilla G. Ínsuficiencia Cardiaca en la Republica Argentina. Variables relacionadas co mortalidad intrahospitalaria. Resultados Preliminares del protocolo. *CONAREC VI* 1999; **67**: 53–62.

Part II

Medical and surgical therapies

5

Pharmacological therapy

KIRKWOOD ADAMS, HERBERT PATTERSON

Introduction

New knowledge relating to drug therapy for heart failure continues to accumulate at a rapid pace. The year 2003 saw the publication of a number of important new trial results, which will be highlighted below.

The Eplerenone Post Myocardial Infarction Heart Failure Efficacy and Survival (EPHESUS) study provides convincing outcome data in support of a new role for aldosterone antagonists, reducing risk in patients with heart failure following acute myocardial infarction. These positive results were seen with a selective aldosterone antagonist, eplerenone, which has a better side effect profile than the non-selective antagonist spironolactone.

The Candesartan in Heart Failure Assessment of Reduction in Mortality and Morbidity (CHARM) study represents a major advance in our understanding of the role of angiotensin receptor blocker (ARB) therapy in patients with heart failure. Designed with three distinct arms to address important clinical questions, the CHARM study provides critical data demonstrating the utility of ARBs in key clinical circumstances in heart failure where their role has been uncertain or clouded. Patients intolerant to angiotensin-converting enzyme (ACE) inhibition were shown to have important outcome benefits when treated with ARBs. Patients taking the combination of ACE inhibitor and β blocker were found to benefit from the addition of candesartan—in distinction to the previous subgroup findings with valsartan. These findings are of substantial clinical importance given the major role for β blockade in the management of heart failure due to left ventricular systolic dysfunction. Finally, CHARM provides the first large-scale randomized controlled trial data supporting a morbidity reduction in patients with heart failure associated with preserved left ventricular ejection fraction (LVEF) with ARB therapy.

The Carvedilol Or Metoprolol European Trial (COMET) provides additional evidence that β blockers shown to be effective in large-scale prospective clinical trials should be utilized in patients with heart failure. This long-awaited study showed that carvedilol therapy was superior to immediate-release metoprolol, dosed as it commonly is in practice, in reducing mortality in patients with heart failure. COMET emphasizes the importance of obtaining adequate β receptor blockade on a 24/7 basis.

The treatment of acute decompensated heart failure remains of significant interest, as this major public health problem continues to present a major morbidity and mortality burden and economic consequence for patients with heart failure. Knowledge concerning nesiritide, one of the few therapies for acute heart failure supported by randomized clinical trial results, continues to accumulate. Several studies on diverse aspects of this drug continue to testify to its clinical utility.

Finally, new data on inotropic agents and a number of investigational pharmaceutical agents are reviewed. Digoxin remains a controversial drug for many, but new data suggest that optimal dosing may help to improve outcomes on this therapy. New results with antagonism of vasopressin and endothelin-1 raise the possibility that inhibition of these neurohormones may produce clinical benefits in patients with heart failure.

All of the above work serves to highlight the continued public health and clinical importance of heart failure, a syndrome which still claims too many lives and impairs quality of life too often. Application of new information reviewed in this section will provide additional strategies for the more effective treatment of this syndrome.

Trial results and clinical studies of specific drugs

Aldosterone antagonists

Although aldosterone activation has been recognized as part of the syndrome of left ventricular dysfunction and heart failure, this hormone has not been regarded as an important therapeutic target until recently |1|. The Randomized Aldactone Evaluation Study (RALES) trial demonstrated that blockade of aldosterone could have important clinical benefits in patients with severe heart failure. Mechanistic studies based on the RALES population suggest that profibrotic activity has adverse effects and correlates with the benefit of aldosterone antagonism |2|. The recently completed EPHESUS study reported the benefits of the selective aldosterone blocker, eplerenone, in another important subset of the syndrome of heart failure, those with symptomatic left ventricular dysfunction after acute myocardial infarction.

Eplerenone, a selective aldosterone blocker, in patients with left ventricular dysfunction after myocardial infarction
Pitt B, Remme W, Zannad F, *et al*. Eplerenone Post-acute Myocardial Infarction Heart Failure Efficacy and Survival Study Investigators. *N Engl J Med* 2003; **348**: 1309–21

BACKGROUND. This trial (EPHESUS) was a double-blind, placebo-controlled study evaluating the effect of eplerenone, a selective aldosterone blocker, on morbidity and mortality among patients with acute myocardial infarction complicated by left ventricular dysfunction and heart failure. Patients were randomly assigned to eplerenone

(25 mg per day initially, titrated to a maximum of 50 mg per day; 3319 patients) or placebo (3313 patients) in addition to optimal medical therapy. The study continued until 1012 deaths occurred. The primary end-points were death from any cause and death from cardiovascular causes or hospitalization for heart failure, acute myocardial infarction, stroke, or ventricular arrhythmia (Fig. 5.1). During a mean follow-up of 16 months there were 478 deaths in the eplerenone group and 554 deaths in the placebo group (relative risk [RR] 0.85; 95% confidence interval [CI] 0.75–0.96; $P = 0.008$). Of these deaths, 407 in the eplerenone group and 483 in the placebo group were attributed to cardiovascular causes (RR 0.83; 95% CI 0.72–0.94; $P = 0.005$). The rate of the other primary end-point, death from cardiovascular causes or hospitalization for cardiovascular events, was reduced by eplerenone (RR 0.87; 95% CI 0.79–0.95; $P = 0.002$), as was the secondary end-point of death from any cause or any hospitalization (RR 0.92; 95% CI 0.86–0.98; $P = 0.02$). There was also a reduction in the rate of sudden death from cardiac causes (RR 0.79; 95% CI 0.64–0.97; $P = 0.03$). The rate of serious hyperkalaemia was 5.5% in the eplerenone group and 3.9% in the placebo group ($P = 0.002$), whereas the rate of hypokalaemia was 8.4% in the eplerenone group and 13.1% in the placebo group ($P < 0.001$).

INTERPRETATION. This study provides important confirmatory evidence of the benefit of aldosterone blockade in patients with left ventricular systolic dysfunction. The addition of eplerenone resulted in important reductions in morbidity and mortality among patients with acute myocardial infarction complicated by left ventricular dysfunction and heart failure. Combined with the data from the RALES trial that showed that spironolactone administration was associated with a 30% reduction in all-cause mortality in patients with severe heart failure, the EPHESUS trial supports the value of aldosterone inhibition in a new subset of the heart failure syndrome.

Comment

It is important to note that the benefit of eplerenone was seen despite the extensive use of other drugs known to reduce mortality after myocardial infarction (86% of the study population were on ACE inhibitors, 75% were on β blockers). The advantages and disadvantages between spironolactone (lower cost but 10% incidence of gynaeco-mastia in RALES) and eplerenone (higher cost but no gynaecomastia) are currently being debated.

ACE inhibitors/ARBs

Drugs that have the potential to inhibit the adverse effects of angiotensin II continue to be of major interest in the treatment of heart failure. ARBs are a very well-tolerated class of drug, but uncertainty about their efficacy in patients with heart failure, including those with symptoms and left ventricular systolic dysfunction, patients with heart failure and preserved LVEF and patients with recent acute myocardial infarction and left ventricular dysfunction, has persisted despite previous studies. Several trials critical to our understanding of the benefits and risks of this class of drug across the spectrum of heart failure were completed and published in 2003. The CHARM trial included three study arms: (1) patients with LVEF ≤40% and

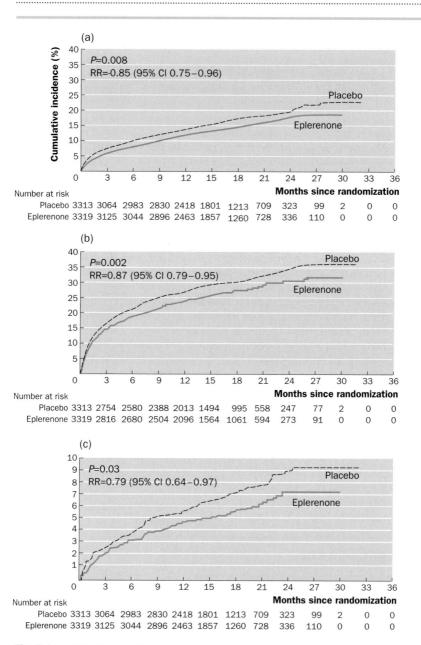

Fig. 5.1 Kaplan–Meier estimates of the rate of death from any cause (a), the rate of death from cardiovascular causes or hospitalization for cardiovascular events (b), and the rate of sudden death from cardiac causes (c). RR, relative risk; CI, confidence interval. Source: Pitt *et al.* (2003).

intolerant to ACE inhibitors (CHARM-Alternative), (2) patients with LVEF ≤40% and on an ACE inhibitor (CHARM-Added) and (3) patients with preserved systolic function (CHARM-Preserved) |3|. In addition, new data on patients treated following an acute myocardial infarction provide more support for the effectiveness of ARB therapy in patients with heart failure and systolic dysfunction.

Effects of candesartan in patients with chronic heart failure and reduced left-ventricular systolic function taking angiotensin-converting-enzyme inhibitors: the CHARM-Added trial

McMurray JJ, Östergren J, Swedberg K, *et al*. CHARM Investigators and Committees. *Lancet* 2003; **362**: 767–71

BACKGROUND. This study enrolled 2548 patients with New York Heart Association functional class II–IV symptoms and an LVEF of 40% or lower who were all being treated with ACE inhibitors. Patients were randomly assigned to candesartan ($n = 1276$, target dose 32 mg once daily) or placebo ($n = 1272$). Baseline therapy included β blockers in 55% and 17% of the patients were treated with spironolactone. The primary outcome of the study was the composite of cardiovascular death or hospital admission for chronic heart failure. During a median follow-up of 41 months, 483 (38%) patients in the candesartan group and 538 (42%) in the placebo group experienced the primary outcome (unadjusted hazard ratio [HR] 0.85; 95% CI 0.75–0.96; $P = 0.011$; covariate adjusted $P = 0.010$). Candesartan significantly reduced both cardiovascular death and the risk of hospital admission for heart failure. The benefits of candesartan versus placebo were similar in all predefined subgroups, including patients receiving baseline β blocker treatment.

INTERPRETATION. This trial demonstrated that the addition of candesartan to ACE inhibitor therapy produced additional clinical benefit in patients with heart failure and reduced LVEF. The effect of the addition of candesartan to patients taking ACE inhibitor and β blocker was of major interest.

Comment

The results of this study refuted an earlier subgroup analysis from the Valsartan in Heart Failure Trial (Val-HeFT) trial that suggested that patients on an ACE inhibitor plus an ARB and a β blocker had a worse outcome. The addition of candesartan to an ACE inhibitor was associated with a significant reduction in the composite end-point of cardiovascular death or heart failure hospitalization in the 55% of patients who were treated with a β blocker. This is a major finding of the CHARM programme, given the critical importance of β blockade in the management of patients with heart failure due to systolic dysfunction.

Effects of candesartan in patients with chronic heart failure and reduced left-ventricular systolic function intolerant to angiotensin-converting-enzyme inhibitors: the CHARM-Alternative trial

Granger CB, McMurray JJ, Yusuf S, *et al.* CHARM Investigators and Committees. *Lancet* 2003; **362**: 772–6

BACKGROUND. This study enrolled 2028 patients with symptomatic heart failure and an LVEF of 40% or less who were not receiving ACE inhibitors because of previous intolerance. The determination of ACE inhibitor intolerance was made on clinical grounds prior to study enrolment, with ACE inhibitor cough (72%) being the most common reason for intolerance, followed by symptomatic hypotension (13%) and renal dysfunction (12%). Patients were randomly assigned candesartan (target dose 32 mg once daily) or matching placebo. The primary outcome of the study was the composite of cardiovascular death or hospital admission for heart failure. During a median follow-up of 33.7 months, 334 (33%) of 1013 patients in the candesartan group and 406 (40%) of 1015 in the placebo group had cardiovascular death or hospital admission for chronic heart failure (unadjusted HR 0.77; 95% CI 0.67–0.89; P = 0.0004). Interestingly, despite a history of ACE inhibitor intolerance, rates of discontinuation of the study drug were similar in the candesartan (30%) and placebo (29%) groups.

INTERPRETATION. This arm of the CHARM trial provides convincing evidence of ARB benefit in patients intolerant to ACE inhibitor by clinical criteria. Candesartan was generally well tolerated in this patient population and reduced cardiovascular mortality and morbidity in patients with symptomatic chronic heart failure and intolerance to ACE inhibitors.

Comment

ACE inhibitors remain major drugs for the treatment of heart failure due to left ventricular systolic dysfunction. Despite known benefits of this therapy, many patients experience sufficient side effects from these agents that they discontinue therapy. ARBs, while known to be better tolerated, had not been demonstrated in prospective outcomes trials to be clearly effective in patients with heart failure who were intolerant to ACE inhibition. CHARM becomes the first study to provide such data for ARB therapy in patients with heart failure. In addition, previous clinical trials with ARBs had shown the incidence of cough or angioedema with these drugs to be no greater than placebo. However, there was still concern about administering an ARB to a patient with a history of ACE inhibitor-induced angioedema. This arm of the CHARM programme included 38 patients with a history of ACE inhibitor-induced angioedema who received candesartan. Of those patients, only four developed angioedema and only one of those had the drug discontinued. Therefore, the results of this study suggest that an ARB can be safely administered to a patient with a history of angioedema (or cough) secondary to an ACE inhibitor.

Effects of candesartan in patients with chronic heart failure and preserved left-ventricular ejection fraction: the CHARM-Preserved Trial

Yusuf S, Pfeffer MA, Swedberg K, *et al.* CHARM Investigators and Committees. *Lancet* 2003; **362**: 777–81

BACKGROUND. Patients were enrolled who had New York Heart Association functional class II–IV symptoms of heart failure and a documented LVEF higher than 40%. In total, 3023 patients were randomized to candesartan ($n = 1514$, target dose 32 mg once daily) or matching placebo ($n = 1509$). The primary study end-point was cardiovascular death or admission to hospital for heart failure. After a median follow-up of 36.6 months there were 333 (22%) patients in the candesartan group and 366 (24%) in the placebo group who experienced the primary study end-point (unadjusted HR 0.89; 95% CI 0.77–1.03; $P = 0.118$; covariate adjusted 0.86; 95% CI 0.74–1.0; $P = 0.051$). Cardiovascular death did not differ between the treatment groups (170 vs 170), but fewer patients had at least one hospital admission for heart failure in the candesartan versus the placebo group (230 vs 279; $P = 0.017$). There was also a beneficial effect on the composite end-point of non-fatal myocardial infarction and non-fatal stroke (388 patients randomized to candesartan versus 429 randomized to placebo; unadjusted 0.88; 95% CI 0.77–1.01; $P = 0.078$; covariate adjusted 0.86; 95% CI 0.75–0.99; $P = 0.037$). Fig. 5.2 demonstrates the significant reduction in the risk of

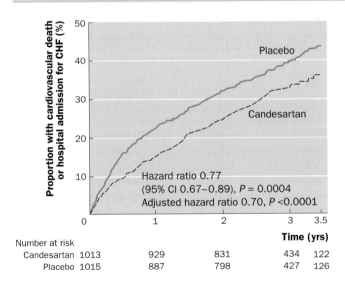

Number at risk				
Candesartan	1013	929	831	434	122
Placebo	1015	887	798	427	126

Fig. 5.2 Kaplan–Meier cumulative event curves for primary outcome. Source: Yusuf *et al.* (2003).

cardiovascular death on hospitalization for heart failure by candesartan compared to placebo in patients with heart failure due to left ventricular systolic dysfunction who were intolerant of ACE inhibitors.

INTERPRETATION. This trial demonstrated an effect of ARB therapy in patients with heart failure associated with preserved LVEF. The study reported a reduction in morbidity related to heart failure with this therapy and showed reduction in other types of cardiovascular event as well.

Comment

Heart failure associated with preserved LVEF is felt to be present in half of all patients with chronic heart failure. Despite the importance of this subset in heart failure, randomized, controlled clinical trials to evaluate the efficacy of key therapies often employed in this patient population have been lacking. This arm of the CHARM trials was designed to provide this information for ARB therapy. Although there was no effect on mortality, there was a clinically important reduction in the risk of heart failure hospitalizations. Although positive, the event rate in patients treated with ARB was still high, supporting continued drug development research in this important subset of patients with heart failure.

Valsartan, captopril, or both in myocardial infarction complicated by heart failure, left ventricular dysfunction, or both

Pfeffer MA, McMurray JJ, Velazquez EJ, et al. for the Valsartan in Acute Myocardial Infarction Trial Investigators. N Engl J Med 2003; **349**: 1893–906 (erratum in N Engl J Med 2004; **350**: 203)

BACKGROUND. This study was designed to prospectively compare the effect of the ARB valsartan (n = 4909), the ACE inhibitor captopril (n = 4909), and their combination (n = 4885) in patients followed after acute myocardial infarction. Patients were randomly assigned to the three arms of the study between 0.5 and 10 days after acute myocardial infarction. The primary end-point was death from any cause. After a median follow-up of approximately 25 months, there were 979 deaths in the valsartan group, 941 deaths in the valsartan-and-captopril group and 958 deaths in the captopril group (HR in the valsartan group as compared with the captopril group, 1.00; 97.5% CI 0.90–1.11; P = 0.98; HR in the valsartan-and-captopril group as compared with the captopril group, 0.98; 97.5% CI 0.89–1.09; P = 0.73). The upper limit of the one-sided 97.5% CI for the comparison of the valsartan group with the captopril group was within the pre-specified margin for non-inferiority with regard to mortality (P = 0.004) and with regard to the composite end-point of fatal and non-fatal cardiovascular events (P <0.001). The group which received the combination of valsartan and captopril were more likely to experience drug-related adverse events. When ARB therapy was compared with ACE inhibitor therapy, hypotension and renal dysfunction were more common in the valsartan group, and cough, rash, and taste disturbance were more common in the captopril group.

INTERPRETATION. This study provides the first confirmatory data that an ARB (valsartan) is equally effective as a proven ACE inhibitor (captopril) in reducing mortality in patients with left ventricular dysfunction post-myocardial infarction. Interestingly, the combination of captopril and valsartan provided no additional efficacy, but was associated with an increase in adverse events, suggesting no role for combination therapy with an ACE inhibitor and ARB in improving outcomes in the post-infarction population.

Comment

This study is very important to clinicians in everyday practice who are trying to maximize the utilization of life-saving therapies in patients after myocardial infarction. ARBs are well known for their excellent tolerability but there is concern that they are not as effective as ACE inhibitors in the post-myocardial infarction setting. This study was adequately powered to evaluate whether valsartan alone was equally effective on the primary end-point as captopril. The results from this large clinical trial suggest that valsartan could be used in place of captopril in this population. Although the ACE inhibitor chosen is not necessarily a common choice, captopril has been proved in the Survival and Ventricular Enlargement (SAVE) study to improve outcomes in patients with left ventricular dysfunction following acute myocardial infarction.

β blockers

Evolution of the clinical data concerning β blockade in patients with heart failure due to systolic dysfunction continues to demonstrate the marked clinical effectiveness of this approach. Much current work focuses on how this therapy may be optimized to achieve as much of the theoretical benefit as possible in everyday patient care. The relative benefits of different β blockers continue to be debated, especially in the context of COMET |4,5|. Investigation of this issue has contributed to our understanding not only of the mechanism of action of these drugs in heart failure, but also the role of pharmacokinetics and dynamics in maximizing response.

Comparison of carvedilol and metoprolol on clinical outcomes in patients with chronic heart failure in the Carvedilol Or Metoprolol European Trial (COMET): randomized controlled trial

Poole-Wilson PA, Swedberg K, Cleland JGF, *et al.* and COMET Investigators.
Lancet 2003; **362**: 7–13

BACKGROUND. This study enrolled patients with chronic heart failure due to left ventricular systolic dysfunction and compared outcomes in 1511 patients randomized to treatment with carvedilol (target dose 25 mg twice daily) with 1518 treated with immediate-release metoprolol (metoprolol tartrate, target dose 50 mg twice daily). Patients had the following inclusion criteria: chronic heart failure (New York Heart Association II–IV), previous admission for a cardiovascular reason, and an ejection fraction (EF) of less than 0.35. Patients were also required to have been previously treated with diuretics and ACE inhibitors unless not tolerated. The primary study end-points were all-cause mortality and the composite end-point of all-cause mortality or all-cause admission. Analysis was performed by intention to treat. After a mean study duration of 58 months, all-cause mortality was 34% (512/1511) for carvedilol and 40% (600/1518) for metoprolol (HR 0.83; 95% CI 0.74–0.93; $P = 0.0017$). The reduction of all-cause mortality was consistent across predefined subgroups. The composite end-point of mortality or all-cause admission occurred in 1116 (74%) of 1511 on carvedilol and in 1160 (76%) of 1518 on metoprolol (HR 0.94; CI 0.86–1.02; $P = 0.122$).

INTERPRETATION. This long-awaited study showed that carvedilol therapy was superior to immediate-release metoprolol, dosed as it commonly is in practice, in reducing mortality in patients with heart failure. Although there was a difference in mortality, there was no difference in the risk of hospitalization between the two agents, as reflected in the results with the composite end-point.

Comment

COMET provides more support for the concept that β blockers shown to be effective in mortality trials should be prescribed at the clinical trial target doses as tolerated, in patients with heart failure. This trial also emphasizes the need for adequate β receptor blockade on a 24/7 basis, as the reduction in heart rate and blood pressure during much of the trial favoured carvedilol. Due to the dosing strategy used with immediate-release metoprolol, different degrees of β blockade seem likely in the two treatment arms. However, whether a higher dose given more frequently would have been tolerated or equally effective is unknown. While it appears that carvedilol is superior to immediate-release metoprolol at the doses used in this trial, these data cannot be extrapolated to other β blockers and formulations.

Clinical outcomes in patients on beta-blocker therapy admitted with worsening chronic heart failure

Gattis WA, O'Connor CM, Leimberger JD, Felker GM, Adams KF, Gheorghiade M. *Am J Cardiol* 2003; **91**: 169–74

BACKGROUND. This study evaluated clinical outcomes in patients from the Outcomes of the Prospective Trial of Intravenous Milrinone for Exacerbations of Chronic Heart Failure (OPTIME-CHF) study, a trial of patients hospitalized with acute decompensated heart failure, who were prescribed β blockers on admission ($n = 212$) compared with patients who were not prescribed β blockers on admission ($n = 737$). Baseline characteristics were similar between these treatment groups, except that patients prescribed β blockers on admission had slightly higher EFs, fewer New York Heart Association class IV symptoms, and lower heart rates. There was no difference in clinical events during hospitalization or 60-day follow-up between patients who were treated with β blockers at the time of admission and those who were not. Exploratory analyses suggested that patients whose β blocker therapy was discontinued had a

higher risk of adverse outcomes, particularly in the subset of patients randomized to milrinone.

INTERPRETATION. Continuation of pre-existing β blocker therapy was not associated with an increased risk of adverse clinical events in patients admitted with worsening heart failure. These results suggest that caution should be taken when withdrawing β blockade in this population.

Comment

Whether to continue patients on β blockade who are hospitalized with decompensated heart failure has been a vexing clinical problem. The advantages of continuing therapy include not having to titrate the patient again in hospital or following discharge and the potential for benefits of β blockade even during periods of decompensation. The concern has been that the antisympathetic effects of continuing β blockade would decrease the effectiveness of acute heart failure treatment, as this syndrome is characterized by haemodynamic deterioration. Unfortunately, no data from a controlled clinical comparison of the management strategy of continuing β blockade in this setting are available. However, this study, based on the OPTIME-CHF population, provides data to support that continuation of β blockade is feasible in these patients. This analysis was the first to show the importance of continuing β blocker therapy even in the face of an exacerbation of heart failure. These findings suggest that every effort should be made to continue β blocker therapy in patients admitted with worsening chronic heart failure.

Endothelin receptor antagonists

Activation of endothelin-1 is known to occur in heart failure, especially in patients with more severe evidence of clinical heart failure. The potential benefits of agents which antagonize this activation have been investigated in a number of studies. Although studies of chronic outpatient therapy have not shown evidence of benefit, the acute haemodynamic effects of these agents make them of potential benefit in patients admitted with acute heart failure |6|. The study below provides evidence concerning the clinical benefits of this approach with the investigational agent tezosentan.

Hemodynamic and clinical effects of tezosentan, an intravenous dual endothelin receptor antagonist, in patients hospitalized for acute decompensated heart failure

Torre-Amione G, Young JB, Colucci WS, *et al. J Am Coll Cardiol* 2003; **42**: 140–7

BACKGROUND. In total, 292 patients with decompensated heart failure were randomized in a double-blind manner to 24 h of intravenous treatment with tezosentan

(50 or 100 mg/h) or placebo. Haemodynamic inclusion criteria were a cardiac index ≤2.5 l/min/m² and pulmonary capillary wedge pressure ≥15 mmHg. The enrolled patients were felt to need intravenous treatment for acute heart failure and to require central haemodynamic monitoring. Measurements of central haemodynamic variables, dyspnoea score, and safety variables were conducted. After 6 h of treatment, significantly greater increases in the cardiac index and decreases in pulmonary capillary wedge pressure were observed with both tezosentan dosages compared with placebo (P <0.0001). A mean decline in pulmonary capillary wedge pressure of 3.9 mmHg was noted for each dose and both doses resulted in similar mean improvement in cardiac index (0.38 and 0.37 l/min/m² with 50 and 100 mg/h). These beneficial haemodynamic effects were maintained during the remainder of the 24-h infusion and were found to continue for at least 6 h after treatment with tezosentan was stopped. A tendency for an improved dyspnoea score and a decreased risk of clinical worsening was observed after 24 h of treatment with each tezosentan dose. In contrast, the following adverse events were more frequent with tezosentan than with placebo: headache, asymptomatic hypotension, early worsening of renal function, nausea, vomiting. There was evidence of an increased risk of these adverse events in the group receiving 100 mg/h tezosentan.

INTERPRETATION. Administration of tezosentan was shown to rapidly improve haemodynamics in patients hospitalized with severe heart failure. A significant reduction in filling pressure and improvements in cardiac output were noted at both doses of the drug. In addition, clinical assessments also provided evidence of benefit. There were significant adverse events at the doses used, including symptomatic hypotension.

Comment

Tezosentan, a dual endothelin receptor antagonist, has been previously shown to improve short-term haemodynamics in patients with stable chronic heart failure. In this trial, the effects of intravenous tezosentan were studied in a group of patients admitted for treatment of acute heart failure. One key issue remains, the proper dose of tezosentan for patients with acute heart failure. This study provides strong evidence that the doses studied to date are probably above the optimal ones. The doses in this study produced similar beneficial effects on haemodynamics. In addition, there was evidence of increased adverse events with the higher dosage, suggesting that further studies with the dose <50 mg/h should be conducted. Nevertheless, this therapy remains a potentially useful one for patients with acute, decompensated heart failure. Additional trials to better define the dose response and clinical effectiveness of tezosentan in this clinical setting are underway.

Inotropes

Ongoing research in patients with heart failure continues to seek to define the benefits and potential harm of positive inotropic agents. These agents continue to have the appeal of improving central haemodynamics, which remain an important part of the pathophysiological scheme of heart failure. The data discussed below reflect some progress in this area of research. The use of digoxin, a time-honoured medication for the treatment of heart failure, remains controversial in heart failure, despite 200 years of use. Although it has been a long-standing suspicion that the dose (equated with serum concentration) might be a key to this therapy, studies have only recently addressed this issue.

Association of serum digoxin concentration and outcomes in patients with heart failure

Rathore SS, Curtis JP, Wang Y, Bristow MR, Krumholz HM. *JAMA* 2003; **289**: 871–8

BACKGROUND. This study reported the results of a post-hoc analysis of the relationship between serum digoxin concentration and outcome based on data from the randomized, double-blind, placebo-controlled Digitalis Investigation Group trial. The main reported analysis was restricted to men with an LVEF of 45% or less ($n = 3782$) who were randomized to placebo or had blind serum digoxin concentration determined at their week 4 visit. The primary end-point reviewed was all-cause mortality, as it had been in the original trial. The main analytical method was a categorical analysis. Patients randomly assigned to receive digoxin were divided into three groups based on serum digoxin concentration at 1 month (0.5–0.8 ng/ml, $n = 572$; 0.9–1.1 ng/ml, $n = 322$; and ≥1.2 ng/ml, $n = 277$) and compared with patients randomly assigned to receive placebo ($n = 2611$). All-cause mortality was determined at a mean follow-up of 37 months. Higher serum digoxin concentrations were associated with increased crude all-cause mortality rates (0.5–0.8 ng/ml, 29.9%; 0.9–1.1 ng/ml, 38.8%; and ≥1.2 ng/ml, 48.0%; $P = 0.006$ for trend). Patients with serum digoxin concentrations of 0.5–0.8 ng/ml had a 6.3% (95% CI 2.1–10.5%) lower mortality rate compared with patients receiving placebo. Digoxin was not associated with a reduction in mortality among patients with serum digoxin concentrations of 0.9–1.1 ng/ml (2.6% increase; 95% CI 3.0–8.3%), whereas patients with serum digoxin concentrations of 1.2 ng/ml and higher had an 11.8% (95% CI 5.7–18.0%) higher absolute mortality rate than patients receiving placebo. The association between serum digoxin concentration and mortality persisted after multivariable adjustment (serum digoxin concentration 0.5–0.8 ng/ml HR 0.80; 95% CI 0.68–0.94; serum digoxin concentration 0.9–1.1 ng/ml HR 0.89; 95% CI 0.74–1.08; serum digoxin concentration ≥1.2 ng/ml HR 1.16; 95% CI 0.96–1.39; and HR of 1.00 [referent] for placebo).

INTERPRETATION. Digoxin therapy has enjoyed a dedicated following among a number of clinicians who care for patients with heart failure. Recently, however, a number of heart failure specialists have questioned this position, given the poor overall results with inotropic therapy in general and the failure of the Digitalis Investigation Group trial to find an overall mortality benefit from digoxin. This important study may provide part of the answer for the persistent use of this drug. One clear finding has emerged from studies of other inotropic agents over the past decade: dose, meaning the serum concentration of active drug in most cases, is important. This retrospective analysis of the Digitalis Investigation Group trial results make a convincing argument that this is true for digoxin as well.

Comment

We have previously published a retrospective analysis of the results of the Prospective Randomized Study of Ventricular Failure and Efficacy of Digoxin (PROVED) and Randomized Assessment of Digoxin on Inhibitors of the Angiotensin-Converting Enzyme (RADIANCE) studies with digoxin |7| that found that serum concentrations from 0.5 to 0.9 ng/ml were as effective at improving short-term clinical end-points as higher concentrations. The number of hard outcomes was insufficient in these studies to determine what the relationship between serum concentrations and important outcomes such as morbidity and mortality would be. The present retrospective study provides convincing data that higher serum digoxin concentrations are associated with increased mortality and suggests that the effectiveness of digoxin therapy in men with heart failure and an LVEF of 45% or less may be optimized in the serum digoxin concentration range of 0.5–0.8 ng/ml. Some limitations concerning the study's findings should be noted. The data upon which the analysis was based came from the Digitalis Investigation Group trial, which was conducted from August 1991 to December 1995. At this time, few patients with heart failure were treated with β blockers, so whether digoxin would have favourable effects at low serum concentrations in patients treated with these critical medications for heart failure is uncertain. Additional studies are needed to assess the effect of serum concentration on the relationship between digoxin and outcomes in women with heart failure. For now, it is prudent to use the same serum concentration targets in women as in men.

Sustained hemodynamic effects of intravenous levosimendan

Kivikko M, Lehtonen L, Colucci WS. *Circulation* 2003; **107**: 81–6

B ACKGROUND. In this study, patients with decompensated heart failure received escalating infusion rates of intravenous levosimendan (*n* = 98) or placebo (*n* = 48) for 6 h. At the end of 6 h, 85 of the levosimendan-treated patients were continued on open-label drug for a total of 24 h, at which time they were randomized 1:1 to an additional 24 h of levosimendan (*n* = 43) or placebo (*n* = 42). Haemodynamic measurements showed that the effects observed at 24 h were maintained at 48 h whether levosimendan was continued or not. Levels of the active metabolite OR-1896 were similar whether levosimendan was continued or not. Concentrations of the active metabolite increased further (3.5-fold to 4-fold) from 24 to 48 h in both groups.

I NTERPRETATION. Levosimendan is a novel inotrope that has among other mechanisms the ability to sensitize myofilaments to calcium, which may allow positive inotropic effects to occur without excessive elevations of intracellular calcium. Although the parent compound is haemodynamically active, its half-life is short. In contrast, there are several metabolites of levosimendan which are haemodynamically active and have much longer half-lives. The proper dosing of this drug probably needs to take these compounds into account. This study provides an excellent profile of the role of these active metabolites. The active metabolite OR-1896 increased for at least 24 h after cessation of drug infusion and its presence is a probable explanation for the prolonged haemodynamic benefits of levosimendan.

Comment

The role of positive inotropes in patients admitted with acute heart failure remains contentious. Levosimendan may be an agent in this class with sufficiently low risk to be effective therapy. The major issue for inotropic drugs appears to be the determination of the optimal dose. Also, benefits on clinical outcomes must be shown. Additional clinical studies are underway to define the optimal dose and clinical utility of this drug in patients with acute decompensated heart failure.

Nesiritide, recombinant human b-type natriuretic peptide

Therapy for acute heart failure which has been demonstrated to be of benefit in randomized controlled clinical trials remains very limited. In addition to lowering wedge pressure at low doses and increasing cardiac output at higher doses, nesiritide has been shown to be effective at relieving symptoms when added to conventional therapy primarily consisting of diuretics. As the recombinant form of human b-type natriuretic peptide, nesiritide mimics the physiological effects of this important cardiovascular hormone |8|. B-type natriuretic peptide appears to function in a counter-regulatory manner to many known toxic hormones involved in heart failure, especially those related to activation of the sympathetic nervous system and the renin–angiotensin–aldosterone system. Although still largely supported by theoretical arguments, these properties make the administration of nesiritide attractive to patients with acute heart failure independent of its direct haemodynamic and diuretic effects. Given these positive results, interest continues in better understanding the effects of this drug in patients with acute heart failure. Areas of interest include the physiological effects of nesiritide, comparison of the effects of nesiritide relative to inotropic agents, and economic assessments of this therapy.

Effects of intravenous nesiritide on human coronary vasomotor regulation and myocardial oxygen uptake
Michaels AD, Klein A, Madden JA, Chatterjee K. *Circulation* 2003; **107**: 2697–701

BACKGROUND. In this study, ten patients underwent right and left heart catheterization with determination of baseline coronary blood flow and myocardial oxygen uptake. The patients then received an intravenous infusion of nesiritide (2 μg/kg bolus followed by 0.01 μg/kg/min infusion) for 30 min. Haemodynamic measurements revealed that right atrial pressure decreased 52% ($P = 0.012$), pulmonary artery mean pressure decreased 19% ($P = 0.03$), pulmonary capillary wedge pressure decreased 46% ($P = 0.002$), and the mean arterial pressure decreased 11% ($P = 0.007$) during the infusion. These changes were accompanied by a 15% increase in

coronary artery diameter from a baseline of 2.6 ± 0.8 to 3.0 ± 0.8 mm at 30 min
(*P* = 0.007). Measurements demonstrated that coronary blood flow increased 35%
(*P* = 0.007) and coronary resistance decreased 23% both at 15 and 30 min (*P* = 0.036)
of infusion. In addition, myocardial oxygen uptake also decreased 8% during the
nesiritide infusion (*P* = 0.043).

INTERPRETATION. This study provides convincing evidence that nesiritide exerts
coronary vasodilator effects on both the coronary conductance and resistance arteries. A
number of favourable effects related to coronary flow and myocardial oxygen consumption
were evident. Despite falling coronary perfusion pressure from the vasodilatory actions of
the drug, coronary artery blood flow increased and coronary resistance decreased while
myocardial oxygen uptake declined.

Comment

Many patients with acute heart failure have underlying ischaemic heart disease and,
in some cases, both ischaemia and decompensated heart failure are present in patients
admitted with acute congestive heart failure. Concern continues that some or all inotropic agents may worsen myocardial oxygen consumption in many of these patients.
The pharmacological effects of nesiritide in an experimental setting suggest that the
actions of this drug would be different, but the effects of intravenous nesiritide on the
human coronary vasculature have not been studied. This study provides important
reassuring data on the effects of nesiritide on myocardial oxygen consumption and
coronary flow in patients with heart failure.

Effects of nesiritide (b-type natriuretic peptide) and dobutamine on ventricular arrhythmias in the treatment of patients with acutely decompensated congestive heart failure: the PRECEDENT study

Burger AJ, Horton DP, LeJemtel T, *et al*. Am Heart J 2002; **144**: 1102–8

BACKGROUND. In this randomized, multicentre trial, the effects of nesiritide
(human b-type natriuretic peptide) on arrhythmia frequency were compared with those of
dobutamine in patients hospitalized with decompensated heart failure. In total,
255 patients were randomized to one of two doses of intravenous nesiritide (0.015 or
0.03 µg/kg/min) or dobutamine (5 µg/kg/min) and stratified by means of an earlier
history of ventricular tachycardia. The frequency of arrhythmia in the various arms of the
study was assessed with 24-h Holter recordings. Dobutamine was found to significantly
increase the mean (1) number of ventricular tachycardia events per 24 h by 48 ± 205
(*P* = 0.001), (2) repetitive ventricular beats per hour by 15 ± 53 (*P* = 0.001), (3)
premature ventricular beats per hour by 69 ± 214 (*P* = 0.006), and (4) heart rate by
5.1 ± 7.7 beats per minute (*P* <0.001). These end-points were significantly decreased
or unchanged in the nesiritide groups. Nesiritide did not increase heart rate, despite a
greater reduction in blood pressure. Both drugs were similarly effective means of
improving signs and symptoms of congestive heart failure.

INTERPRETATION. This randomized clinical trial provides convincing evidence that nesiritide in acute decompensated heart failure does not increase arrhythmia frequency. In addition, the study showed that dobutamine administration is associated with substantial proarrhythmic and chronotropic effects in patients with decompensated heart failure.

Comment

Dobutamine, a positive inotropic agent due to β adrenergic stimulation, continues to be commonly used in the treatment of patients with severe decompensated congestive heart failure. Despite improving haemodynamics in most patients, dobutamine therapy is associated with increased risk of arrhythmia, including ventricular tachycardia. In contrast, experimental studies have suggested that nesiritide would not increase the likelihood of ventricular arrhythmias in this setting, but human data were lacking. These findings, taken together with experimental results, indicate that nesiritide will be safer, from an arrhythmia point of view, than dobutamine in patients with heart failure.

Economic implications of nesiritide versus dobutamine in the treatment of patients with acutely decompensated congestive heart failure

de Lissovoy G, Stier DM, Ciesla G, Munger M, Burger AJ. *Am J Cardiol* 2003; **92**: 631–3

BACKGROUND. Pooled data from trials comparing nesiritide with dobutamine for the treatment of acute decompensated congestive heart failure were combined with national hospital cost data to produce an economic assessment of the cost of nesiritide versus dobutamine. The study calculated the cost for the acute admission and for subsequent re-admissions in patients treated with each drug. Although the cost of nesiritide is significantly greater than dobutamine and results in somewhat higher costs for the initial admission for decompensated heart failure, the use of nesiritide was associated with a decreased risk of re-admission compared with dobutamine.

INTERPRETATION. The study analysis demonstrated that the costs of nesiritide, compared with dobutamine, were completely offset by decreased hospital costs related to re-admission.

Comment

Given the number of admissions each year for acute heart failure (over one million per year with an expectation for additional increases), the cost of the syndrome is staggering, with estimates of over $20 billion in direct expenses each year. Clearly, any therapy for the condition will be examined from the perspective of cost as well as benefit. This study provides some initial data on the economic impact of the utilization of nesiritide, illustrates the complexity of cost assessment and gives some perspective on the high initial cost of nesiritide.

Tumour necrosis factor-α inhibition

Heart failure has many faces and recent work has convincingly demonstrated that a pro-inflammatory state exists in many patients, especially those with more advanced symptoms. A number of cytokines and other inflammatory molecules are known to be elevated in heart failure. Experimental studies suggest that a reduction in the degree of inflammatory activity may have beneficial effects on haemodynamics and the heart failure state.

Randomized, double-blind, placebo-controlled, pilot trial of infliximab, a chimeric monoclonal antibody to tumor necrosis factor-alpha, in patients with moderate-to-severe heart failure: results of the Anti-TNF Therapy Against Congestive Heart Failure (ATTACH) trial

Chung ES, Packer M, Lo KH, Fasanmade AA, Willerson JT. Anti-TNF Therapy Against Congestive Heart Failure Investigators. *Circulation* 2003; **107**: 3133–40

BACKGROUND. This study enrolled 150 patients who had symptoms consistent with stable New York Heart Association function class III or IV and reduced LVEF (≤35%). Patients were randomly assigned to receive placebo ($n = 49$), infliximab 5 mg/kg ($n = 50$), or infliximab 10 mg/kg ($n = 51$) at 0, 2 and 6 weeks after randomization and were followed-up prospectively for 28 weeks. The primary end-point of the study was clinical status. No improvement in clinical status was noted at 14 weeks. Interestingly, there was suppression of inflammatory markers (C-reactive protein and interleukin-6) and a modest increase in EF in the patients receiving 5 mg/kg ($P = 0.013$). In addition, after 28 weeks of therapy, some disturbing trends were noted in the high-dose infliximab group. There were 13 patients hospitalized in the placebo group versus ten in the 5 mg/kg infliximab group and 20 in the 10 mg/kg infliximab group. An adverse effect on the combined risk of death from any cause or hospitalization for heart failure was also seen at 28 weeks in patients randomized to 10 mg/kg infliximab (HR 2.84; 95% CI 1.01–7.97; nominal $P = 0.043$).

INTERPRETATION. This study provides very convincing evidence against the use of infliximab, a chimeric monoclonal antibody to tumour necrosis factor-α. Short-term tumour necrosis factor-α antagonism with this drug did not improve patients clinically at the low dose studied, while at the high dose (10 mg/kg) adverse clinical effects were noted in patients with moderate-to-severe chronic heart failure.

Comment

There has been substantial interest in the possible therapeutic benefits of cytokine inhibition in heart failure. Despite the negative nature of this trial, interest in drugs with anti-inflammatory potential in heart failure persists, in part because of the complexities of the cytokine system and the likelihood that drugs which block only one mediator, like tumour necrosis factor-α, may not be effective. Additional studies of approaches with more generalized anti-inflammatory actions are underway as this hypothesis continues to be tested.

Vasopressin antagonists

Vasopressin is known to be activated or inappropriately elevated in many patients with heart failure. The hyponatraemia that occurs in heart failure appears to be mediated to a major extent by vasopressin and patients with this finding may be particularly likely to benefit from blockade of this hormone. Whether inhibition of vasopressin will result in therapeutic benefit in broad populations of patients with heart failure has been under active investigation for some time |9|. One agent in this class in particular, tolvaptan, a selective V2 receptor antagonist, is showing promise. One of the initial studies with this investigational compound is reviewed below.

Vasopressin v2-receptor blockade with tolvaptan in patients with chronic heart failure

Gheorghiade M, Niazi I, Ouyang J, et al. for the Tolvaptan Investigators.
Circulation 2003; **107**: 2690–6

BACKGROUND. This study was a double-blind trial investigating the effects of three doses of tolvaptan and placebo in patients with chronic heart failure. In total, 254 patients were randomized after a run-in period to placebo ($n = 63$) or tolvaptan (30 mg [$n = 64$], 45 mg [$n = 64$], or 60 mg [$n = 63$]) once daily for 25 days. Patients were not fluid restricted and were maintained on stable doses of furosemide. A decrease in body weight was noted at day 1 in all three active groups compared with baseline (–0.79 ± 0.99, –0.96 ± 0.93, and –0.84 ± 0.02 kg in the 30, 45, and 60 mg tolvaptan groups, respectively) while there was an increase in body weight of +0.32 ± 0.46 kg in the placebo group (P <0.001 for all treatment groups versus placebo). No further reduction in body weight was observed after the first day of the study, but the initial decline in body weight was maintained throughout the study. A substantial increase in urine volume was observed with tolvaptan when compared with placebo (3.9 ± 0.6, 4.2 ± 0.9, 4.6 ± 0.4, and 2.3 ± 0.2 l/24 h at day 1 for 30, 45, and 60 mg tolvaptan groups, and placebo, respectively; P <0.001). A decrease in oedema and a normalization of serum sodium in patients with hyponatraemia were observed in the tolvaptan group but not in the placebo group. No significant changes in heart rate, blood pressure, serum potassium, or renal function were observed in response to tolvaptan therapy.

INTERPRETATION. In patients with heart failure, tolvaptan reduced body weight and oedema and normalized serum sodium in the hyponatraemic patients. The drug was well tolerated overall, despite a substantial increase in urine volume. The reduction in body weight was modest and the clinical relevance of this degree of change remains to be defined.

Comment

Vasopressin antagonists represent a new approach to the relief of congestion in patients with heart failure. One of the potential advantages of these agents is the possibility that congestion may be relieved without a number of deleterious effects associated with diuretic therapy, including electrolyte depletion and worsening renal function. Weight loss was achieved in the above study without these side effects. Additional studies of tolvaptan are underway in patients with acute heart failure where more extensive volume overload is expected to be present and the opportunity for beneficial effects of vasopressin antagonism may be enhanced in this setting.

Diuretics

Although non-potassium-sparing diuretics remain important for symptom relief, concern continues that they may have adverse long-term effects through a variety of mechanisms, including electrolyte depletion and neurohormonal activation. Randomized trials to investigate this possibility have not been forthcoming, but some insight can be gained from retrospective studies.

Diuretic use, progressive heart failure, and death in patients in the Studies Of Left Ventricular Dysfunction (SOLVD)

Domanski M, Norman J, Pitt B, Haigney M, Hanlon S, Peyster E. Studies of Left Ventricular Dysfunction. *J Am Coll Cardiol* 2003; **42**: 705–8

BACKGROUND. This retrospective work investigated the risk of hospitalization for, or death from, heart failure between patients taking a potassium-sparing diuretic and those who were not, adjusting for known covariates. The study population was comprised of the 6797 patients in the Studies Of Left Ventricular Dysfunction (SOLVD) study which included both symptomatic and asymptomatic patients with left ventricular systolic dysfunction (LVEF ≤35%). The risk of hospitalization from worsening heart failure in those taking a potassium-sparing diuretic relative to those taking only a non-potassium-sparing diuretic was 0.74 (95% CI 0.55–0.99; $P = 0.047$). The relative risk for cardiovascular death was 0.74 (95% CI 0.59–0.93; $P = 0.011$), for death from all causes 0.73 (95% CI 0.59–0.90; $P = 0.004$), and for hospitalization for, or death from, heart failure 0.75 (95% CI 0.58–0.97; $P = 0.030$). Compared with patients not taking any diuretic, the risk of hospitalization or death due to worsening heart failure in patients taking non-potassium-sparing diuretics alone was significantly increased (risk ratio = 1.31; 95% CI 1.09–1.57; $P = 0.0004$); this was not observed in patients taking potassium-sparing diuretics with or without a non-potassium-sparing diuretic (risk ratio = 0.99; 95% CI 0.76–1.30; $P = 0.95$).

INTERPRETATION. This retrospective study provides new evidence concerning the relative effects of diuretics that waste potassium versus those that do not. A review of data from hard outcomes suggested that potassium-sparing diuretics are associated with better outcomes. In this study, the use of potassium-sparing diuretics versus non-potassium-sparing diuretics was associated with a reduced risk of death from, or hospitalization for, progressive heart failure or all-cause or cardiovascular death.

Comment

This study had a number of important limitations. The specific drugs given and the dose used were not given. The analysis was retrospective and the modelling may not have completely accounted for differences in risk that led to the administration of a non-potassium-sparing diuretic in some patients versus potassium sparing in others. Nevertheless, concern continues that, despite their favourable effects on symptoms, diuretics may result in long-term adverse effects. There has been continued interest in the possibility that potassium-sparing diuretics may be associated with better outcomes because they lack some of these properties. Data from the randomized, placebo-controlled RALES trial has established the benefits of spironolactone in patients with severe heart failure. It is interesting that the dose employed in this study was not associated with a significant diuretic effect, highlighting the fact that inhibition of aldosterone is probably important. Whether the use of potassium-sparing diuretics would be associated with benefit in a broader population of patients with heart failure has not been determined.

Conclusion

Despite the advent of device therapy, pharmacological management remains the most critical part of heart failure therapeutics for most patients. The important studies in 2003 continue to emphasize that the use of multiple drugs at the right dose and frequency and in the correct subset of patients with heart failure continues to be essential for the successful treatment of this life-threatening and disabling syndrome. Although the achievement of multiple drug therapy can be challenging, ongoing clinical experience has revealed a number of strategies to enhance the likelihood that adequate pharmacological management will occur. Acute heart failure persists as a therapeutic dilemma, but continued clinical experience with nesiritide and new studies of novel agents offer significant promise in this important subset of patients with heart failure.

References

1. Pitt B. Aldosterone blockade in patients with systolic left ventricular dysfunction. *Circulation* 2003; **108**: 1790–4.

2. Zannad F, Alla F, Dousset B, Perez A, Pitt B, on behalf of RALES Investigators. Limitation of excessive extracellular matrix turnover may contribute to survival benefit of spironolactone therapy in patients with congestive heart failure. Insights from the Randomized Aldactone Evaluation Study (RALES). *Circulation* 2000; **102**: 2700–6.

3. Pfeffer MA, Swedberg K, Granger CB, Held P, McMurray JJV, Michelson EL, Olofsson B, Ostergren J, Yusuf S, for the CHARM Investigators Committees. Effects of candesartan on mortality and morbidity in patients with chronic heart failure: the CHARM-Overall programme. *Lancet* 2003; **362**: 759–66.

4. Bristow MR, Feldman AM, Adams Jr KF, Goldstein S. Selective versus non-selective beta-blockade for heart failure therapy: are there lessons to be learned from the COMET trial? *J Card Fail* 2003; **9**: 444–53.

5. Packer M. Do beta-blockers prolong survival in heart failure only by inhibiting the beta1-receptor? A perspective on the results of the COMET trial. *J Card Fail* 2003; **9**: 429–43.

6. Cotter G, Kiowski W, Kaluski E, Kobrin I, Milovanov O, Marmor A, Jafari J, Reisin L, Krakover R, Vered Z, Caspi A. Tezosentan (an intravenous endothelin receptor A/B antagonist) reduces peripheral resistance and increases cardiac power therefore preventing a steep decrease in blood pressure in patients with congestive heart failure. *Eur J Heart Fail* 2001; **3**: 457–61.

7. Adams KF Jr, Gheorghiade M, Uretsky BF, Patterson JH, Schwartz TA, Young JB. Clinical benefits of low serum digoxin concentrations in heart failure. *J Am Coll Cardiol* 2002; **39**: 946–53.

8. Adams Jr KF, Mathur VS, Gheorghiade M. B-type natriuretic peptide: from bench to bedside. *Am Heart J* 2003; **145**(2 Suppl): S34–46.

9. Lee CR, Watkins ML, Patterson JH, Gattis W, O'Connor CM, Gheorghiade M, Adams Jr KF. Vasopressin: a new target for the treatment of heart failure. *Am Heart J* 2003; **146**: 9–18.

6

Cell replacement strategies for heart failure

JAMES YOUNG

Introduction

Cell replacement therapies for heart failure have become alluring over the past decade |**1–6**|. This sexy strategy is rooted in the concept that the replacement of lost contractile cardiac elements can bolster the heart's ability to contract and relax more normally and, thus, address the basic evil of heart failure. The concept is intuitively pleasing. Obviously, a gross example of cardiac cell transplantation for the treatment of heart failure is heterologous orthotopic cardiac transplantation. Because of the inherent limitations of this radical therapy, great attention has been focused on embryonic stem cell and autologous cell transplantation for the treatment of damaged myocardium. In order to put current knowledge of this important therapeutic strategy into perspective, reviewing the last several years' background materials becomes important.

Table 6.1 summarizes the sources of cells that can either be directly implanted or mobilized such that they move to the damaged myocardium. As nicely overviewed in a review by Lee *et al.* |**6**|, inherent advantages and disadvantages of each type of cell are listed in this table. Obviously, there is a spectrum of donor cells that might be used to replace damaged or dead myocytes, but the bottom line is using these donor cells to create more normal systolic and diastolic cardiac pump muscle function. Which specific approach is best is unclear today.

Stem cells (Table 6.1), which are the present focus of attention, are undifferentiated but pleuripotent cells with the capability of recapitulation and differentiation into cardiomyocytes. Obviously, the use of these cells to replace or stimulate cardiomyocyte regeneration offers an extraordinary treatment option that might ameliorate deleterious haemodynamic consequences in patients with congestive heart failure, particularly heart failure caused by ischaemic myocardial necrosis of the heart. As Table 6.1 summarizes, there are five basic cell types available that are potential donor cells in heart failure.

Fetal cardiomyocytes may, perhaps, be the ideal cells to use because, phenotypically, they are smooth muscle cell contractile elements. Fetal cardiomyocytes compared with adult or paediatric cardiomyocytes have superior growth potential

Table 6.1 Donor cells that might be useful in heart failure

Cell type	Advantages	Potential problems
Fetal cardiomyocytes	Differentiated pump cell Contractility ensured	Allogeneic May need immunosuppression Largely unavailable Short survival Ethical proscriptions
Skeletal myoblasts	Readily available Can be autologous homografts Slow twitch fibres (resist fatigue and ischaemia) Divide readily in cell culture	Heterogenic considerations Lack gap junctions Perhaps arrhythmogenic Need expansion in tissue culture
Endothelial progenitor cells	Can be autologous homograft Focus on revascularization Cells can transdifferentiate into cardiomyocytes	May result more in revascularization than contracting myocardium Need expansion in tissue culture
Embryonic stem cells	Pleuripotent Rapidly expandable	Ethical proscription Largely unavailable Oncogenic potential Need expansion in tissue culture
Adult mesenchymal stem cells	Pleuripotent Can be autologous homograft Cryopreservable Absence of ethical proscription	Functional properties unclear Electrical properties unclear Difficult to isolate/purify Need expansion in tissue culture

Modified from |6|.

and animal models have found that fetal cardiomyocytes transplanted into the heart can form gap junctions with, arguably, appropriate electrical-conducting pathways. Furthermore, utilization of fetal cardiomyocytes has been demonstrated to induce new blood vessel formation, to remove cellular debris, and to form new cardiac tissue while preventing post-myocardial infarct heart failure. Because these cells are more developed, allosensitivity could occur with inflammatory-based destruction developing and these cells will, in all likelihood, require immunosuppression after implantation. Perhaps this is the major disadvantage of this approach noted to date. Also important is the ethical, and now political, proscription against the utilization of these cell lines in both basic and clinical research. These disadvantages have driven exploration of alternative autologous cell transplantation techniques.

Skeletal myoblasts are precursors for new and contracting skeletal muscle cells and are present within the muscle tissue itself. Myotubular formation can be seen in skeletal myoblasts when they are implanted into smooth muscle myocardium. From an access standpoint, skeletal myoblasts can be harvested from muscle biopsy specimens and, after selection and replication in culture, can be transplanted into the myocardium. These cells, with their fatigue- and ischaemia-resistant slow twitch fibres, might survive and even contract, although perhaps not synergistically, when implanted into ischaemic areas of the heart after myocardial infarction. A major limitation of using these cells might be ventricular tachyarrhythmias, which have been noted in some patients undergoing autologous skeletal myoblast transfer experiments. Perhaps these arrhythmias are related to the fact that skeletal muscle cells, unlike adult cardiomyocytes, do not form gap junctions. Perhaps this leads to a redirecting of electrical conduction in the heart, which could create a situation where these cells do not contract or relax synchronously with the heart *in toto*.

Endothelial progenitor cells are an interesting potential cell donor because they may stimulate neovascularization and can salvage hibernating myocardium in ischaemic heart models. Endothelial progenitor cells circulate in peripheral blood. There appears to be acute mobilization of these cells from the bone marrow into the peripheral circulation in patients with acute myocardial infarction. This may be dependent on the release of vascular endothelial growth factor (VEGF), which is upregulated in these ischaemic events. An attractive hypothesis is to deliver concentrated slurries of endothelial progenitor cells directly into infarct-related arteries to ameliorate ischaemic disasters. Autologous harvesting from bone marrow makes these cells particularly feasible because of their lack of immunogenicity and their availability. Nonetheless, a great challenge exists to isolate, purify and expand these cells. Tissue culture expansion is, indeed, required and a challenge.

Embryonic stem cells are the most primitive of the stem cells studied for myocardial regeneration. They are pleuripotent and have the ability to undergo multiple cell doublings and can differentiate into specific cell types such as cardiomyocytes. Embryonic stem cells harvested from blastocysts and then expanded in tissue culture with subsequent injection directly into the myocardium can reduce experimental infarct size with subsequent improvement in cardiac contractility. Embryonic stem cells also appear to release other important factors such as VEGF. Presently, because of political constraints prompted by some ethical concerns, embryonic stem cells are not utilized in humans or, generally, in experimental preparations. Another disadvantage is the major biological concern that the pleuripotent genetics of these cells might set the stage for cancerous transformations.

Because of the constraints surrounding research with and the utilization, in general, of human embryonic stem cells, alternative stem cell sources have been sought and, in particular, adult mesenchymal stem cells are currently the focus of great attention. Mesenchymal stem cells are also referred to as bone marrow stromal cells and are a form of rare progenitor cells that have the ability to home to different tissues that have been injured. They then replicate and possess the ability to differentiate into specialized tissues such as cardiomyocytes, endothelial cells, and smooth muscle cells. Autologous bone marrow harvesting and subsequent expansion of selected cells followed by transplantation of these cells solves the problem of allosensitization with cell rejection and makes these mesenchymal stem cells attractive to use after myocardial infarction. Because there is only a small number of stem cells that can be harvested from bone marrow aspirations, some have used stimulating factors to increase their number (and even the likelihood of mobilization to injured tissue). Table 6.2, for example, summarizes stimulating factors that can initiate stem cell mobilization, migration and distant damaged tissue infiltration. At the present time, however, these cells appear to require *ex vivo* tissue culture expansion with subsequent myocardial injection or coronary artery infusion. Other disadvantages include the fact that the cells are difficult to isolate and purify and there remain ill-characterized functional and electrophysiological properties of this cell line.

Once cells have been procured, three modes of delivery have received attention, intramyocardial injection, intracoronary infusion and intravenous infusion. For intramyocardial injections to be performed, an operative procedure is necessary. However, the advantages are that smaller numbers of cells are needed to achieve engraftment compared with intracoronary or intravenous administration. Further-more, this is a relatively simple procedure that can be performed after direct inspection of scarred areas of the heart with specific placement of the cells. A disad-vantage is the fact that a patchy network of cells might develop, providing the nidus for potentially unstable ventricular arrhythmias. The concept behind intracoronary injection is that one can deliver the maximum concentration of cells to the specific site of infarcted or peri-infarct tissue during the first post-infusion blood flow passage. Intracoronary injection may allow stem cells to be taken up in areas border-ing the infarct zone more homogeneously. Intravenous injection is obviously the simplest and least invasive method of delivering stem cells to an injured heart, par-ticularly after myocardial infarction. However, stem cells may migrate to other organs, diluting the number of cells ultimately reaching the zone of interest.

A historic overview of ten seminal papers related to stem cell transplants for heart failure was published in 2003 [7]. This outstanding overview pointed out that Leor *et al.* [8] demonstrated the feasibility of using rat fetal and human myocardial tissue transplantation in an infarction model in 1996. Fetal myocardial tissue was obtained from human fetuses at 7–12 weeks of gestation and from 14-day-old rat embryos. Fetal myocytes developed with consistent ultrastructural morphology and there was significant engraftment into infarct zones. This work used β-galactosidase-transfected cells, which, according to the report, may have prompted an adverse

Table 6.2 Soluble factors mediating stem cell mobilization

Factor	Results
Granulocyte colony stimulating factor (GCSF)	Moves bone marrow stem cells into circulation
Stem cell factor (SCF)	Moves bone marrow stem cells into circulation
Vascular endothelial growth factor (VEGF)	Induces new blood vessel formation 'Homing' signal for circulating progenitor cells
Stromal cell-derived factor-1 (SCDF-1)	'Homing' signal for circulating progenitor cells

Modified from [6].

immune reaction. This seminal study suggested, however, that fetal cardiomyocytes could be successfully implanted into infarct zones with the cells surviving. The Leor overview also highlighted the report of Murry *et al.* |9|. This paper detailed an experiment where a cell suspension of fibroblasts and myoblasts cultured from the limb muscles of 1–3-day-old Fischer rats developed into muscle tissue when injected into hearts of a rodent infarct model. Donor cells were identified using an immunofluorescence technique and an appearance of mature myofibres with myotubules was noted by 14 days. This study suggested that the technique of injecting skeletal myoblasts directly into myocardium was reasonable and laid the groundwork for subsequent more detailed experiments and, specifically, human clinical trials involving transplantation of skeletal muscle cells into scarred myocardium.

A third highlighted work was that of Taylor *et al.* |10| who, in 1998, demonstrated that, in intact animals, chronic improvement in diastolic and systolic myocardial function could be attained by transplanting autologous skeletal myoblasts into myocardial infarction areas.

This background leads, then, to the seminal publications in 2003 detailing stem cell transplant results, which have greatly excited the clinical community. One of the first reports of autologous skeletal myoblast transplantation for severe post-infarction left ventricular dysfunction was a summary of ten cases by Menasché *et al.* |11|. The ten patients had severe irreversible left ventricular dysfunction with extensive scarring noted by positron emission tomography. The infarcts were remote and angiographically demonstrated to be in cardiac territories served by completely occluded and non-revascularizable coronary arteries. Skeletal muscle biopsies were taken autologously from the vastus lateralis muscle with myoblasts harvested and recapitulated in tissue culture. Cultures contained at least 0.5 billion cells, with over 60% being myoblasts, and appeared viable over a 2–3-week period. The patients, during coronary artery bypass grafting, had the cell suspension directly injected within and around the myocardial scar tissue during cardioplegic arrest. The report indicates that no peri-operative complications occurred secondary to the injections. A small needle and syringe were used. The same cell suspension was injected into irradiated diabetic severe combined immunodeficient mice to evaluate macroscopic tumour formation and none was seen. In this report, all patients had reasonable post-operative courses, with the exception of one who succumbed to a mesenteric infarction. This study was, however, the first to suggest that this particular method of cell transplantation might be associated with problematic arrhythmias. Four patients developed clinically tolerable, but sustained, monomorphic ventricular tachycardia by a 3-week follow-up period. Automatic internal cardioverter defibrillators were placed in these individuals. Three of the four patients were noted to have significant ventricular arrhythmias pre-operatively. Most important, the authors of this report suggested that clinical benefits accrued as an echocardiographic analysis with interpreters blind to the therapeutic intervention suggested improved systolic function in the region of treatment. Follow-up at almost 1 year indicated improvement in New York Heart Association functional class and an increase in mean ejection fraction (EF). Furthermore, positron emission tomographic studies demonstrated new myocardial tissue viability in the region of the injected cells. Concern has been raised regarding the interpretation of these results because of the potential benefit of concomitant coronary artery bypass graft surgery performed in these individuals. Still, this is largely regarded as the first and a pioneering study that suggested that autologous skeletal myoblast transplantation could be done safely and is, perhaps, efficacious. The risk of ventricular arrhythmias has been raised and must be sorted out, but this study clearly set the stage for subsequent clinical trials.

Perin *et al.* |**12**|, in 2003, reported a non-randomized study in 14 patients with chronic ischaemic heart disease juxtaposed to seven control patients. Trans-endocardial injections of autologous bone marrow mononuclear cells to induce neovascularization was attempted. Patients were required to have a left ventricular ejection fraction (LVEF) less than 40%, chronic coronary artery disease and a revers-ible perfusion defect as detected by simple photon emission computed tomography (SPECT). Prior infarctions were at least 3 months old. Bone marrow was aspirated and mononuclear cells isolated. Characterization of the cells suggested that less than 3% were haematopoetic progenitor cells, with the largest percentage, almost one-third, being CD4-positive T cells. Electromechanical mapping was performed immediately prior to and during the procedure, with biplane left ventricular angio-graphy to match areas of reversible ischaemia identified by SPECT and to determine target injection areas. Subsequently, approximately 25 million cells were injected into each patient using a mapping–injection catheter. A mean of 15 injections was performed. Seven control patients received no injections. There was one death in each group, with the one treatment death showing 'improvement' in cardiac func-tion at the 2-month follow-up. Unfortunately, a post-mortem examination of this treated heart was not carried out. The report indicates that the patients treated with cell injection experienced fewer anginal symptoms and showed an improvement in maximum VO_2 consumption during exercise. A 6% improvement in EF was noted in the cell-treated group. Accompanying this seeming contractility improvement was a reduction in cardiac volume. This report, then, suggests that a percutaneous technique of delivering bone marrow cells could safely be performed with, arguably, functional cardiac benefit. The control group, however, did not have placebo injec-tions and the test group was small. In contrast to the Menasché report, arrhythmias post-treatment did not appear significant.

Another catheter-based intramyocardial injection of autologous skeletal myoblasts protocol was reported by Smits *et al.* |**13**|. In this study, five patients with symptom-atic heart failure after large anterior wall myocardial infarctions underwent cell injection. Autologous skeletal myoblasts were obtained from a quadricep muscle biopsy and then expanded in tissue culture. Approximately 300 million cells were harvested and then utilizing electromechanical NOGA mapping (NOGASTAR catheter), target areas were identified as infarct zones and the cells were injected. Electrocardiographic monitoring during the procedure and subsequent ambulatory arrhythmia monitoring was carried out to assess pro-arrhythmia. A series of func-tional tests was performed to determine physiological outcomes and included radionuclear cardiography, dobutamine stress echocardiography and magnetic resonance imaging. The authors reported that all cell transplant procedures were uneventful and that no serious adverse events occurred during follow-up. One patient did receive an implantable cardioverter defibrillator device after cell implantation because of asymptomatic non-sustained ventricular tachycardia. In this uncontrolled case series, the EF increased significantly from baseline (36 ± 11% to 41 ± 9% at 3 months; $P = 0.009$). Furthermore, the EF at 6 months was 45 ± 8%. Magnetic resonance imaging regional wall motion analysis suggested significant wall thickening in the targeted areas of cell injection, with less thickening noted in remote scar tissue areas. This study was a seminal one and the first to demonstrate the potential and feasibility of percutaneous skeletal myoblast delivery as a 'stand-alone' procedure for myocardial repair in patients with post-infarction ventricular remodelling and heart failure. The numbers were small, though, and similar to the report by Menasché et al., ventricular arrhythmias were noted and may be problematic.

In an accompanying editorial by Makkar et al. |14|, this arrhythmogenic concern with cell transplantation was addressed more extensively. Perhaps as many as 40% of patients with post-autologous myoblast injection will have potentially problematic ventricular arrhythmias. The type and severity of the arrhythmia may be related to the cell type used and the dose, the method of cell delivery, or worsening of the underlying heart failure in a setting of an operative procedure. Of course, patients undergoing cell transplantation at a time that other cardiac procedures are being performed would be at risk of post-procedure arrhythmias ordinarily. Sorting out the real observation from one impacted by other comorbidities is difficult in these early observation non-randomized trials. Nonetheless, pro-arrhythmia after stem cell therapy, as noted in the Smits et al. and Menasché et al. reports, is concerning. Makkar et al. point out that pro-arrhythmias in this setting might be related to a variety of factors, including heterogeneity between native myocytes and injected stem cells, an intrinsic arrhythmic potential of the injected cells themselves, 'nerve sprouting' induced by stem cell injection, or simply local myocardial injury induced by the injection. The potential for arrhythmia risk must be carefully weighed during clinical trial design and, perhaps, these studies would best be performed in individuals with defibrillators already in place.

Because the challenge of direct cell injection is great and potential toxicity, particularly pro-arrhythmia, possibly identified, enhancing myocardial regeneration via stem cell mobilization at the time of acute myocardial injury is also attractive. Askari et al. |15| focused on this issue in a rat myocardial infarction model. In this model, the effects of stem cell mobilization by using granulocyte colony stimulating factor (GCSF) with or without direct transplantation of syngeneic cells were evaluated. Shortening fraction and myocardial strain determined by quantitative tissue Doppler echocardiographic study were the study end-points. Stem cell mobilization with GCSF alone did not lead to engraftment with bone marrow-derived cells. However, when stromal cell-derived factor-1 (SCDF-1) was added, stem cell homing to the infarct site from bone marrow was upregulated immediately after the infarction and subsequently downregulated in approximately 1 week. Whether this approach alone would lead to improved cardiac function is not known. Eight weeks after myocardial infarction, however, transplantation of syngeneic cardiac fibroblasts transfected to express SCDF-1 into the peri-infarct zone induced the movement of CD117-positive stem cells into injured myocardial zones after GCSF administration. This approach resulted in greater left ventricular mass and improved shortening fraction. These authors suggested that SCDF-1 is sufficient to induce therapeutic stem cell homing to injured myocardium and delineates an approach for directed stem cell engraftment in the injured heart tissue. Some insight has been gained into, arguably, a technique of progenitor cell mobilization that could be used with or without additional cell delivery techniques.

More recently, two stem cell transplantation studies have raised concerns about complications of intracoronary cell infusion techniques. Kang et al. |16| studied ten patients who had received peripheral blood stem cells mobilized by GCSF given by intracoronary injection post-percutaneous angioplasty. This was actually a randomized study of 27 patients, with ten receiving cell infusion, ten receiving GCSF alone, and seven randomized to the control group. End-points were changes in left ventricular systolic function and dobutamine stress echocardiography, with treadmill exercise testing also carried out at a 6-month follow-up point. Combined GCSF injection and intracoronary infusion of mobilized peripheral blood stem cells did not aggravate inflammation or ischaemia in the peri-procedural period. Exercise capacity, myocardial perfusion and LVEF improved significantly in patients who received cell infusion. However, the observation of an unexpectedly high rate of in-stent restenosis at the culprit lesion site in patients who received GCSF therapy during subsequent angiographic study was disconcerting. Although in this study GCSF therapy with intracoronary infusion of peripheral blood stem cells showed improved cardiac function with resolution of ischaemia, restenosis of stented lesions (or worsening of native coronary disease) could be a substantive problem.

A second study by Vulliet et al. |17| evaluated the effect of intracoronary arterial injection of mesenchymal stromal cells in a dog ischaemic heart disease model. These investigators injected approximately 500 000 mesenchymal stromal stem cells per kilogram of body weight into the left circumflex coronary artery of an anaesthetized dog. During administration of the cells, ST segment elevation and T wave changes characteristic of acute ischaemia were noted. Macroscopic and microscopic evidence of myocardial infarction was seen at an evaluation 7 days later, with histological sections of myocardium demonstrating regions of dense fibroplasia with macrophage infiltration only in areas where mesenchymal stromal cells were seen. The authors concluded that these findings showed acute myocardial ischaemia and subsequent myocardial 'microinfarction' after intracoronary injection of mesenchymal stromal cells.

In a commentary accompanying the publication of these two observations, Matsubara |18| suggested that before randomized double-blind clinical trials of GCSF cytokine therapy or intracoronary injections of cell slurries were more routinely carried out, further exploration of the safety of these techniques would be necessary. It should be emphasized that both studies were in remarkably few subjects.

Table 6.3 summarizes the available reports to date of clinical trials utilizing myocardial injection or direct coronary infusion of stem cell therapies to address heart failure in the setting of ischaemic heart disease. Common to all of the reports is the limited number of patients studied. Additionally, the follow-up was quite short. Nonetheless, outcomes have suggested, although not with extraordinarily compelling evidence, that stem cell therapies in this setting could be helpful. Complications, particularly arrhythmias, raise concern and might temper unbridled enthusiasm.

Table 6.3 Clinical trials of stem cell therapy for heart failure from ischaemic heart disease

Study	Year	No. of patients	Procedure	Follow-up period	Donor cell	Complications
Hamano et al. [19]	2001	5	Myocardial injection during CABG	1 year	Bone marrow cells	None
Strauer et al. [20]	2002	10	Intracoronary infusion during PTCA	3 months	Bone marrow cells	None
Assmus et al. [21]	2002	20	Intracoronary infusion during PTCA	4 months	Progenitor cells	None
Menasché et al. [11]	2003	10	Myocardial injection during CABG	10.9 months	Skeletal myoblasts	1 death
Stamm et al. [22]	2003	6	Myocardial injection during CABG	3–9 months	Bone marrow cells	2 patients experienced SVT
Pagani et al. [23]	2003	5	Myocardial injection during LVAD	68–191 days	Skeletal myoblasts	Four patients experienced arrhythmias; 1 LVAD death
Tse et al. [24]	2003	8	Myocardial injection during cath	3 months	Bone marrow cells	None
Perin et al. [12]	2003	14	Myocardial injection during cath	4 months	Bone marrow cells	1 death; no arrhythmias
Wollert et al. [25]	2003	30	Intracoronary infusion during PTCA	6 months	Bone marrow cells	None
Brehm et al. [26]	2003	20	Intracoronary infusion during PTCA	3 months	Bone marrow cells	None
Smits et al. [13]	2003	5	Myocardial injection during cath	6 months	Skeletal myoblasts	1 patient experienced VT
Kang et al. [16]	2004	10	Intracoronary infusion during PTCA	6 months	Peripheral blood stem cells with and without PTCA	High restenosis rate with GCSF

CABG, coronary artery bypass graft; GCSF, granulocyte colony stimulating factor.
PTCA, percutaneous coronary angioplasty; LVAD, left ventricular assist device; cath, catherization;
SVT, supraventricular tachycardia; VT, ventricular tachycardia.
Modified from [6].

Nonetheless, these observations should encourage continued work in this potentially fruitful arena and, ultimately, properly powered and designed, randomized, controlled, clinical trials will tell the tale.

References

1. Penn MS, Francis GS, Ellis SG, Young JB, McCarthy PM, Topol EJ. Autologous cell transplantation for the treatment of damaged myocardium. *Prog Cardiovasc Dis* 2002; **45**(1): 21–32.

2. Hassink RJ, de la Riviere AB, Mummery CL, Coevendans PA. Transplantation of cells for cardiac repair. *J Am Coll Cardiol* 2003; **41**: 711–17.

3. Straver BE, Kornowski R. Stem cell therapy in perspective. *Circulation* 2003; **107**: 929–34.

4. Perin EC, Geng YJ, Willerson JT. Adult stem cell therapy in perspective. *Circulation* 2003; **107**: 935–8.

5. Kereiakes DJ. Stem cells; the chameleon fountain of youth. *Circulation* 2003; **107**: 939–40.

6. Lee MS, Lill M, Makkar RR. Stem cell transplantation in myocardial infarction. *Rev Cardiovasc Med* 2004; **5**(2): 82–93.

7. Dighe K, Kanaganagagam GS, Marber MS. Stem cells: summaries of ten seminal papers. *Dialog Cardiovas Med* 2003; **8**(3): 163–73.

8. Leor J, Patterson M, Quinones MJ, Kedes LH, Kloner RA. Transplantation of fetal myocardial tissue into the infarcted myocardium of rat; a potential method for repair of infarcted myocardium? *Circulation* 1996; **94**(suppl): II332–6.

9. Murry CE, Wiseman RW, Schwartz SM, Hauschka SD. Skeletal myoblast transplantation for repair of myocardial necrosis. *J Clin Invest* 1996; **98**: 2512–23.

10. Taylor DA, Atkins BZ, Hungspreugs P, Jones TR, Reedy MC, Hutcheson KA, Glower DD, Kraus WE. Regenerating functional myocardium: improved performance after skeletal myoblast transplantation. *Nat Med* 1998; **4**: 929–33.

11. Menasché P, Hagege AA, Vilquin JT, Desnos M, Abergel E, Pouzet B, Bel A, Sarateanu S, Scorsin M, Schwartz K, Bruneval P, Benbunan M, Marolleau JP, Duboc D. Autologous skeletal myoblast transplantation for severe postinfarction left ventricular dysfunction. *J Am Coll Cardiol* 2003; **41**: 1078–83.

12. Perin EC, Dohmann HF, Borojevic R, Silva SA, Sousa AL, Mesquita CT, Rossi MI, Carvalho AC, Dutra HS, Dohmann HJ, Silva GV, Belem L, Vivacqua R, Rangel FO, Esporcatte R, Geng YJ, Vaughn WK, Assad JA, Mesquita ET, Willerson JT. Transendocardial, autologous bone marrow cell transplantation for severe, chronic ischemic heart failure. *Circulation* 2003; **107**: 2294–302.

13. Smits PC, van Geuns RM, Poldermans D, Bountioukos M, Onderwater EEM, Lee CH, Maat APWM, Serruys PW. Catheter-based intramyocardial injection of autologous skeletal myoblasts as a primary treatment of ischemic heart failure. *J Am Coll Cardiol* 2003; **42**: 2063–9.

14. Makkar RR, Lill M, Chen P-S. Stem cell therapy for myocardial repair; is it arrhythmogenic? *J Am Coll Cardiol* 2003; **42**(12): 2070–2.

15. Askari AT, Brovic ZB, Goldman CK, Forudi F, Kiedrowski M, Rovner A, Ellis SG, Thomas JD, DiCorleto PE, Topol EJ, Penn MS. Effect of stromal-cell-derived factor-1 on stem cell homing and tissue regeneration in ischemic cardiomyopathy. *Lancet* 2003; **362**: 697–703.

16. Kang HJ, Kim HS, Zhang SY, Park KW, Hyun-Jai C, Koo BK, Yong-Jin K, Dong SL, Sohn DW, Kyou-Sup H, Byung-Hee O, Myoung-Mook L, Young-Bae P. Effects of intracoronary infusion of peripheral blood stem cells mobilized with granulocyte-colony stimulating factor on left ventricular systolic function and restenosis after coronary stenting in myocardial infarction: the MAGIC cell randomized clinical trial. *Lancet* 2004; **363**: 751–6.

17. Vulliet PR, Greeley M, Halloran SM, MacDonald KA, Kittleson MD. Intra-coronary arterial injection of mesenchymal stromal cells and micro-infarction in dogs. *Lancet* 2004; **363**: 783–4.

18. Matsubara K. Risk to the coronary arteries of intra-coronary stem cell infusion and G-CSF cytokine therapy. *Lancet* 2004; **363**(9411): 746–7.

19. Hamano K, Nishida M, Hirata K, Mikamo A, Li TS, Harada M, Miura T, Matsuzaki M, Esato K. Local implantation of autologous bone marrow cells for therapeutic angiogenesis in patients with ischemic heart disease: clinical trial and preliminary results. *Jpn Circ J* 2001; **65**: 845–7.

20. Strauer BE, Brehm M, Zeus T, Kostering M, Hernandez A, Sorg RV, Kogler G, Wernet P. Repair of infarcted myocardium by autologous intracoronary mononuclear bone marrow cell transplantation in humans. *Circulation* 2002; **106**: 1913–18.

21. Assmus B, Schachinger V, Teupe C, Britten M, Lehmann R, Dobert N, Grunwald F, Aicher A, Urbich C, Martin H, Hoelzer D, Dimmeler S, Zeiher AM. Transplantation of progenitor cells and regeneration enhancement in acute myocardial infarction (TOPCARE-AMI). *Circulation* 2002; **106**: 3009–17.

22. Stamm C, Westphal B, Kleine HD, Petzsch M, Kittner C, Klinge H, Schumichen C, Nienaber CA, Freund M, Steinhoff G. Autologous bone-marrow stem-cell transplantation for myocardial regeneration. *Lancet* 2003; **361**: 45–6.

23. Pagani FP, DerSimonian H, Zawadzka A, Wetzel K, Edge AS, Jacoby DB, Dinsmore JH, Wright S, Aretz TH, Eisen HJ, Aaronson KD. Autologous skeletal myoblasts transplanted to ischemia-damaged myocardium in humans. *J Am Coll Cardiol* 2003; **41**: 879–88.

24. Tse HF, Kwong YL, Chan JK, Lo G, Ho CL, Lau CP. Angiogenesis in ischemic myocardium by intraomyocardial autologous bone marrow mononuclear cell implantation. *Lancet* 2003; **361**: 47–9.

25. Wollert KC, Meyer GP, Lotz J, Ringes-Lichtenberg S, Lippolt P, Breidenbach C, Fichtner S, Korte T, Hornig B, Messinger D, Arseniev L, Hertenstein B, Ganser A, Drexler H, for the American Heart Association. Bone marrow transfer to enhance ST-elevation infarct regeneration (BOOST) trial. Late Breaking Clinical Trials. *Circulation* 2003; **108**: 2723.

26. Brehm M, Zeus T, Kostering M. Angiogenesis and myogenesis after intracoronary transplantation of autologous bone marrow cells in patients with acute myocardial infarction (abstract). *Circulation* 2003; **108** (Suppl IV): IV–418.

7

Surgical treatments and approaches

JAMES O'NEILL, PATRICK MCCARTHY

Introduction

Only a minority of surgical practice is governed by data from randomized clinical trials [1]. In contra-distinction to the overwhelming barrage of well-designed, prospective, randomized, multicentre controlled trials that guide the application of pharmacological therapy, there are few randomized data available pertaining to the surgical management of patients with advanced heart failure. Studies of surgical procedures are challenging to perform for a multitude of reasons (Table 7.1). A

Table 7.1 Why are there so few randomized controlled trials of surgical procedures?

1. Technical limitations
    Technical proficiency may vary widely within and among institutions, and differences tend to increase according to the complexity of the procedure.
    This also hampers the performance of multicentre trials.
    Surgical techniques and associated technology evolve quickly, usually before a trial can be completed.
2. Non-controllability
    Unethical to perform sham or control operations (with rare exceptions*).
    Strong placebo effect of surgical intervention.
    How to handle multiple procedures, e.g. coronary artery bypass grafting ± valve surgery ± ventricular reconstruction.
3. Patient preference
    Patients are often reluctant to be randomized to a control group, especially if they are highly motivated. This is especially true of patients with advanced disease and poor quality of life.
4. Funding
    In the absence of a novel device or medication, there is no incentive for industry to fund a study which examines a technique, e.g. the Batista procedure.
5. Not everything *needs* to be randomized
    Some interventions are accepted practice, even in the absence of randomized, controlled data e.g. aortic valve replacement for aortic stenosis, permanent pacemaker insertion for complete heart block, radiofrequency ablation for accessory pathway mediated re-entrant supraventricular tachycardias.

*A recent *New England Journal of Medicine* randomized trial of arthroscopy in chronic knee pain [2].
Source: Moseley *et al.* (2002) [2].

---

particularly difficult problem to circumvent is the competing interest of cardiac transplantation as a censor in studies which examine mortality.

When reviewing late survival following surgical procedures for heart failure, one needs to consider the confounding variables of changes in medical and device therapy over time, as well as changes in peri-operative care. For example, a patient undergoing surgery in 2004 is at a lower risk than the one operated on in 1984 and has the potential benefit of angiotensin-converting enzyme inhibitors, β blockers and implantable cardioverter defibrillators that have been introduced and have proliferated since then |3|.

Much clinical decision-making must be made on the basis of non-randomized field data. The adage 'bad data require good statistics' is particularly applicable in this respect. Thus, the literature contains many observational studies, complex multi-variate analyses and computer intensive techniques, including propensity matching |4|, bootstrapping |5| and jack-knifing |6|. Against this challenging backdrop, the Surgical Treatment for Ischaemic Cardiomyopathy (STICH) trial (see below), is attempting to evaluate coronary artery bypass grafting (CABG), with and without left ventricular reconstruction, in the setting of a prospective multicentre controlled clinical trial.

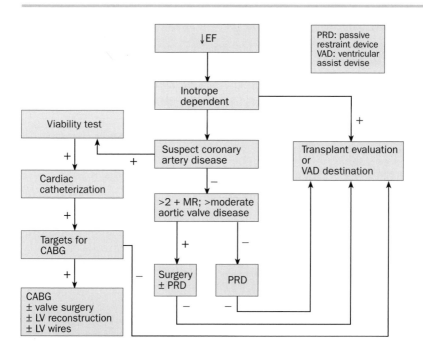

Fig. 7.1 Schema for the evaluation of patients with advanced heart failure. Source: Moseley *et al.* (2002) |2|.

There is an extensive surgical armamentarium available to the modern heart fail-ure practitioner which may be applied to the failing heart. These approaches include: conventional revascularization, valve repair (or replacement), left ventricular recon-struction, maze procedure, epicardial left ventricular lead implantation for cardiac synchronization therapy, endocardial resection, cryoablation, ventricular assist devices and passive cardiac restraint devices. To deploy these strategies appropriately requires a comprehensive pre-operative evaluation by the cardiologist and surgeon, in a logical sequence (Fig. 7.1), careful patient selection, and meticulous intra-opera-tive and post-operative management. While cardiac transplantation has a median 10-year survival, and is often the best or only option for patients with advanced dis-ease, those with medical insurance coverage and, in addition, donor supply will always trail demand, creating a continuing necessity for non-transplant surgical alternatives.

As with many medical interventions, patient selection and clinical judgement are of paramount importance to achieve optimal outcomes. In addition, the approaches work best in the milieu of a tailored, evidence-based, pharmacological regimen.

Coronary artery bypass grafting and infarct exclusion

CABG and left ventricular reconstruction

Coronary heart disease is the leading cause of left ventricular dysfunction, and is the predominant aetiological factor in >50% of patients with heart failure in indus-trialized societies [7]. About 22% of male and 46% of female survivors of myocardial infarction are disabled with heart failure within 6 years (Heart Disease and Stroke Statistics 2003 Update, American Heart Association). The prognosis for patients with heart failure due to an ischaemic cardiomyopathy is poor and may be as high as 50% at 1 year in certain subgroups [8,9]. Orthotopic cardiac transplantation, in some senses, offers the best surgical treatment option for patients with end-stage cardio-myopathy, but due to donor shortage, it is limited to approximately 2000 patients a year in the USA. Furthermore, the risks of rejection, infection, transplant vascu-lopathy and the complications of complex immunosuppressive drug regimens, make transplant less appealing. These factors have prompted a resurgence of non-transplant surgical alternatives to be developed. Advances in surgical techniques, anaesthesiology, pharmacological agents and, in particular, the application of newer imaging modalities, have allowed improved patient selection and targeted multidis-ciplinary therapy for the treatment of ischaemic cardiomyopathy.

As indicated above, no data exist from randomized, controlled clinical trials regarding the outcome of CABG in advanced ischaemic cardiomyopathy [10]. The three major randomized clinical trials of CABG surgery versus medical management, the European Coronary Surgery Study [11], the Veterans Administration Cooperative Study [12], and the Coronary Artery Surgery Study [13], excluded patients with HF or

Table 7.2 Selected recent studies reporting survival in patients with severe left ventricular dysfunction following coronary artery bypass grafting

Year	Authors (ref.)	Era	Type of study	Definition low ejection fraction	n	Perioperative mortality	Survival		
							Short-term	Intermediate-term	Long-term
2003	McCarthy et al. (unpublished data)	1997–2003	Prospective Observational	≤35%	728	2.6%	91% 1 year	81% 3 year	72% 5 year
2003	Ascione et al. |14|	1996–2002	Prospective Observational Propensity subgroup	<30%	250	4%	90% 1 year	84% 3 year	–
2003	Shah et al. |15|	1989–1994	Prospective Observational	<35%	57	1.7%*	83% 1 year	–	56% 5 year, 24% 10 year
2003	Selim et al. |16|	1996–2001	Retrospective Observational	≤30%	212		94% 1 year	80% 3 year	–
1995	Langenburg et al. |17|	1983–1993	Observational	≤25%	96	8.3%	–	–	–
1995	Mickleborough et al. |18|	1982–1993	Observational	<20%	79	3.8%	–	–	67.5% 5 year
1994	Hausmann et al. |19|	1986–1992	Observational	Mean 24%	265	7.6 %	–	87% 3 year	–
1993	Elefteriades et al. |20|	1986–1992	Observational	Mean 25%	83	8.4%	–	80% 3 year	–

severely depressed ejection fractions (EFs). However, significant observational data exist favouring a comprehensive hunt for targets for revascularization (Table 7.2). Approximately half of the patients awaiting cardiac transplantation have ischaemic heart disease as the aetiology of their heart failure, and about one-quarter will die on the waiting list. An aggressive revascularization policy can remove patients from the waiting list and may provide similar survival in selected patients.

CABG improves survival in patients with demonstrated myocardial viability (see Allman *et al.*). Despite this, patients with the greatest left ventricular volumes do not show an improvement in outcomes. Surgical reconstruction results in an improved stress–strain relationship and favourable myocardial remodelling |21|. This improvement in ventricular anatomy may lead to improved survival and better quality of life.

The modern era of left reconstruction was heralded by a greater understanding of the complex geometry of the left ventricle, and in particular the changes it undergoes following myocardial infarction |22|. Localized infarction and ischaemia result in regional fibrosis and produce areas of scarring, akinesis or dyskinesis. Remote areas of the myocardium therefore, according to the Law of Laplace, experience increased wall tension and undergo initial physiological eccentric hypertrophy, which eventually leads to pathological remodelling. The final result is dilatation of the left ventricle, and the conversion from a rugby ball (normal shape) into a soccer ball-shaped (spherical, dilated) heart. The clinical corollary of Laplace's law is seen by the fact that ventricular dilatation increases the risk of death after myocardial infarction |23|. The Global Utilization of Streptokinase and t-PA for Occluded Coronary Arteries (GUSTO-1) trial examined the effect of streptokinase and tissue-type plasminogen activator on ventricular size immediately after reperfusion therapy and found that a left ventricular end-systolic volume index >40 ml/m$_2$ was associated with an increased risk of mortality at 1 year |24|.

The aim of surgical remodelling is to alter the natural history of patients following myocardial infarction by excising the akinetic or dyskinetic, infarcted segment and prevent progressive dilatation—in short, to maintain a rugby ball-shaped heart. The Reconstructive Endoventricular Surgery, Returning Torsion Original Radius Elliptical Shape to the Left Ventricle (RESTORE) group was a multicentre registry, established to evaluate surgical anterior ventricular endocardial restoration (SAVER) in an observational study of 439 patients with post-infarction ischaemic cardiomyopathy |25|. The SAVER procedure was performed with CABG and/or mitral valve surgery as indicated. The mean pre-operative EF was $29 \pm 10\%$ and increased postoperatively to $39 \pm 12.4\%$. Concomitant CABG was performed in 89% and mitral valve surgery in 26% (mainly mitral valve repair). The pre-operative left ventricular end-systolic volume index averaged 109 ± 71 ml/m$_2$ and decreased post-operatively to 69 ± 42 ml/m$_2$. The safety and efficacy of this procedure was fundamental to the subsequent development of the STICH trial.

Funded by the National Institutes of Health in the USA, the STICH study is an ambitious multicentre, randomized, controlled trial which aims to recruit 2300 patients in 15 countries and 90 centres (http://www.stichtrial.org). The inclusion criteria are: New York Heart Association functional class III and IV, left ventricular EF <35% and targets for revascularization. The exclusion criteria include: valvular disease requiring repair or replacement, inotrope dependence and more than one prior cardiac surgery. Patients are randomized to optimal medical management, optimal medical management plus CABG or optimal medical management, medications and left ventricular reconstruction with CABG. End-points include all-cause mortality and quality of life outcomes. This is the largest ever National Institutes of Health funded study. Recruitment is progressing slowly and is expected to take some years.

Myocardial viability testing and impact of revascularization on prognosis in patients with coronary artery disease and left ventricular dysfunction: a meta-analysis

Allman KC, Shaw LJ, Hachamovitch R, Udelson JE. *J Am Coll Cardiol* 2002; **39**: 1151–8

BACKGROUND. This important meta-analysis sought to determine the prognostic value of myocardial viability studies in ischaemic cardiomyopathy and also which technique for viability (thallium perfusion imaging, dobutamine stress echocardiography or positron emission tomography) is optimal.

INTERPRETATION. The authors identified 24 studies between 1966 and 1999 which reported on long-term follow-up of patients undergoing myocardial viability imaging studies. Overall, this meta-analysis included 3088 patients (2228 men) with a mean age of 61 years and a mean left ventricular EF of 32 ± 8%. The mean New York Heart Association functional class was 2.8. A majority of patients (65%) were treated medically, while 35% were revascularized. Myocardial viability was present in 42% of the cohort. Over a mean follow-up of 25 ± 10 months, 12% of patients died. Among patients who had myocardial viability (irrespective of the imaging modality utilized), mortality was 16% in the medically treated group and 3.2% in the revascularized group (*P* <0.0001, relative risk reduction 79.6%). In those patients without viability, mortality was 6.2% in the medically treated group and 7.7% in those revascularized (*P* = NS). Interestingly, in patients treated medically, those with viability had 158% higher mortality than those without viability (16 vs 6.2%, *P* = 0.001) (Fig. 7.2). Using multivariate modelling, in patients with viability, revascularization was a strong determinant of improved survival. Patients with the lowest EFs benefited most by revascularization, provided viability was present. No imaging modality proved superior at predicting outcome. The use of angina as a clinical indicator of myocardial viability is insensitive |26|. These data support the use of formal viability testing in patients with heart failure and coronary disease. The choice modality employed appears to be a less important factor. Once viability has been identified, the data here indicate that it behoves us to implement an aggressive revascularization policy. This meta-analysis indicates excellent 2-year survival in patients undergoing revascularization with viability, despite severe impairment of left ventricular systolic function.

Comment

While the data provided here are valuable, the study was a meta-analysis. Of importance, data regarding magnetic resonance imaging are missing. Yet this is a modality which is being increasingly used to identify myocardial scar and viability. The higher mortality in patients with viability who were treated medically may be related to the fact that these patients had comorbidities that made them unsuitable candidates for revascularization. Alternatively, patients with viability and severe left ventricular dysfunction may have more substrate for myocardial ischaemia, arrhythmias and

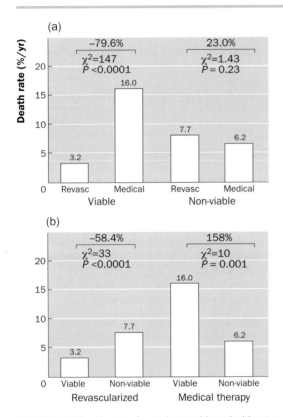

Fig. 7.2 (a) Death rates for patients with and without myocardial viability treated by revascularization or medical therapy. There was a 79.6% reduction in mortality for patients with viability treated by revascularization ($P < 0.0001$). In patients without myocardial viability, there was no significant difference in mortality with revascularization versus medical therapy. (b) Same data as (a) with comparisons based on treatment strategy in patients with and without viability. Annual mortality was lower in revascularized patients when viability was present versus absent (3.2 vs 7.7%, $P < 0.0001$). Annual mortality was significantly higher in medically treated patients when viability was present versus absent (16 vs 6.2%, $P = 0.001$). Revasc, revascularization. Source: Allman *et al.* (2002).

sudden death. Nonetheless, the data indicate that prior to undertaking revascularization, a viability study (irrespective of the modality) must be performed. That said, if one study is negative, because the sensitivity of each testing modality is upwards of 80%, should that prompt us to perform a second, or even a third viability study, in a hunt for surgical substrate?

Positron emission tomography and recovery following revascularization (PARR-1): the importance of scar and the development of a prediction rule for the degree of recovery of left ventricular function

Beanlands RS, Ruddy TD, deKemp RA, *et al. J Am Coll Cardiol* 2002; **40**(10): 1735–43

BACKGROUND. While the prognostic significance of myocardial viability in patients undergoing CABG is widely accepted (see Allman *et al.*), the influence of the extent of myocardial scar on outcomes in these patients has not been well characterized. This was a prospective, multicentre observational study, designed to ascertain the power of the extent of myocardial scar, as assessed by F-18 FDG positron emission tomography scanning, to predict an improvement in EF at 3 months in patients undergoing CABG. The included patients were all referred for CABG, with suitable distal targets, EF ≤35% and could not be scheduled for valve or left ventricular reconstructive surgery. The authors concluded that the extent of scar was a strong and independent predictor of an improvement in EF (Fig. 7.3). For patients with left ventricular scars of 0–16, 16–27.5 and 27.5–47%, EFs improved by 9, 3.7 and 1.3%, respectively. Interestingly, increased age, diabetes and previous revascularization were all independently associated with an increased degree of recovery. The authors attributed this to possible collateral circulation in these patients or, alternatively, selection bias, in that these high-risk patients would have been more likely to have been sent for viability studies.

INTERPRETATION. No randomized controlled data exist to support the use of positron emission tomography imaging in patients with severe left ventricular dysfunction. The data presented here indicate that increased scar content may be a significant determinant of failure to improve EF following CABG alone.

Comment

This was a small, non-controlled study which could not address mortality. It excluded patients undergoing left ventricular reconstruction, which might have been a therapeutic target for many with moderate scars. In addition, as previously mentioned, the RESTORE group, which included patients with extensive myocardial scar, showed that left ventricular reconstruction resulted in a significant improvement in left ventricular EF (from 29 to 39%) [25]. Improvement in EF may not necessarily equate with improved survival, and failure to improve EF following CABG has been shown not to result in worsened survival, in selected cases [27]. In addition, revascularization,

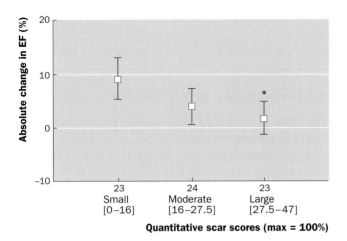

Fig. 7.3 Absolute change in EF versus scar scores: small (0–16% of left ventricle), moderate (16–27.5% of left ventricle), and large (27.5–47% of left ventricle); $P = 0.002$, small versus large scar score. Source: Beanlands *et al.* (2002).

even with extensive myocardial scar, may reduce the potential for developing late ventricular arrhythmias |**28**|.

Early and midterm clinical outcomes in patients with severe left ventricular dysfunction undergoing coronary artery surgery

Ascione R, Narayan P, Rogers CA, Lim KH, Capoun R, Angelini GD. *Ann Thorac Surg* 2003; **76**: 793–9

B A C K G R O U N D . Historically, many patients have been turned down as candidates for CABG, because of fears regarding high peri-operative mortality. No randomized controlled trials exist for revascularization of patients with severely depressed left ventricular systolic function (see STICH). Thus, the data regarding the outcomes of CABG in these patients are largely based on field, registry-based data. Revascularization of these patients is occurring at an increasing rate. This paper reported on the outcome of a large prospectively studied cohort of 5195 consecutive patients who underwent CABG at a single centre between 1996 and 2002. Of these, only 250 had a pre-operative left ventricular EF <30%. Most patients had severely debilitating symptoms of heart failure (58% New York Heart Association functional class III–IV) and angina (70% Canadian Cardiovascular Society III–IV). The mean age was 65 years. Patients undergoing emergency surgery or surgery within 24 h of an acute myocardial infarction were excluded.

INTERPRETATION. This study used propensity matching to compare the outcome of on-pump versus off-pump CABG. Unadjusted survival at 3 years was higher with on-pump surgery (87 vs 73%), but this was not statistically significant after adjusting for baseline variables utilizing propensity matching techniques. In-hospital mortality was 4%, peri-operative myocardial infarction occurred in 4% and acute renal failure requiring renal replacement therapy occurred in 5%. The requirement for inotropic use was significantly less frequent in the off-pump cohort (odds ratio 5.1, confidence interval 2.55–10.2).

Comment

This study is important as it indicated a very low mortality (4% at 30 days) in patients with severe, ischaemic cardiomyopathy. The 3-year survival reported is similar to that of patients undergoing cardiac transplantation. The potential advantage of off-pump CABG in these patients was not realized, but the number who had this modality of surgery was small, only 74, and inferences are limited.

Survival after myocardial revascularization for ischemic cardiomyopathy: a prospective ten-year follow-up study
Shah PJ, Hare DL, Raman JS, *et al. J Thorac Cardiovasc Surg* 2003; **126**: 1320–7

BACKGROUND. This is another contemporary outcomes paper in patients with ischaemic cardiomyopathy who underwent CABG. It addressed the survival of patients who underwent elective revascularization, and importantly the authors excluded unstable angina, recent (<4 weeks) myocardial infarction, repeat CABG, valvular operations, aneurysmectomy and patients with left main coronary disease. The authors prospectively followed 57 patients with left ventricular EFs (by contrast left ventriculography) ≤35%. All patients underwent stress thallium single photon emission computed tomography (SPECT) imaging pre-operatively. Rather incongruously, 20 studies were missing or uninterpretable. The major end-points were all-cause mortality at 30 days, 1 year and 10 years and patients were actively followed in the clinic or by telephone assessment. Patients were also tracked actively for worsening symptoms, admission for heart failure, cardiac transplantation and other cardiac procedures.

INTERPRETATION. The mean age was 67 years, 93% were male, 65% were New York Heart Association functional class III or IV, and the mean left ventricular EF (LVEF) was 28%. One patient died in the early post-operative phase (these were all elective cases). Over the 10 years for which these patients were studied, 40 died and two underwent cardiac transplantation. The 1-, 5- and 10-year survival rates were 83, 56 and 24% Repeat radionucleotide ventriculography was performed in 47 of the 49 patients who survived 12 months. The mean LVEF did not differ significantly from before the operation (30 ± 9 vs 28 ± 4, *P* = 0.09). Mean EFs did increase, however, in the patients who had large reversible defects pre-operatively (40 ± 5 vs 30 ± 3, *P* = 0.01). Short-term survival and event-free survival were independently and positively correlated with large reversible perfusion defects pre-operatively. Long-term survival was not predicted by the presence of large reversible defects.

Comment

Although a single centre, with small numbers in a non-randomized observational study, the data presented here are important in that they indicate that elective CABG can be performed with very low (<2%) mortality in patients with advanced ischaemic cardiomyopathy. Myocardial viability is a predictor of good short-term outcome and the lack of long-term utility may be a function of the small numbers of patients included with viability data available. The average age of these patients at the time of the operation was 67 years, so their survival over 10 years should be made with reference to life expectancy at this age in the general population (13 years for a man aged 67 years and 17 years for a woman aged 67 years: National Center for Health Statistics US Decennial Life Tables for 1979–1981). Morbidity was also reduced in these patients and, of interest, at 10 years, all eleven patients who survived were in New York Heart Association functional class II.

CABG conclusion

CABG should be considered in all patients with left ventricular dysfunction and targets for revascularization. There is currently sufficient data to mandate viability studies in all patients and those without viability should be treated medically. CABG should be performed on these patients in centres of excellence, with high surgical volumes and, ideally, with left ventricular assist device backup available.

The recent blossoming of the drug-eluting stent field further complicates management decisions. Percutaneous revascularization, with minimal restenosis, has become a reality |29|. How this will potentially impact on revascularization of patients with ischaemic cardiomyopathy remains to be elucidated.

Extensive experience in the use of left ventricular reconstruction has confirmed that it carries a low peri-operative mortality and excellent intermediate and long-term survival |25,30–35|. Left ventricular reconstruction should be considered in centres proficient in this technique, when there are discrete akinetic or dyskinetic regions. Surgery should generally be combined with a multifaceted approach and peri-operative evaluation should include viability studies.

Mitral valve surgery

Mitral regurgitation is common in patients with heart failure and may arise from any combination of four main mechanisms:

- Ischaemic: in ischaemic cardiomyopathy, due to prior infer-posterior myocardial infarction or ischaemia and papillary muscle dysfunction.

- 'Functional': may occur in all forms of cardiomyopathy. Arises from alteration of left ventricular geometry, which causes apical displacement of the papillary muscles and failure of leaflet coaptation. This may be accompanied by varying degrees of mitral annular dilatation.

- Systolic anterior motion of the mitral valve apparatus: occurs in hypertrophic cardiomyopathy and causes displacement of the anterior mitral valve leaflet with resultant late systolic mitral regurgitation.

- Intrinsic valve disease: may include myxomatous, rheumatic, congenital, degenerative causes, etc.

Irrespective of aetiology, mitral regurgitation imposes volume overload on the failing ventricle and may accelerate progressive adverse remodelling. It imparts an adverse prognosis proportional to its severity (see Koelling *et al.*). Patients with ≥2+ mitral regurgitation on their surface echocardiogram, who are undergoing cardiac surgery for another reason, are offered mitral valve repair at our institution. We perform intra-operative transoesophageal echocardiography on patients undergoing CABG. Intra-operatively, pharmacological manipulation to elevate blood pressure and provoke regurgitation should be utilized. If ≥2+ mitral regurgitation is identified, either on the pre-operative surface study, or on the intra-operative study, mitral valve repair is performed, although this is somewhat controversial. There is widespread agreement that, in cases with intrinsic valve disease, repair should be performed. Some centres do not perform mitral valve repair in pure 'ischaemic' mitral regurgitation, arguing that the problem is with the ventricle and not with the valve. Valve repair is superior to replacement in ischaemic mitral regurgitation |36|. At our centre, we employ an aggressive policy of mitral valve repair in patients undergoing CABG with ≥2+ mitral regurgitation.

Mitral valve surgery in patients with non-ischaemic cardiomyopathy is even more contentious. Traditionally, undertaking mitral valve surgery in these patients was avoided, because of high peri-operative mortality |37|. Archaic techniques involving excision of the sub-valvular apparatus adversely affected ventricular geometry and left ventricular performance.

The use of small annuloplasty rings and mitral valve replacement with chordal preservation has been successfully applied to small numbers of patients with non-ischaemic dilated cardiomyopathy with reasonable results. Bach and Bolling |38| reported on 20 patients with dilated cardiomyopathy and severe symptoms of heart failure. Seventy per cent were alive at 18 months. Badhwar and Bolling |39| subsequently reported on a larger series of 125 patients, which included ischaemic and non-ischaemic cases. All had severe mitral regurgitation and underwent mitral valve reconstruction, at a single institution. There were no intra-operative deaths. One- and 2-year actuarial survival was 80 and 70%, respectively. Surviving patients showed echocardiographic evidence for reverse ventricular remodelling, with LVEF increasing from 16 ± 5% to 26 ± 8% and left ventricular end-diastolic volumes decreasing from 281 ± 86 ml to 206 ± 88 ml at 2 years.

We reported on 44 patients at the Cleveland Clinic with severe mitral regurgitation and LVEF <35% who underwent isolated mitral valve surgery. Most patients (35/44) had repair. All had severe symptoms of heart failure and were New York Heart Association functional class III or IV. Peri-operative mortality was 2%. The 1-, 2- and 5-year survival rates were 89, 86 and 67%, respectively, and freedom from re-admission for heart failure was 88, 82 and 72% during the same follow-up |40|. It should be noted, however, that this was a markedly heterogeneous cohort, and only 30% of these patients had non-ischaemic dilated cardiomyopathy and functional mitral regurgitation.

Whether isolated mitral valve repair should be offered to patients with severe mitral regurgitation and non-ischaemic cardiomyopathy cannot currently be inferred, due to insufficient data. The Acorn® trial (see p. 117) included 167 patients who underwent mitral valve repair/replacement, in addition to a myocardial restraint device.

Prognostic significance of mitral regurgitation and tricuspid regurgitation in patients with left ventricular systolic dysfunction

Koelling TM, Aaronson KD, Cody RJ, Bach DS, Armstrong WF. *Am Heart J* 2002; **144**(3): 524–9

BACKGROUND. Heart failure is characterized by complex geometrical changes in all four cardiac chambers. Among the consequences of this are atrio-ventricular valve leaflet tethering, impaired coaptation, which along with varying degrees of annular dilatation and increased vascular resistance result in mitral and tricuspid regurgitation. Isolated valvular regurgitation may itself result in volume overload and consequent adverse ventricular remodelling (as in the case of aortic regurgitation, for example). The failing ventricle is particularly susceptible to increased volume loading, and this study sought to assess the prognostic significance of 'functional' mitral and tricuspid regurgitation on survival in patients with left ventricular systolic dysfunction.

INTERPRETATION. This was a single-centre, retrospective, registry-based study of 1617 patients with LVEFs ≤35% and without intrinsic valve disease who underwent echocardiography between 1995 and 1998. The outcome was all-cause mortality as assessed by reference to the Social Security Death Index or urgent cardiac transplantation. Multivariable stepwise Cox proportional hazards analysis was used to identify independent predictors of survival. The majority of patients (68%) were male and most (59%) had ischaemic cardiomyopathy. Overall, there was significant mortality and 463 (32%) patients were dead or had undergone urgent transplantation during a mean follow-up of 368 ± 368 days. Functional valvular regurgitation was common; 272 patients (18.9%) had severe and 427 (30%) had moderate mitral regurgitation. Tricuspid regurgitation was also common; 171 patients (12%) had severe and 325 (23%) had moderate tricuspid regurgitation. Logically enough, increased age, left atrial enlargement, left ventricular end-diastolic dimension, EF and the severity of tricuspid regurgitation correlated with the severity of mitral regurgitation. The presence of atrial fibrillation was strongly associated with tricuspid regurgitation. Not surprisingly, overall predictors of tricuspid regurgitation severity were generally the same as for mitral regurgitation. Multivariable predictors of mortality or urgent transplantation included increasing mitral and tricuspid regurgitation grade, cancer, coronary artery disease, LVEF, and increased heart rate. Kaplan–Meier survival curves (Fig. 7.4a, b) for mitral and tricuspid regurgitation severity showed markedly reduced survival in patients with higher grades of regurgitation.

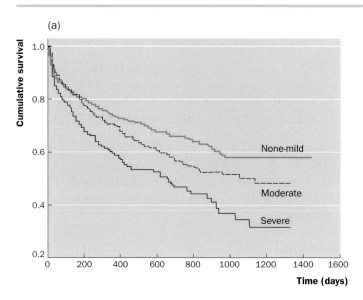

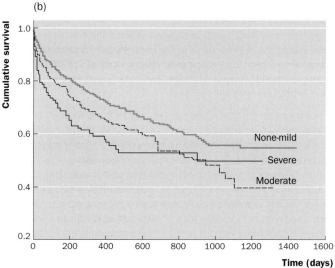

Fig. 7.4 Effect of (a) mitral regurgitation grade and (b) tricuspid regurgitation grade on cumulative survival rate for patients with left ventricular systolic dysfunction. None to mild, moderate and severe regurgitation are depicted separately. With log-rank analysis: (a) pooled over strata, $P < 0.0001$; none to mild versus moderate, $P = 0.09$; none to mild versus severe, $P < 0.0001$; and moderate versus severe, $P = 0.003$; (b) pooled over strata, $P = 0.0003$; none to mild versus moderate, $P = 0.007$; none to mild versus severe, $P < 0.0003$; and moderate versus severe, $P = 0.22$. Source: Koelling et al. (2002).

The 1- and 3-year survival rates for patients with severe mitral regurgitation were 59 and 39%, respectively, and the corresponding survival rates for patients with severe tricuspid regurgitation were 59 and 49%, respectively.

Comment

These data are retrospective, but the mortality is high and comparable with other studies of patients with severe HF. It would have been interesting to know the impact of combined severe mitral and tricuspid regurgitation on outcome. These and other data strongly indicate that atrio-ventricular regurgitation heralds a poor prognosis. Unfortunately, we do not definitively know if restoring competence to the regurgitant valves improves outcome. However, most recent reports of mitral valve repair in patients with severe left ventricular dysfunction demonstrate improved survival |39,40|.

Mitral valve repair in patients with end stage cardiomyopathy: who benefits?

Gummert JF, Rahmel A, Bucerius J, *et al*. *Eur J Cardiothorac Surg* 2003; **23**: 1017–22

BACKGROUND. This was a retrospective analysis of 66 patients with advanced heart failure who underwent isolated mitral valve repair at a single centre. The mean age of the patients was 59 years. All had LVEFs <30% (mean 23%) and 53/66 had non-ischaemic cardiomyopathy.

INTERPRETATION. Overall 30-day mortality was 6.1% (12.5% for patients over 60 years). Event-free survival is shown in Fig. 7.5. During follow-up, an additional 16 patients died 9 ± 10 months following surgery. Three patients required repeat mitral valve surgery, two early, one late (at 800 days). In survivors, the median New York Heart Association functional class improved from a median of III to II during long-term follow-up (P <0.001). LVEF improved from 25 ± 6 to 34 ± 15% during long-term follow-up (18 months). Cardiac transplantation was performed in seven patients. Transplant-free survival was only 40% at 5 years. Mean transplant-free survival in the 13 patients with ischaemic cardiomyopathy was particularly poor (17 ± 4 months) compared with the non-ischaemic group (51 ± 5 months; P <0.001).

Comment

The authors reached the conclusion that '….[mitral valve repair] is a feasible therapeutic option for most patients with significant mitral valve incompetence'. This may be an over-optimistic interpretation of the data. They also concluded that older patients and patients with ischaemic cardiomyopathy fare worse. The inherent weakness in these data is that, due to the small numbers involved, multivariable analysis or complex modelling was not possible. Thus, it is possible that the increased mortality

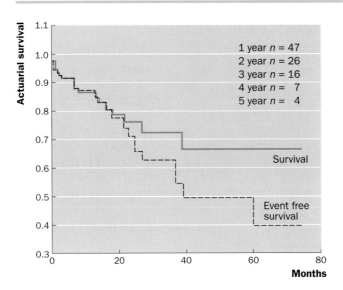

Fig. 7.5 Survival and event-free survival after mitral valve repair. Event-free survival was defined as survival without heart transplantation. The mean survival rate was 55 ± 4 months, the event-free survival rate was 40 ± 11 months. Source: Gummert *et al.* (2003).

in the patients with ischaemic cardiomyopathy was a function of their age. The overall age of the patients was younger than the general heart failure population. It is likely that the transplanted patients constituted a greater number of relatively younger patients, and, as this was a censoring point, this further impairs the ability to make any inferences about which patients do best. An attempt to identify historical controls for propensity matching may have proved more valuable.

Mitral valve surgery conclusion

Mitral regurgitation is common and is associated with a worse prognosis in patients with advanced left ventricular systolic dysfunction. It appears prudent to repair mitral regurgitation of ≥2+ severity at the time of CABG. The decision of whether to perform isolated mitral valve repair on patients with dilated cardiomyopathy (ischaemic or non-ischaemic) is not so clear-cut. The studies presented here are fuelling the ongoing debate. These data suggest that in patients with ischaemic cardiomyopathy, isolated mitral valve repair appears to impart less survival benefit than in non-ischaemics or in patients undergoing concomitant CABG. However, this difference may potentially be explained by advanced age and other comorbidities in this cohort.

Non-transplant surgical alternatives

In the never-ending battle to palliate an increasing number of heart failure patients, non-transplant surgery (including CABG, ventricular reconstruction, mitral valve repair, as previously discussed) is being aggressively pursued in many centres. This involves the application of conventional surgery in patients who may have heretofore been refused an operation. In addition, the development of mechanical assist devices continues, while the field of passive mechanical restraint devices is coming of age.

Thanks to pharmacological, surgical and anaesthetic advances, aortic valve replacement can now be performed in patients with severely depressed left ventricular function, with low peri-operative mortality. There is convincing evidence that valve replacement may be performed safely, with good intermediate-term results in patients with severely depressed left ventricular function and low-gradient aortic stenosis (see Pereira *et al.*).

Classic teaching was that in the case of chronic aortic regurgitation, symptomatic patients with advanced left ventricular dysfunction and left ventricular end-systolic dimension >6 cm may have irreversible adverse remodelling, which may not respond to volume overload reduction by replacing the valve. However, at the Cleveland Clinic, we recently reviewed our experience with valve surgery for aortic incompetence with severe left ventricular dysfunction. From 1972 to 1999, 88 patients with LVEFs ≤30% underwent isolated aortic valve replacement for chronic aortic regurgitation. Survival at 5, 10, 15, 20 and 25 years in patients with severe left ventricular dysfunction was 68, 46, 41, 18 and 9%, respectively. This is comparable with cardiac transplantation. Since 1990, 1- and 5-year survival in patients with severe left ventricular dysfunction who underwent aortic valve replacement for aortic regurgitation has been 97 and 85%, respectively |**41**|.

Despite great technological developments, the total artificial heart is only in phase 1 studies |**42**|. Left ventricular assist devices (LVADs) currently provide only a 23% 2-year survival when used as destination therapy |**43–5**|. The Federal Drug Administration in the USA has approved the use of LVADs as 'destination therapy'.

LVADs have become an essential safety net for centres that undertake high-risk non-transplant surgery. In our centre, some operations are performed with 'LVAD backup', and patients undergo preliminary cardiac transplant evaluation prior to surgery.

Lessons from the now abandoned latissimus dorsi dynamic cardiomyoplasty inspired the development of passive restraint devices, of which two are in clinical trials. The Myocor Myosplint® consists of splints which are placed through the left ventricle and reduce the stress–strain relationship of the failing ventricle by effectively reducing the diameter of one sphere, by making two hemispheres |**46**|.

The Acorn® CorCap™ is a sock-shaped mesh that is applied to the heart to limit dilatation in patients with advanced non-ischaemic cardiomyopathy |**47**|. It is currently the subject of a prospective, multicentre, randomized clinical trial, which has enrolled 300 patients. Initial results are promising, but results are not expected until late 2004.

Survival after aortic valve replacement for severe aortic stenosis with low transvalvular gradients and severe left ventricular dysfunction

Pereira JJ, Lauer MS, Bashir M, *et al. J Am Coll Cardiol* 2002; **39**: 1356–63

BACKGROUND. Severe, uncorrected aortic stenosis leads initially to hypertrophy and eventually to adverse left ventricular remodelling, with dilatation and function, with resultant development of the heart failure syndrome. With progressive pump failure, gradients across the stenosed valve fall and hence may not be a reliable indicator of the severity of aortic stenosis. Historically, these patients had 21% peri-operative mortality. This study used propensity matching to determine whether aortic valve replacement in patients with severe left ventricular dysfunction (≤35%) and low transvalvular gradients (≤30 mmHg) results in improved survival over medical 'therapy'.

INTERPRETATION. The authors identified 68 patients with severe left ventricular dysfunction, an aortic valve area ≤0.75 cm₂ and low transvalvular gradients who underwent aortic valve replacement between 1990 and 1998. A control group of 89 patients was identified who had identical echocardiographic criteria, but did not undergo surgery. Using complicated statistical techniques, the authors used propensity scoring techniques to create two matched groups—39 in the surgical cohort and 56 in the non-surgical, control group. The mean age of patients was 70 years in the surgical group and 77 years in the control group and the overall mean LVEF was 22%. Concomitant CABG was performed in 60% of the surgical group. Aortic valve replacement was associated with significantly better outcomes—during the follow-up of 2.7 ± 2.3 years, 32% of those patients treated surgically died, compared with 83% of the control group. Kaplan–Meier survival curves are shown in Fig. 7.6. Aortic valve surgery was associated with 8% in-hospital mortality. Only 2% of survivors in the surgical group had severely debilitating HF symptoms.

Comment

These data should encourage an aggressive approach to the management of low-gradient, severe aortic stenosis in patients with severe left ventricular dysfunction. The mortality was overwhelming in the group who did not undergo surgery. Peri-operative mortality was acceptable (8%) and long-term survival was greatly enhanced. A particular weakness of the study relates to the fact that, despite careful matching techniques, the surgically treated group was younger, more likely to be male, had a better New York Heart Association functional class pre-operatively and had lower pre-operative serum creatinine levels.

Non-transplant surgical alternatives conclusion

Non-transplant surgical alternatives are essential to provide reduced mortality and morbidity to this ever-expanding pool of patients with heart failure. All of these

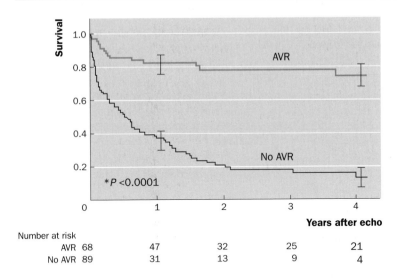

Fig. 7.6 Survival by Kaplan–Meier analysis among all patients in the aortic valve replacement (AVR) and control (no AVR) groups ($P < 0.0001$). The number of patients at risk during follow-up is shown on the x-axis. Echo, echocardiography. Source: Pereira *et al.* (2002).

approaches require systematic evaluation, ideally, although rarely feasible, with randomized controlled trials. In the absence of these, we will continue to rely on well-conducted observational studies and complex statistical techniques to guide clinical practice.

References

1. Horton R. Surgical research or comic opera: questions, but few answers. *Lancet* 1996; 347(9007): 984–5.

2. Moseley JB, O'Malley K, Petersen NJ, Menke TJ, Brody BA, Kuykendall DH, Hollingsworth JC, Ashton CM, Wray NP. A controlled trial of arthroscopic surgery for osteoarthritis of the knee. *N Engl J Med* 2002; 347(2): 81–8.

3. McCarthy PM. Ventricular aneurysms, shock, and late follow-up in patients with heart failure. *J Thorac Cardiovasc Surg* 2003; 126(2): 323–5.

 4. Rubin DB. Estimating causal effects from large data sets using propensity scores. *Ann Intern Med* 1997; **127**(8 Pt 2): 757–63.

 5. Altman DG, Andersen PK. Bootstrap investigation of the stability of a Cox regression model. *Stat Med* 1989; **8**(7): 771–83.

 6. Ludbrook J. Issues in biomedical statistics: comparing means by computer-intensive tests. *Aust N Z J Surg* 1995; **65**(11): 812–19.

 7. Sutton GC. Epidemiologic aspects of heart failure. *Am Heart J* 1990; **120**(6 Pt 2): 1538–40.

 8. Franciosa JA, Wilen M, Ziesche S, Cohn JN. Survival in men with severe chronic left ventricular failure due to either coronary heart disease or idiopathic dilated cardio-myopathy. *Am J Cardiol* 1983; **51**(5): 831–6.

 9. Levy D, Kenchaiah S, Larson MG, Benjamin EJ, Kupka MJ, Ho KK, Murabito JM, Vasan RS. Long-term trends in the incidence of and survival with heart failure. *N Engl J Med* 2002; **347**(18): 1397–402.

10. Jones RH. Is it time for a randomized trial of surgical treatment of ischemic heart failure? *J Am Coll Cardiol* 2001; **37**(5): 1210–13.

11. Varnauskas E. Twelve-year follow-up of survival in the randomized European Coronary Surgery Study. *N Engl J Med* 1988; **319**(6): 332–7.

12. The Veterans Administration Coronary Artery Bypass Surgery Cooperative Study Group. Eleven-year survival in the Veterans Administration randomized trial of coronary bypass surgery for stable angina. *N Engl J Med* 1984; **311**(21): 1333–9.

13. Killip T, Passamani E, Davis K. Coronary Artery Surgery Study (CASS): a randomized trial of coronary bypass surgery. Eight years follow-up and survival in patients with reduced ejection fraction. *Circulation* 1985; **72**(6 Pt 2): V102–9.

14. Ascione R, Narayan P, Rogers CA, Lim KH, Capoun R, Angelini GD. Early and midterm clinical outcome in patients with severe left ventricular dysfunction undergoing coronary artery surgery. *Ann Thorac Surg* 2003; **76**(3): 793–9.

15. Shah PJ, Hare DL, Raman JS, Gordon I, Chan RK, Horowitz JD, Rosalion A, Buxton BF. Survival after myocardial revascularization for ischemic cardiomyopathy: a prospective ten-year follow-up study. *J Thorac Cardiovasc Surg* 2003; **126**(5): 1320–7.

16. Selim Isbir C, Yildirim T, Akgun S, Civelek A, Aksoy N, Oz M, Arsan S. Coronary artery bypass surgery in patients with severe left ventricular dysfunction. *Int J Cardiol* 2003; **90**(2–3): 309–16.

17. Langenburg SE, Buchanan SA, Blackbourne LH, Scheri RP, Sinclair KN, Martinez J, Spotnitz WD, Tribble CG, Kron IL. Predicting survival after coronary revascularization for ischemic cardiomyopathy. *Ann Thorac Surg* 1995; **60**(5): 1193–6; discussion 1196–7.

18. Mickleborough LL, Maruyama H, Takagi Y, Mohamed S, Sun Z, Ebisuzaki L. Results of revascularization in patients with severe left ventricular dysfunction. *Circulation* 1995; **92**(9 Suppl): II73–9.

19. Hausmann H, Ennker J, Topp H, Schuler S, Schiessler A, Hempel B, Friedel N, Hofmeister J, Hetzer R. Coronary artery bypass grafting and heart transplantation in end-stage coronary artery disease: a comparison of hemodynamic improvement and ventricular function. *J Card Surg* 1994; **9**(2): 77–84.

20. Elefteriades JA, Tolis G Jr, Levi E, Mills LK, Zaret BL. Coronary artery bypass grafting in severe left ventricular dysfunction: excellent survival with improved ejection fraction and functional state. *J Am Coll Cardiol* 1993; **22**(5): 1411–17.

21. Artrip JH, Oz MC, Burkhoff D. Left ventricular volume reduction surgery for heart failure: a physiologic perspective. *J Thorac Cardiovasc Surg* 2001; **122**(4): 775–82.

22. Buckberg GD. The structure and function of the healthy helical and failing spherical heart. Overview: the ventricular band and its surgical implications. *Semin Thorac Cardiovasc Surg* 2001; **13**(4): 298–300.

23. White HD, Norris RM, Brown MA, Brandt PW, Whitlock RM, Wild CJ. Left ventricular end-systolic volume as the major determinant of survival after recovery from myocardial infarction. *Circulation* 1987; **76**(1): 44–51.

24. Migrino RQ, Young JB, Ellis SG, White HD, Lundergan CF, Miller DP, Granger CB, Ross AM, Califf RM, Topol EJ. End-systolic volume index at 90 to 180 minutes into reperfusion therapy for acute myocardial infarction is a strong predictor of early and late mortality. The Global Utilization of Streptokinase and t-PA for Occluded Coronary Arteries (GUSTO)-I Angiographic Investigators. *Circulation* 1997; **96**(1): 116–21.

25. Athanasuleas CL, Stanley AW Jr, Buckberg GD, Dor V, DiDonato M, Blackstone EH. Surgical anterior ventricular endocardial restoration (SAVER) in the dilated remodeled ventricle after anterior myocardial infarction. RESTORE group. Reconstructive Endoventricular Surgery, returning Torsion Original Radius Elliptical Shape to the LV. *J Am Coll Cardiol* 2001; **37**(5): 1199–209.

26. Auerbach MA, Schoder H, Hoh C, Gambhir SS, Yaghoubi S, Sayre JW, Silverman D, Phelps ME, Schelbert HR, Czernin J. Prevalence of myocardial viability as detected by positron emission tomography in patients with ischemic cardiomyopathy. *Circulation* 1999; **99**(22): 2921–6.

27. Samady H, Elefteriades JA, Abbott BG, Mattera JA, McPherson CA, Wackers FJ. Failure to improve left ventricular function after coronary revascularization for ischemic cardiomyopathy is not associated with worse outcome. *Circulation* 1999; **100**(12): 1298–304.

28. Veenhuyzen GD, Singh SN, McAreavey D, Shelton BJ, Exner DV. Prior coronary artery bypass surgery and risk of death among patients with ischemic left ventricular dysfunction. *Circulation* 2001; **104**(13): 1489–93.

29. Moses JW, Leon MB, Popma JJ, Fitzgerald PJ, Holmes DR, O'Shaughnessy C, Caputo RP, Kereiakes DJ, Williams DO, Teirstein PS, Jaeger JL, Kuntz RE; SIRIUS Investigators. Sirolimus-eluting stents versus standard stents in patients with stenosis in a native coronary artery. *N Engl J Med* 2003; **349**(14): 1315–23.

30. McCarthy PM, Young JB, Hoercher KJ, Smedira NG, Blackstone EH, Starling RC. *Surgical LV reconstruction for end-stage heart disease: outcomes and effect on NYHA class and rehospitalizations for heart failure.* 74th Scientific Session of the American Heart Association. November, 2001.

31. McCarthy PM. Synergistic approaches in the surgical treatment of heart failure: complex solutions for complex problems. *Semin Thorac Cardiovasc Surg* 2002; **14**(2): 187–9.

32. Di Donato M, Sabatier M, Dor V, Toso A, Maioli M, Fantini F. Akinetic versus dyskinetic postinfarction scar: relation to surgical outcome in patients undergoing endoventricular circular patch plasty repair. *J Am Coll Cardiol* 1997; **29**(7): 1569–75.

33. Di Donato M, Sabatier M, Montiglio F, Maioli M, Toso A, Fantini F, Dor V. Outcome of left ventricular aneurysmectomy with patch repair in patients with severely depressed pump function. *Am J Cardiol* 1995; **76**(8): 557–61.

34. Di Donato M, Toso A, Maioli M, Sabatier M, Stanley AW Jr, Dor V. Intermediate survival and predictors of death after surgical ventricular restoration. *Semin Thorac Cardiovasc Surg* 2001; **13**(4): 468–75.

35. Dor V, Di Donato M, Sabatier M, Montiglio F, Civaia F. Left ventricular reconstruction by endoventricular circular patch plasty repair: a 17-year experience. *Semin Thorac Cardiovasc Surg* 2001; **13**(4): 435–47.

36. Grossi EA, Goldberg JD, LaPietra A, Ye X, Zakow P, Sussman M, Delianides J, Culliford AT, Esposito RA, Ribakove GH, Galloway AC, Colvin SB. Ischemic mitral valve reconstruction and replacement: comparison of long-term survival and complications. *J Thorac Cardiovasc Surg* 2001; **122**(6): 1107–24.

37. Lee SJ, Bay KS. Mortality risk factors associated with mitral valve replacement: a survival analysis of 10 year follow-up data. *Can J Cardiol* 1991; **7**(1): 11–18.

38. Bach DS, Bolling SF. Improvement following correction of secondary mitral regurgitation in end-stage cardiomyopathy with mitral annuloplasty. *Am J Cardiol* 1996; **78**(8): 966–9.

39. Badhwar V, Bolling SF. Mitral valve surgery in the patient with left ventricular dysfunction. *Semin Thorac Cardiovasc Surg* 2002; **14**(2): 133–6.

40. Bishay ES, McCarthy PM, Cosgrove DM, Hoercher KJ, Smedira NG, Mukherjee D, White J, Blackstone EH. Mitral valve surgery in patients with severe left ventricular dysfunction. *Eur J Cardiothorac Surg* 2000; **17**(3): 213–21.

41. McCarthy PM. Aortic valve surgery in patients with left ventricular dysfunction. *Semin Thorac Cardiovasc Surg* 2002; **14**(2): 137–43.

42. Dowling RD, Etoch SW, Stevens KA, Johnson AC, Gray LA Jr. Current status of the AbioCor implantable replacement heart. *Ann Thorac Surg* 2001; **71**(3 Suppl): S147–9; discussion S183–4.

43. Rose EA, Gelijns AC, Moskowitz AJ, Heitjan DF, Stevenson LW, Dembitsky W, Long JW, Ascheim DD, Tierney AR, Levitan RG, Watson JT, Meier P, Ronan NS, Shapiro PA, Lazar RM, Miller LW, Gupta L, Frazier OH, Desvigne-Nickens P, Oz MC, Poirier VL; Randomized Evaluation of Mechanical Assistance for the Treatment of Congestive Heart Failure (REMATCH) Study Group. Long-term mechanical left ventricular assistance for end-stage heart failure. *N Engl J Med* 2001; **345**(20): 1435–43.

44. Delgado DH, Rao V, Ross HJ, Verma S, Smedira NG. Mechanical circulatory assistance: state of art. *Circulation* 2002; **106**(16): 2046–50.

45. McCarthy PM. Mechanical assist devices. *J Card Surg* 2001; **16**(3): 177.

46. McCarthy PM, Takagaki M, Ochiai Y, Young JB, Tabata T, Shiota T, Qin JX, Thomas JD, Mortier TJ, Schroeder RF, Schweich CJ Jr, Fukamachi K. Device-based change in left ventricular shape: a new concept for the treatment of dilated cardiomyopathy. *J Thorac Cardiovasc Surg* 2001; **122**(3): 482–90.

47. Konertz WF, Shapland JE, Hotz H, Dushe S, Braun JP, Stantke K, Kleber FX. Passive containment and reverse remodeling by a novel textile cardiac support device. *Circulation* 2001; **104**(12 Suppl 1): I270–5.

8

Is too much neurohormonal blockade harmful?

INDER ANAND

This chapter first appeared under the reference *Curr Cardiol Rep* 2004; 6(3): 169–75 and is reproduced with kind permission of the publishers.

Introduction

Chronic heart failure is characterized by haemodynamic abnormalities |1|, impaired exercise capacity |2|, neurohormonal and cytokine activation |3,4| and a relentless progression with a high mortality |5|. The event that initiates the syndrome of heart failure is, of course, damage to the heart that reduces cardiac output and threatens the arterial blood pressure. The body responds to this threat via a baroreceptor-mediated activation of two sets of neurohormones, with opposing effects |6|. In the short term, these responses are compensatory and adaptive, helping to maintain homeostasis. Eventually, however, excessive production of neurohormones becomes maladaptive, leading to progression of heart failure through a variety of mechanisms. Vasoconstrictor hormones such as norepinephrine, angiotensin II, vasopressin and endothelin (ET) are antinatriuretic and antidiuretic, and have growth-promoting properties. In contrast, vasodilator hormones such as the natriuretic peptides, prostaglandins and the kinin system that are also activated have natriuretic, diuretic and antimitogenic effects. In heart failure, the natriuretic and vasodilator effects are overwhelmed by influences that lead to vasoconstriction, salt and water retention, necrotic and apoptotic myocyte death, and abnormal cellular growth with left ventricular remodelling |7,8|.

Although the mechanisms are not entirely clear, increasing data suggest that heart failure progresses through a process of structural remodelling of the heart, to which neurohormonal and cytokine activation make an important contribution |8|. Several lines of evidence support the role of neurohormones in the progression of heart failure: norepinephrine |9|, angiotensin II |10| and cytokines |11| are directly toxic to cardiac myocytes; the degree of neurohormonal activation in heart failure is proportional to disease severity, increases with the progression of heart failure, and is related to prognosis |12|. Moreover, changes in neurohormonal activation over time, occurring either spontaneously or in response to pharmacological therapy, are associated with proportional changes in subsequent mortality and morbidity |**13**|. These findings led to the hypothesis that blocking the deleterious effects of the vasoconstrictive hormones and stimulating the vasodilators would have beneficial effects. The spectacular success in reducing heart failure morbidity and mortality by inhibiting the sympathetic and renin–angiotensin–aldosterone systems with β blockers, angiotensin-converting enzyme (ACE) inhibitors and aldosterone receptor blockers further underscored the importance of neurohormonal activation in the progression of heart failure |**14–18**| and strengthened the conviction that more complete blockade of the neurohormonal system would provide incremental benefit. However, in recent clinical trials evaluating strategies of stacking additional neurohormonal blockers on top of ACE inhibitors, β blockers and aldosterone antagonists, this has not been successful and in some cases even shown to be deleterious |**19–22**|. Do these findings suggest that neurohormonal blockade in patients with heart failure has reached a ceiling? Is this because ACE inhibitor and β blocker therapy has attenuated the progression of heart failure to such an extent that further improvement in these patients may be difficult to detect? Or are there data to show that excessive neurohormonal inhibition with newer add-on therapies is harmful because they undermine the body's compensatory homeostatic mechanisms?

It must be recognized that because of the remarkable success of ACE inhibitors and β blockers in reducing heart failure mortality and morbidity, all new add-on therapies have to be tested on top of this 'standard of care'. There is, therefore, no way to assess whether newer therapies are as effective, or indeed, even more effective, than either ACE inhibitors or β blockers. Hence, the disappointing results of recent heart failure trials are no reflection on the soundness of the neurohormonal hypothesis or on the drug being tested, but rather on the strategy of stacking newer drugs on top of the standard of care. Whereas it is fairly straightforward to assess whether a new 'add-on' therapy produces incremental benefits, it is more difficult to conclude whether a lack of incremental benefit on mortality and morbidity is due to excessive neurohormonal inhibition. Few of the clinical trials that have reported disappointing or adverse effects on mortality and morbidity measured neurohormones to confirm whether they were excessively blocked. Moreover, β blockers do not appear to work by decreasing norepinephrine. It is not even clear whether levels of circulating neurohormones accurately reflect the body's ability to maintain homeostasis. Nor is it clear which measurements point to excessive blockade of the sympathetic or renin–angiotensin–aldosterone system. Finally, only a few of the surrogates of excessive neurohormonal blockade, such as heart rate and blood pressure, are routinely measured in clinical trials. Despite these limitations, this review attempts to analyse some of the recent heart failure trials with newer neurohormonal inhibitors that have reported disappointing results.

Excessive blockade of the sympathetic nervous system

Beta blockers reduce mortality in patients with New York Heart Association class II–IV heart failure by 34–35% |**16,17,23**|. The association between the degree of sympathetic activation and mortality |**3,13**|, and dose-dependent favourable effects of β blockers on heart failure mortality and morbidity |**24**| raised the possibility that 'more complete' adrenergic blockade might produce even greater benefit on outcomes. Moxonidine, a centrally acting α agonist that greatly reduces circulating catecholamines |**25**|, was used to test this hypothesis in the Moxonidine in Congestive Heart Failure (MOXCON) trial |**26**|. The study had to be terminated early, with only 1934 of the 4533 patients randomized, because of a 38% higher mortality in the moxonidine group. Hospitalizations for heart failure and myocardial infarctions were also increased. The increase in mortality and morbidity was accompanied by a significant decrease in plasma norepinephrine by moxonidine (−18.8%) as compared with placebo (+6.9%) |**26**|. An earlier study had shown that moxonidine produced marked sympatholytic effects in the target dose of the MOXCON trial, and that this was accompanied by serious adverse effects |**25**|. Although the mechanisms for the increase in mortality and morbidity in the MOXCON trial are not entirely clear, the marked sympatholytic effects of moxonidine could have produced severe myocardial depression, bradycardia or hypotension. However, these effects could not be documented in the patients who died. Alternatively, premature discontinuation of the drug or non-compliance with the use of higher doses of moxonidine could have resulted in rebound excessive sympathetic discharge that might have been responsible for the serious adverse effects observed in the MOXCON trial. Again, evidence to support this possibility is also not available.

Another example of the association between marked sympatholytic effect and adverse outcomes was seen in a subgroup of patients in the Beta-blocker Evaluation of Survival Trial (BEST) |**27**|. BEST was the only β blocker heart failure trial that did not show a mortality benefit. This might be related to the marked sympatholytic effects of bucindolol, not seen with carvedilol or metoprolol. In the BEST trial, patients ($n = 153$) receiving the sympatholytic β blocker bucindolol who had a decrease in norepinephrine of >224 pg/ml from baseline to 3 months, had a 169% increase in mortality as compared with patients who had no significant change in norepinephrine (relative risk 1.69; 95% confidence interval [CI] 1.22–2.34) |**28**|.

These two examples underscore the fact that a severe decrease in adrenergic support may render the body devoid of any compensatory mechanisms, resulting in adverse outcomes.

Further blockade of the renin–angiotensin–aldosterone system

Effect of high-dose versus low-dose ACE inhibitor in heart failure

Two trials have compared the effects of low-dose versus high-dose ACE inhibitor in patients with moderate to severe heart failure, to test the hypothesis that more effective blockade of ACE may produce incremental benefits. The Assessment of Treatment with Lisinopril and Survival (ATLAS) randomized 3164 patients with New York Heart Association class II–IV heart failure to either low-dose (2.5–5.0 mg/day, average 4.5 ± 1.1 mg) or high-dose (32.5–35 mg/day, average 33.2) lisinopril for a median of 45.7 months. The high-dose group had a non-significant, 8% decrease in mortality as compared with the low-dose group ($P = 0.128$). The risk of death or hospitalization was, however, 12% lower ($P = 0.002$) and hospitalizations for heart failure 24% lower ($P = 0.002$) in the high-dose group. The second study was much smaller and investigated a very high dose of enalapril (60 mg/day, average 42 ± 19.3 mg) compared with usual dose (average 17.9 ± 4.3 mg/day) and could not find any benefit of high-dose ACE inhibitor [29]. This relative lack of beneficial effect with 'excessive' blockade of ACE could be related to the phenomenon of 'angiotensin II and aldosterone escape' seen with ACE inhibitor use despite complete blockade of ACE. Indeed, Tang et al. [30] have shown that whereas high-dose enalapril (40 mg/day) caused a much greater suppression of serum ACE activity, levels of angiotensin and aldosterone remained elevated to the same extent in both the high- and low-dose ACE inhibitor groups. Thus, high doses of ACE inhibitor produce only a minimal or no incremental benefit but are associated with more adverse side effects.

Effect of dual ACE inhibitor and angiotensin receptor blocker (ARB) in heart failure

Because physiologically active levels of angiotensin II persist despite chronic ACE inhibitor therapy [31,32], three separate studies, the Valsartan Heart Failure Trial (Val-HeFT) [19], Candesartan in Heart Failure–Assessment of Reduction in Mortality and Morbidity (CHARM) [33–36], and Valsartan in Acute Myocardial Infarction (VALIANT) [37], were undertaken to determine whether ARBs could further reduce morbidity and mortality in patients already receiving an ACE inhibitor. Val-HeFT was the first large-scale trial to evaluate the ARB valsartan added to an ACE inhibitor. The results showed that the addition of valsartan did not affect mortality but significantly reduced morbidity, and that this effect was largely due to a 28% reduction in hospitalizations for HF. In 35% of the patients who were receiving β blockers, in addition to an ACE inhibitor, the use of valsartan was associated with an unfavourable trend to increased mortality and morbidity. This finding raised concerns that excessive blockade of the renin–angiotensin system might have been responsible for the unfavourable effects of triple therapy.

Whether the result of this *post hoc* subgroup analysis of Val-HeFT is just a statistical play of chance or can be explained scientifically remains unclear and needs some discussion. In the Metoprolol CR/XL Randomized Intervention Trial in Congestive Heart Failure (MERIT-HF) trial |16|, the annual mortality in patients with New York Heart Association class II–III heart failure with an average ejection fraction (EF) of 28% was only 7.2% in patients receiving the β blocker metoprolol and an ACE inhibitor or ARB (Table 8.1). In contrast, the annual mortality was 9.1% in the placebo group of Val-HeFT that randomized a very similar population of patients but only 35% of whom were receiving a β blocker |19|. However, in the subgroup of patients who were all on β blockers and ACE inhibitors, the annual mortality was only 5.7%. Thus, in the setting of clinical trials, the effective use of β blockers and ACE inhibitors has reduced the mortality of patients with moderate to severe heart failure to a remarkably low level, considering that the annual mortality rate in the population of average white American males aged 65 years, without heart failure, is approximately 3.0%. It would, therefore, be very difficult to show any further improvement in mortality with newer add-on therapies. However, even a small difference in the number of deaths between the placebo and active therapy groups would result in a large percentage increase in mortality. In the Val-HeFT triple therapy group, 129 of 791 patients receiving valsartan died (16.3%) against 97 of 815 patients receiving placebo (11.9%), a significant 37% increase in mortality. The difference in the number of deaths between the groups was only 32 from a total of 1606 patients.

A careful analysis of several determinants of heart failure mortality and morbidity, such as left ventricular EF, brain natriuretic peptide, norepinephrine, blood urea nitrogen (BUN), serum creatinine and potassium, systolic blood pressure and heart

Table 8.1 Annual mortality rate in some recent heart failure clinical trials

Trial	NYHA class (II/III/IV)	Ejection fraction (%)	Use of ACE inhibitor/ARB	Use of β blockers	Annual mortality (%)
MERIT-HF (β blocker group, $n = 2001$)	53/44/3	28	95%	100%	7.2
Val-HeFT (placebo group, $n = 2499$)	62/36/1.7	27	93%	35%	9.1
Val-HeFT ACE inhibitor/ β blocker group, $n = 815$	63/37	27	100%	100%	5.7
National Vital Statistics Report: 65-year-old male					3.0

NYHA, New York Heart Association; ACE, angiotensin-converting enzyme; ARB, angiotensin receptor blocker; MERIT-HF, Metoprolol CR/XL Randomized Intervention Trial in Congestive Heart Failure; VAL-HeFT, Valsartan Heart Failure Trial.

rate, did not show any difference in the valsartan or placebo groups of patients who died or were alive at the end of the Val-HeFT study |38|. The only exception was a paradoxical greater beneficial effect of valsartan on brain natriuretic peptide in patients who died. Therefore, changes in the physiological markers of heart failure mortality and morbidity do not appear to explain the unexpected adverse outcome observed in patients with heart failure receiving valsartan in addition to concomitant therapy with ACE inhibitors and β blockers. It is therefore likely that the increased mortality seen in the triple therapy group could be due to a play of chance.

In contrast, in the CHARM |33| and VALIANT |37| trials, no adverse effect of candesartan or valsartan was seen in patients receiving both an ACE inhibitor and β blockers, despite a much higher baseline use of β blockers (over 50%) than in the Val-HeFT. Indeed, these patients received the same benefit as those not taking ACE inhibitors and/or β blockers at baseline. Thus, the initial concern regarding excessive neurohormones with triple therapy does not seem to have been substantiated with later studies. It should be noted, however, that the populations studied in VALIANT and CHARM were different, with the former being a post-myocardial infarction group and the latter a chronic heart failure group.

Role of endothelin antagonists

Like norepinephrine and angiotensin II, endothelin-1 (ET-1) also plays a pivotal role in cardiovascular regulation |39,40|. Plasma concentrations of ET-1 and big ET-1 are elevated in heart failure |41,42| and are strong independent predictors of mortality |43|. In advanced chronic heart failure, ET_A receptors and ET-converting enzyme-1 are upregulated |44|. Therefore, like ACE inhibitors, β blockers and aldosterone antagonists, ET receptor antagonists might also improve prognosis in heart failure. In a rat model of heart failure, ET_A blockade improved survival |45|. These data encouraged the clinical development of ET receptor antagonists in heart failure. Both ET_A selective (darusentan) and mixed $ET_{A/B}$ receptor antagonists (bosentan) appeared promising, as single-dose administration of these agents increased cardiac output and reduced systemic and pulmonary vascular resistance in patients with severe chronic heart failure |46,47|. The long-term effects of the mixed ET blocker, bosentan, in heart failure were reported in the Research on Endothelin Antagonism in Chronic Heart Failure (REACH-1) trial |21| and the Endothelin Antagonist Bosentan for Lowering Cardiac Events in Heart Failure (ENABLE) study |20|. In REACH-1, bosentan caused early worsening of heart failure, but tended to improve symptoms at 6 months, suggesting a possible long-term benefit. REACH-1 was terminated prematurely because of a reversible increase in liver transaminases. In the ENABLE study, a lower dose of bosentan did not improve clinical outcome. In these studies, neurohormonal measurements were not made and, hence, it is not possible to comment on whether excessive neurohormonal blockade had occurred. No adverse effect on blood pressure or heart rate was reported.

As the non-selective $ET_{A/B}$ receptor antagonist bosentan did not show any long-term beneficial effects in heart failure |20|, and because selective ET_B receptor blockade worsens haemodynamics in patients with heart failure |48|, it was suggested that the selective ET_A receptor antagonists may be more effective than the mixed $ET_{A/B}$ ones. The Endothelin A Receptor Antagonist Trial in Heart Failure (EARTH) |49| investigated the chronic effects of different doses of the orally active ET_A antagonist darusentan in 642 patients with New York Heart Association class II–IV heart failure. Over 98% of these patients were receiving ACE inhibitors or ARB and 80% β blockers. The primary end-point was a change in left ventricular end-systolic volume at 24 weeks, compared with baseline, as measured using magnetic resonance imaging. Secondary end-points included changes in left ventricular mass, left ventricular end-diastolic volume, EF, neurohormones (norepinephrine, aldosterone, atrial natriuretic peptide (ANP), brain natriuretic peptide, ET-1 and big ET-1), exercise capacity as assessed by a 6-min walk test, quality of life, and New York Heart Association class. Darusentan did not provide any clinical benefit, and there was no significant change seen in the primary end-point of left ventricular end-systolic volume or any of the secondary end-points. Worsening heart failure was observed in 11.1% of patients, and only 4.7% of patients died during the 6-month study, with no difference between groups. Darusentan had no adverse effects on neurohormones, heart rate or blood pressure |49|. Thus, the use of selective or non-selective ET receptor inhibitors also does not seem to add any incremental benefit in patients adequately treated with β blockers and ACE inhibitors.

Dual ACE and neutral endopeptidase inhibition

The neurohormonal model of the progression of heart failure suggests that blocking the deleterious effects of the vasoconstrictive hormones and stimulating the vasodilators would have beneficial effects, not only on haemodynamics but also on ventricular remodelling and survival. The clinical development of the dual ACE and neutral endopeptidase inhibitor omapatrilat provided the opportunity to test this hypothesis. The Omapatrilat Versus Enalapril Randomized Trial of Utility in Reducing Events (OVERTURE) compared the effects of enalapril (20 mg/day) and omapatrilat (40 mg/day) in 5770 patients with New York Heart Association class II–IV heart failure over 14.5 months who were optimally treated (50% on β blockers, 40% spironolactone, and 60% digoxin) |22|. The primary end-points of death and hospitalization for heart failure were not different in the enalapril and omapatrilat groups (hazard ratio 0.94; 95% CI 0.86–1.03; $P = 0.187$), but the study fulfilled the pre-specified criteria of non-inferiority for omapatrilat. Omapatrilat, however, did reduce the combined risk of cardiovascular deaths or hospitalization by 9% ($P = 0.024$). Although the event rate in these high-risk patients was high, the lack of incremental benefit may have been related to significant episodes of hypotension during the period of drug up-titration. A *post hoc* analysis of the role of baseline systolic blood pressure on the response to omapatrilat showed that omapatrilat had favourable effects in patients with systemic hypertension, and that the magnitude of its effect fell as the blood pressure decreased, so that there was no benefit of oma–patrilat over enalapril in patients with systolic blood pressures <110 mmHg. Thus, in OVERTURE the addition of neutral endopeptidase and ACE inhibition is another example of how excessive use of neurohormonal inhibition that results in significant hypotension may be more effective than the use of ACE inhibitors alone in reducing events.

Role of cytokine inhibition

There is growing evidence that pro-inflammatory cytokines, including tumour necrosis factor (TNF), interleukin-1 and -6, are expressed in heart failure, approximately in proportion to the severity of the disease, and may be involved in the progression of the disease |50|. There also exists an imbalance between pro-inflammatory and anti-inflammatory cytokines in heart failure, similar to the imbalance between vasoconstrictor and vasodilator hormones described above |51|. These led to strategies being devised to antagonize the pro-inflammatory cytokines in patients with heart failure. Two approaches have been used.

Soluble TNF receptors

The first approach involved the use of etanercept (Enbrel), a genetically engineered recombinant human TNF receptor protein that binds to circulating TNF, and thereby prevents TNF from binding to TNF receptors on the target cell surface. Early pre-clinical studies with etanercept were shown to reverse the deleterious negative inotropic effects of TNF *in vivo* |52| and in a series of phase I clinical studies in patients with moderate to advanced heart failure. These early short-term studies in small numbers of patients showed improvements in quality of life, 6-min walking distance and left ventricular EF after 3 months of treatment with etanercept |53,54|. These encouraging findings led to the design of two multicentre clinical trials in patients with New York Heart Association class III–IV heart failure, the Randomized Etanercept North American Strategy to Study Antagonism of Cytokines (RENAISSANCE, $n = 900$) in the USA, and the Research into Etanercept Cytokine Antagonism in Ventricular Dysfunction (RECOVER, $n = 900$), in Europe and Australia. Both trials had parallel study designs, but differed in the doses of etanercept used: RENAISSANCE used doses of 25 mg twice a week (biw) and 25 mg three times a week (tiw), whereas RECOVER used doses of 25 mg once a week (qw) and 25 mg biw. The primary end-point of these trials was a clinical composite. A third trial, Randomized Etanercept Worldwide Evaluation (RENEWAL, $n = 1500$), pooled the data from RENAISSANCE (biw and tiw dosing) and RECOVER (biw dosing only), and had all-cause mortality and hospitalization for heart failure as the primary end-points. The Data Monitoring Safety Board stopped the trials early, because it was felt that the trials were unlikely to show a benefit in the primary end-points if allowed to complete |55|. Preliminary analysis of the data showed no benefit for etanercept on the clinical composite end-point in RENAISSANCE and RECOVER, nor a benefit for etanercept on all-cause mortality and heart failure hospitalization in RENEWAL |**55,56**|. In a *post hoc* analysis, however, the hazard ratio for death/hospitalization for worsening heart failure in patients taking the biw dose of etanercept in RECOVER was 0.87 against 1.21 and 1.23 for patients in RENAISSANCE receiving etanercept biw and tiw, respectively. These disparities in trial findings were considered to be related to the different length of follow-up in the two trials. Patients in RECOVER received etanercept for a median time of 5.7 months, whereas patients in RENAISSANCE received etanercept for 12.7 months |**11**|. This would suggest that the longer the exposure to the drug, the worse the outcome.

Monoclonal antibodies

The second approach involved the use of a genetically engineered monoclonal antibody, infliximab (Remicade), in the Anti-TNFα Therapy Against CHF (ATTACH) phase II study in 150 patients with moderate to advanced heart failure. The primary end-point of the ATTACH trial was also the clinical composite score. Patients were randomized to receive three separate intravenous infusions of infliximab (5 or 10 mg/kg) at baseline, 2 and 4 weeks. Assessment of the clinical composite was made at 14 and 28 weeks. Analysis of the completed trial data showed that there was a 21% dose-related increase in death and heart failure hospitalizations with infliximab compared with placebo at 14 weeks and a 26% increase at 28 weeks |**57**|.

Therefore, a careful examination of these two studies (RECOVER and RENAISSANCE) shows that anticytokine strategies targeting TNF-α were not neutral, but the results are indeed consistent with a trend to an increase in mortality and morbidity. Two possible explanations have been offered to clarify these findings |**11**|. The first is that infliximab and etanercept have intrinsic cytotoxicity. Infliximab exerts its effects, at least in part, by fixing complement in cells that express TNF. As myocytes express TNF on the sarcolemma, complement fixation in the heart could lead to myocyte lysis and further deterioration of cardiac function. Etanercept may also be toxic under certain settings. It has been shown that, in human studies, etanercept binds to TNF in the peripheral circulation, but this binding is not tight and may dissociate at an extremely fast rate. Rapid dissociation of TNF from etanercept can lead to a paradoxical increase in the duration of TNF bioactivity, opposite to what the therapy was intended to do. The second explanation for worsening heart failure may be related to the fact that physiological levels of TNF are cytoprotective and play an important role in tissue remodelling and repair. Excessive antagonism of TNF may, therefore, result in the loss of one or more of its beneficial effects, with consequent loss of homeostasis and resulting worsening of heart failure.

Conclusion

Inhibiting the deleterious consequences of activated renin–angiotensin–aldosterone and sympathetic systems with ACE inhibitors, β blockers and aldosterone receptor antagonists has had an enormous impact in reducing heart failure mortality and morbidity. These drugs are now the standard of care. However, extending this paradigm to other activated neurohormonal and cytokine systems, by stacking multiple neurohormonal blockers together, has not shown any incremental benefit, and in some cases has had deleterious consequences. These findings have led to the suggestion that we may have reached a therapeutic ceiling for the neurohormonal approach. However, in many cases these results are based on studies carried out in patients who, because of being on ACE inhibitors and β blockers, have a very low mortality rate, which may be difficult to improve upon. Testing these agents in higher risk patients may have yielded different results. This notwithstanding, there are numerous examples where clear-cut deleterious consequences of excessive neurohormonal and cytokine inhibition are seen. These findings underscore the fact that not all the body's responses in heart failure are harmful and need to be blocked. Thus, further improvement in the status of heart failure patients may require new paradigms.

References

1. Wilson JR, Schwartz JS, Sutton MS, Ferraro N, Horowitz LN, Reichek N, Josephson ME. Prognosis in severe heart failure and relation to hemodynamic measurements and ventricular ectopic activity. *J Am Coll Cardiol* 1983; 2: 403–10.

2. Szlachcic J, Massie BM, Kramer BL, Topic N, Tubau J. Correlates and prognostic implication of exercise capacity in chronic congestive heart failure. *Am J Cardiol* 1985; 55: 1037–42.

3. Cohn JN, Levine TB, Olivari MT, Garberg V, Lura D, Francis GS, Simon AB, Rector T. Plasma norepinephrine as a guide to prognosis in patients with chronic congestive heart failure. *N Engl J Med* 1984; 311: 819–23.

4. Swedberg K, Eneroth P, Kjekshus J, Wilhelmsen L. Hormones regulating cardiovascular function in patients with severe congestive heart failure and their relation to mortality. CONSENSUS Trial Study Group. *Circulation* 1990; 82: 1730–6.

5. Massie BM, Conway M. Survival of patients with congestive heart failure: past, present, and future prospects. *Circulation* 1987; 7: IV11–19.

6. Anand IS, Chugh SS. Mechanisms and management of renal dysfunction in heart failure. *Curr Opin Cardiol* 1997; 12: 251–8.

7. Anand IS. Pathogenesis of salt and water retention in the syndrome of congestive heart failure. In: Poole-Wilson PA, Chatterjee K, Coates AJS, Colucci WS, Massie BM (eds). *Heart Failure; Scientific Principles and Clinical Practice.* London: Churchill Livingstone, 1996.

8. Anand IS, Florea VG. Alterations in ventricular structure: role of left ventricular remodeling. In: Mann DL (ed.). *Heart Failure: Companion to Braunwald's Heart Disease*. Philadelphia: Saunders, 2002.

9. Mann D, Kent R, Parsons B, Cooper G. Adrenergic effects on the biology of the adult mammalian cardiocyte. *Circulation* 1992; **85**: 790–804.

10. Tan LB, Jalil JE, Pick R, Janicki JS, Weber KT. Cardiac myocyte necrosis induced by angiotensin II. *Circ Res* 1991; **69**: 1185–95.

11. Mann DL. Inflammatory mediators and the failing heart: past, present, and the foreseeable future. *Circ Res* 2002; **91**: 988–98.

12. Anand IS, Chandrashekhar Y. Neurohormonal responses in congestive heart failure: effect of ACE inhibitors in randomized controlled clinical trials. In: Dhalla NS, Singhal PK, Beamish RE (eds). *Heart Hypertrophy and Failure*. Boston: Kluwer, 1996; pp 487–501.

13. Anand IS, Fisher LD, Chiang YT, Latini R, Masson S, Maggioni AP, Glazer RD, Tognoni G, Cohn JN. Changes in brain natriuretic peptide and norepinephrine over time and mortality and morbidity in Val-HeFT. *Circulation* 2003; **107**: 1276–81.

14. CONSENSUS Trial Study Group. Effects of enalapril on mortality in severe congestive heart failure. Results of the Cooperative North Scandinavian Enalapril Survival Study (CONSENSUS). *N Engl J Med* 1987; **316**: 1429–35.

15. The SOLVD Investigators. Effect of enalapril on survival in patients with reduced left ventricular ejection fractions and congestive heart failure. *N Engl J Med* 1991; **325**: 293–302.

16. The MERIT-HF Investigators. Effect of metoprolol CR/XL in chronic heart failure: Metoprolol CR/XL Randomized Intervention Trial in Congestive Heart Failure (MERIT-HF). *Lancet* 1999; **353**: 2001–7.

17. Packer M, Coats AJ, Fowler MB, Katus HA, Krum H, Mohacsi P, Rouleau JL, Tendera M, Castaigne A, Roecker EB, Schultz MK, DeMets DL. Effect of carvedilol on survival in severe chronic heart failure. *N Engl J Med* 2001; **344**: 1651–8.

18. Pitt B, Zannad F, Remme WJ, Cody R, Castaigne A, Perez A, Palensky J, Wittes J. The effect of spironolactone on morbidity and mortality in patients with severe heart failure. Randomized Aldactone Evaluation Study Investigators. *N Engl J Med* 1999; **341**: 709–17.

19. Cohn JN, Tognoni G. A randomized trial of the angiotensin-receptor blocker valsartan in chronic heart failure. *N Engl J Med* 2001; **345**: 1667–75.

20. Packer M. The ENABLE (Endothelin Antagonist Bosentan for Lowering Cardiac Events in Heart Failure) Study. Preliminary data presented at ACC March 2002.

21. Packer M. Multicenter, double-blind, placebo-controlled study of long-term endothelin blockade with bosentan in congestive heart failure—results of the REACH–1 trial. *Circulation* 1998; **98**(Suppl S).

22. Packer M, Califf RM, Konstam MA, Krum H, McMurray JJ, Rouleau JL, Swedberg K. Comparison of omapatrilat and enalapril in patients with chronic heart failure: the Omapatrilat Versus Enalapril Randomized Trial of Utility in Reducing Events (OVERTURE). *Circulation* 2002; **106**: 920–6.

23. The CIBIS II Investigators. The Cardiac Insufficiency Bisoprolol Study II (CIBIS-II): a randomised trial. *Lancet* 1999; **353**: 9–13.

24. Bristow MR, Gilbert EM, Abraham WT, Adams KF, Fowler MB, Hershberger RE, Kubo SH, Narahara KA, Ingersoll H, Krueger S, Young S, Shusterman N. Carvedilol produces

dose-related improvements in left ventricular function and survival in subjects with chronic heart failure. MOCHA Investigators. *Circulation* 1996; **94**: 2807–16.

25. Swedberg K, Bristow MR, Cohn JN, Dargie H, Straub M, Wiltse C, Wright TJ. Effects of sustained-release moxonidine, an imidazoline agonist, on plasma norepinephrine in patients with chronic heart failure. *Circulation* 2002; **105**: 1797–803.

26. Cohn JN, Pfeffer MA, Rouleau J, Sharpe N, Swedberg K, Straub M, Wiltse C, Wright TJ. Adverse mortality effect of central sympathetic inhibition with sustained-release moxonidine in patients with heart failure (MOXCON). *Eur J Heart Fail* 2003; **5**: 659–67.

27. Beta-Blocker Evaluation of Survival Trial Investigators. A trial of the beta-blocker bucindolol in patients with advanced chronic heart failure. *N Engl J Med* 2001; **344**: 1659–67.

28. Bristow M, Krause-Steinrauf H, Abraham WT, Liang CS, Hattler B, Krueger S, Lindenfeld J, Lowes BD, Olson B, Thaneemit-Chen S, Zelis R. Sympatholytic effect of bucindolol adversely affected survival, and was disproportionately observed in the class IV subgroup of BEST. *Circulation* 2001; **104**: II-755.

29. Nanas JN, Alexopoulos G, Anastasiou-Nana MI, Karidis K, Tirologos A, Zobolos S, Pirgakis V, Anthopoulos L, Sideris D, Stamatelopoulos SF, Moulopoulos SD. Outcome of patients with congestive heart failure treated with standard versus high doses of enalapril: a multicenter study. High Enalapril Dose Study Group. *J Am Coll Cardiol* 2000; **36**: 2090–5.

30. Tang WH, Vagelos RH, Yee YG, Benedict CR, Willson K, Liss CL, Fowler MB. Neurohormonal and clinical responses to high- versus low-dose enalapril therapy in chronic heart failure. *J Am Coll Cardiol* 2002; **39**: 70–8.

31. Kawamura M, Imanashi M, Matsushima Y, Ito K, Hiramori K. Circulating angiotensin II levels under repeated administration of lisinopril in normal subjects. *Clin Exp Pharmacol Physiol* 1992; **19**: 547–53.

32. Jorde UP, Ennezat PV, Lisker J, Suryadevara V, Infeld J, Cukon S, Hammer A, Sonnenblick EH, Le Jemtel TH. Maximally recommended doses of angiotensin-converting enzyme (ACE) inhibitors do not completely prevent ACE-mediated formation of angiotensin II in chronic heart failure. *Circulation* 2000; **101**: 844–6.

33. Pfeffer MA, Swedberg K, Granger CB, Held P, McMurray JJ, Michelson EL, Olofsson B, Ostergren J, Yusuf S, Pocock S. Effects of candesartan on mortality and morbidity in patients with chronic heart failure: the CHARM-Overall programme. *Lancet* 2003; **362**: 759–66.

34. Yusuf S, Pfeffer MA, Swedberg K, Granger CB, Held P, McMurray JJ, Michelson EL, Olofsson B, Ostergren J. Effects of candesartan in patients with chronic heart failure and preserved left-ventricular ejection fraction: the CHARM-Preserved Trial. *Lancet* 2003; **362**: 777–81.

35. Granger CB, McMurray JJ, Yusuf S, Held P, Michelson EL, Olofsson B, Ostergren J, Pfeffer MA, Swedberg K. Effects of candesartan in patients with chronic heart failure and reduced left-ventricular systolic function intolerant to angiotensin-converting-enzyme inhibitors: the CHARM-Alternative trial. *Lancet* 2003; **362**: 772–6.

36. McMurray JJ, Ostergren J, Swedberg K, Granger CB, Held P, Michelson EL, Olofsson B, Yusuf S, Pfeffer MA. Effects of candesartan in patients with chronic heart failure and reduced left-ventricular systolic function taking angiotensin-converting-enzyme inhibitors: the CHARM-Added trial. *Lancet* 2003; **362**: 767–71.

37. Pfeffer MA, McMurray JJ, Velazquez EJ, Rouleau JL, Kober L, Maggioni AP, Solomon SD, Swedberg K, Van de Werf F, White H, Leimberger JD, Henis M, Edwards S, Zelenkofske S, Sellers MA, Califf RM. Valsartan, captopril, or both in myocardial infarction complicated by heart failure, left ventricular dysfunction, or both. *N Engl J Med* 2003; **349**: 1893–906.

38. Anand IS, Glazer R, Chiang YT, Hester A, Aknay N, Cohn J. A retrospective analysis of major determinants of heart failure mortality in patients receiving both ACE inhibitors and beta-blockers in Val-HeFT. *J Card Fail* 2003; **5**: P304.

39. Yanagisawa M, Kurihara H, Kimura S, Tomobe Y, Kobayashi M, Mitsui Y, Yazaki Y, Goto K, Masaki T. A novel potent vasoconstrictor peptide produced by vascular endothelial cells. *Nature* 1988; **332**: 411–15.

40. Haynes WG, Webb DJ. Contribution of endogenous generation of endothelin-1 to basal vascular tone. *Lancet* 1994; **344**: 852–4.

41. Stewart DJ, Cernacek P, Costello KB, Rouleau JL. Elevated endothelin-1 in heart failure and loss of normal response to postural change. *Circulation* 1992; **85**: 510–17.

42. McMurray JJ, Ray SG, Abdullah I, Dargie HJ, Morton JJ. Plasma endothelin in chronic heart failure. *Circulation* 1992; **85**: 1374–9.

43. Omland T, Lie RT, Aakvaag A, Aarsland T, Dickstein K. Plasma endothelin determination as a prognostic indicator of 1-year mortality after acute myocardial infarction. *Circulation* 1994; **89**: 1573–9.

44. Fukuchi M, Giaid A. Expression of endothelin-1 and endothelin-converting enzyme-1 mRNAs and proteins in failing human hearts. *J Cardiovasc Pharmacol* 1998; **31**(Suppl 1): S421–3.

45. Sakai S, Miyauchi T, Kobayashi M, Yamaguchi I, Goto K, Sugishita Y. Inhibition of myocardial endothelin pathway improves long-term survival in heart failure. *Nature* 1996; **384**: 353–5.

46. Sutsch G, Kiowski W, Yan XW, Hunziker P, Christen S, Strobel W, Kim JH, Rickenbacher P, Bertel O. Short-term oral endothelin-receptor antagonist therapy in conventionally treated patients with symptomatic severe chronic heart failure. *Circulation* 1998; **98**: 2262–8.

47. Luscher TF, Enseleit F, Pacher R, Mitrovic V, Schulze MR, Willenbrock R, Dietz R, Rousson V, Hurlimann D, Philipp S, Notter T, Noll G, Ruschitzka F. Hemodynamic and neurohumoral effects of selective endothelin A (ET(A)) receptor blockade in chronic heart failure: the Heart Failure ET(A) Receptor Blockade Trial (HEAT). *Circulation* 2002; **106**: 2666–72.

48. Wada A, Tsutamoto T, Fukai D, Ohnishi M, Maeda K, Hisanaga T, Maeda Y, Matsuda Y, Kinoshita M. Comparison of the effects of selective endothelin ETA and ETB receptor antagonists in congestive heart failure. *J Am Coll Cardiol* 1997; **30**: 1385–92.

49. Anand IS, McMurray JJ, Cohn JN, Konstam MA, Notter T, Quitzau K, Ruschitzka F, Luscher TF; EARTH investigators. Long-term effects of darusentan on left-ventricular remodelling and clinical outcomes in the Endothelin A Receptor Antagonist Trial in Heart Failure (EARTH): randomised, double-blind, placebo-controlled trial. *Lancet* 2004; **364**(9431): 347–54.

50. Mann DL. Mechanisms and models in heart failure: a combinatorial approach. *Circulation* 1999; **100**: 999–1008.

51. Aukrust P, Ueland T, Lien E, Bendtzen K, Muller F, Andreassen AK, Nordoy I, Aass H, Espevik T, Simonsen S, Froland SS, Gullestad L. Cytokine network in congestive heart failure secondary to ischemic or idiopathic dilated cardiomyopathy. *Am J Cardiol* 1999; **83**: 376–82.

52. Kapadia S, Torre-Amione G, Yokoyama T, Mann DL. Soluble TNF binding proteins modulate the negative inotropic properties of TNF-alpha in vitro. *Am J Physiol* 1995; **268**: H517–25.

53. Deswal A, Bozkurt B, Seta Y, Parilti-Eiswirth S, Hayes FA, Blosch C, Mann DL. Safety and efficacy of a soluble P75 tumor necrosis factor receptor (Enbrel, etanercept) in patients with advanced heart failure. *Circulation* 1999; **99**: 3224–6.

54. Bozkurt B, Torre-Amione G, Warren MS, Whitmore J, Soran OZ, Feldman AM, Mann DL. Results of targeted anti-tumor necrosis factor therapy with etanercept (ENBREL) in patients with advanced heart failure. *Circulation* 2001; **103**: 1044–7.

55. Wood S. RENEWAL trial: no improvement in CHF with etanercept. *HeartWire News* 2002 (http://www.theheart.org).

56. Mann DL, Swedberg K, Packer M, Fleming TR, Djian J, Warren MS, McMurray JJ. Effects of cytokine antagonism with etanercept on morbidity and mortality in patients with chronic heart failure: results of the RENAISSANCE, RECOVERY, and RENEWAL trials. Paper presented at the Annual Meeting of HFSA, 25 September 2002.

57. Packer M, Chung E, Batra S, Lo K, Kereiakes D, Willerson J. *Randomized placebo-controlled dose-ranging trial of infliximab, a monoclonal antibody to tumor necrosis factor-alpha, in moderate to severe heart failure.* Paper presented at the Annual Meeting of HFSA, 25 September 2002.

Part III

Innovative therapies,
special populations

9

Sleep apnoea in heart failure

MARK DUNLAP

Introduction

While the term 'heart failure' implies a condition due to primary myocardial disease, in fact it is a systemic condition with the involvement of multiple organ systems. Many of these other manifestations have previously been thought to be merely the result of haemodynamic consequences of poor perfusion due to a low cardiac output. However, it is clear that this pure 'haemodynamic model' of heart failure progression is not only overly simplistic, but inaccurate as well. Proof of the shortfall of this approach is the evidence from clinical trials showing that therapy directed towards increasing cardiac output has either not improved prognosis or resulted in an even worse prognosis, whereas therapy directed towards blocking neurohormonal mechanisms has met with marked reductions in morbidity and mortality.

Sleep apnoea has long been recognized as being associated with heart failure. Indeed, in his original description of abnormal patterns of ventilation, John Cheyne [1] observed periods of hyperpnoea alternating with apnoea in a patient with probable alcoholic cardiomyopathy (CM). More recent has been the recognition that heart failure patients who demonstrate sleep apnoea carry a worse prognosis, and that the apnoea may actually contribute to worsening heart failure. For further reading, the reader is directed to these recent excellent reviews of sleep apnoea and heart failure: Bradley TD, Floras JS. Sleep apnoea and heart failure. Part I: obstructive sleep apnea. *Circulation* 2003; **107**: 1671–8. Bradley TD, Floras JS. Sleep apnoea and heart failure. Part II: central sleep apnea. *Circulation* 2003; **107**: 1822–6.

Syndromes of sleep apnoea occur in approximately 50% of patients with heart failure. The prevalence is somewhat lower in women, a potential explanation of improved prognosis in female patients with heart failure compared to males. While syndromes of both central (CSA) and obstructive sleep apnoea (OSA) occur, CSA, often referred to as Cheynes–Stokes respiration CSA, is the most common manifestation of the apnoea syndromes seen in patients with heart failure. OSA also occurs, although less often than CSA. Heart failure patients in whom sleep apnoea should be considered are those with the typical symptoms of the syndrome, such as snoring, daytime somnolence, and excessive fatigue. Other patients in whom the diagnosis should be considered are those with nocturnal dyspnoea, persistent hypertension,

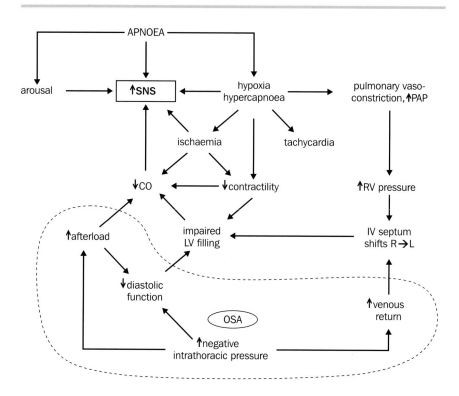

Fig. 9.1 Pathophysiology of apnoea leading to activation of the sympathetic nervous system (SNS). Apnoeas emanating from either central or obstructive origins result in sympathoexcitation via both direct and indirect mechanisms. The direct mechanism involves withdrawal of the normal sympathoinhibitory influence of lung inflation reflexes. Indirect pathways include arousals from sleep leading to increased SNS activity, as well as the combined effects of hypoxia and hypercapnoea. Hypoxia and hypercapnoea activate chemoreceptors, which reflexively increase SNS activity. These combined effects also cause vagal withdrawal with attendant tachycardia, as well as ischaemia. Hypoxia and hypercapnoea also result in vasoconstriction of the pulmonary vasculature, increases in right-sided pressures, shifts of the intraventricular septum leading to impaired filling of the left ventricle, reductions in cardiac output and further sympathoexcitation. When an apnoea is obstructive in origin, the additive effects are shown in the lower portion of the figure (hatched area) (enclosed in dashed line). An obstructive apnoea causes increased negative intrathoracic pressure leading to right-sided overload, worsening diastolic function, increased afterload, impaired left ventricular filling, and reduction in cardiac output, culminating in further activation of the SNS. Note that along with activation of the SNS, other deleterious effects include tachycardia, ischaemia, decreased contractility and cardiac output, and pulmonary hypertension.

and those with signs of persistent pulmonary hypertension, including peripheral oedema and ascites.

Heart failure patients with sleep apnoea have a worse prognosis compared with heart failure patients who do not have this finding. While it is possible that CSA simply represents a marker of worse prognosis, accumulating evidence suggests that there may be an important pathophysiological link between sleep apnoea and the progression of left ventricular dysfunction and heart failure. Moreover, this association has given rise to the speculation that treatment of sleep apnoea might improve prognosis in patients with heart failure.

While it has long been known that the sympathetic nervous system (SNS) is activated in heart failure, it is now clear that this activation plays an important role in the progression of left ventricular dysfunction and heart failure. Proof of this hypothesis has been provided by clinical trials showing the profoundly beneficial effects of blocking the renin angiotensin system and the SNS in patients with heart failure. Sleep apnoea contributes significantly to the activation of the SNS by a variety of mechanisms (Fig. 9.1), and appears to be the predominant pathophysiological mechanism to explain the link between sleep apnoea and the progression of left ventricular dysfunction and heart failure. In addition to activation of the SNS, studies suggest that there are abnormalities of vascular endothelial dysfunction, oxidative stress, inflammation, coagulation, and metabolic dysregulation, all of which may play a role in the pathophysiological syndrome of heart failure.

Epidemiology of sleep apnoea in heart failure

Central sleep apnea in left ventricular dysfunction: prevalence and implications for arrhythmic risk
Lanfranchi PA, Somers VK, Braghiroli A, Corra U, Eleuteri E, Giannuzzi P.
Circulation 2003; **107**: 727–32

BACKGROUND. While it is known that approximately 50% of patients with heart failure have sleep apnoea, the prevalence of sleep apnoea in a population of patients with left ventricular dysfunction without clinical heart failure is not known. In 47 patients with left ventricular ejection fraction (LVEF) ≤40% referred for cardiac evaluation, it was found that CSA was present in 55% of patients, most of whom exhibited severe CSA (apnoea–hypopnoea index [AHI] ≥30/h). OSA was present in 11% of patients. Patients with ischaemic CM had a higher prevalence and severity of CSA than those with non-ischaemic CM. The patients with CSA did not have haemodynamic abnormalities compared with those with left ventricular dysfunction without CSA, but indices of vagal control (heart rate variability) were markedly abnormal. Ambient ventricular arrhythmias (non-sustained ventricular tachycardia) were also present to a greater degree in patients with CSA.

INTERPRETATION. This study extends previous observations regarding the prevalence of sleep apnoea in patients with heart failure to a population of patients at an earlier stage of the disease process, i.e. in the presence of left ventricular dysfunction but prior to the onset of clinical heart failure. The investigators found that sleep apnoea occurred in approximately the same proportion of patients with left ventricular dysfunction without overt heart failure as in patients with frank heart failure, and that the distribution of CSA and OSA was approximately the same in both groups. This suggests that the association between heart failure and sleep apnoea is not a result of more advanced stages of heart failure, but rather that it occurs early in the development of left ventricular dysfunction. Furthermore, neither echocardiographic parameters nor measures of exercise testing (VO_2 peak) were associated with the presence of CSA.

Comment

CSA is as prevalent in patients with left ventricular dysfunction as in fully developed heart failure, and while the patients had not yet developed haemodynamic abnormalities, the association with abnormalities of autonomic dysfunction suggests that these patients carry a worse prognosis. As peak VO_2 is still considered the 'gold standard' for the evaluation of prognosis in patients with heart failure, it is unknown whether these patients with left ventricular dysfunction and CSA carry a worse prognosis than those who do not show CSA. While it seems likely that left ventricular dysfunction patients with CSA might represent a group of patients with a worse prognosis, more prolonged follow-up of larger numbers of patients will be required to determine whether the presence of CSA in patients with left ventricular dysfunction predisposes these patients to more rapid progression of left ventricular dysfunction, heart failure, and higher mortality.

Pathophysiology of sleep apnoea in heart failure

The relationship between congestive heart failure, sleep apnea, and mortality in older men

Ancoli-Israel S, DuHamel ER, Stepnowsky C, Engler R, Cohen-Zion M, Marler M. *Chest* 2003; **124**: 1400–5

BACKGROUND. In order to examine the association between sleep apnoea and outcome in patients with cardiac disease, 353 randomly selected patients hospitalized at a Veterans Affairs Medical Center were followed. Patients with heart failure plus CSA had shorter survival than those with just heart failure, just sleep apnoea (OSA or CSA), or neither. Survival for those with OSA or CSA and no heart failure was no different than for those with neither disorder (Fig. 9.2). A follow-up analysis showed that for those with no heart failure, neither CSA nor OSA shortened survival. For those with heart failure, the presence of CSA shortened the life span, with a hazard ratio of 1.66 ($P = 0.012$), but having OSA had no effect. Patients with heart failure had more severe sleep apnoea than those with no heart disease.

INTERPRETATION. This study showed that the presence of CSA but not OSA shortened survival in patients with heart failure. Furthermore, the presence of sleep apnoea of either type did not confer a worse prognosis in the absence of heart failure.

Comment

The value of this study was the length of the follow-up in these randomly selected hospitalized patients, up to 17 years. As it was a relatively large cohort with death occurring in over 80% of the patients over the course of the study, the prognostic information is particularly valuable. While the data do not clarify issues related to cause and effect between sleep apnoea and heart failure, the data do reinforce the strong associations between sleep apnoea and heart failure in elderly men. It is interesting that OSA did not portend a worse prognosis when present in heart failure patients. The reasons for this are not clear, although it may be that whereas CSA may be both a marker of worse disease and leads to a worse prognosis, OSA represents a distinct clinical entity that by itself does not confer a poorer prognosis.

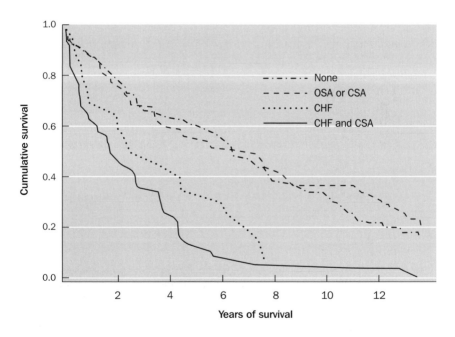

Fig. 9.2 Survival curves for those with heart failure (HF) with or without sleep apnoea. Patients with HF plus central sleep apnoea (CSA) had significantly worse survival compared with those with just HF, or just obstructive sleep apnoea (OSA) or CSA.
Source: Ancoli-Israel *et al.* (2003).

Relationship of systolic BP to obstructive sleep apnea in patients with heart failure

Sin DD, Fitzgerald F, Parker JD, *et al. Chest* 2003; **123**: 1536–43

BACKGROUND. OSA is an independent risk factor for hypertension in the general population, and is an important risk factor for the development and progression of heart failure. This cross-sectional study sought to determine whether OSA would be associated with elevated daytime blood pressure in medically treated patients with chronic heart failure. In total, 301 consecutive patients with heart failure were seen in tertiary care, university-affiliated sleep disorder and heart failure clinics. OSA was

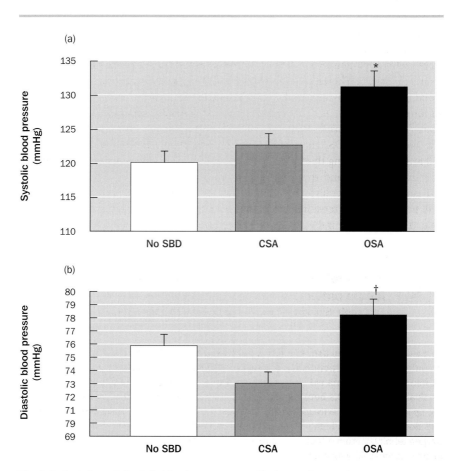

Fig. 9.3 Systolic and diastolic blood pressure stratified according to sleep apnoea status. *$P \geq 0.05$ compared with both other groups; †$P \geq 0.05$ compared with the central sleep apnoea (CSA) group only. Source: Sin *et al.* (2003).

present in 121 patients (40%) and their systolic blood pressure was significantly higher than in patients without OSA. Patients with OSA were 2.9 times more likely to have systolic hypertension than those without OSA, after controlling for other risk factors including obesity (Fig. 9.3). The degree of systolic blood pressure elevation was directly related to the frequency of obstructive apnoeas and hypopnoeas.

INTERPRETATION. In medically treated patients with heart failure, daytime systolic blood pressure and the prevalence of systolic hypertension were significantly increased in patients with OSA, compared with those without OSA. OSA may, therefore, have contributed to the presence of systolic hypertension in these patients.

Comment

OSA is known to be associated with hypertension, and proper treatment can lead to reductions in blood pressure. These investigators confirmed this relationship in patients with heart failure, in whom higher blood pressure persisted despite treatment with angiotensin-converting enzyme inhibitors, β blockers and calcium channel blockers. Therefore, it seems likely that the OSA contributed to the higher blood pressure, probably mediated through higher sympathetic tone. While the 'optimum' blood pressure in patients has not yet been defined, most clinical trials in heart failure have enrolled patients with blood pressures in the 120 mmHg range. The patients with OSA in this study had average systolic blood pressures over 130 mmHg, suggesting that these patients deserve special attention to the possibility of coexistent OSA, and that the elevated blood pressure in these patients may be resistant to pharmacological treatment alone. Additionally, heart failure patients with persistent hypertension should be screened carefully for concomitant OSA, and treated appropriately if the diagnosis is confirmed.

Apnea-related heart rate variability in congestive heart failure patients

Tateishi O, Shouda T, Sakai T, Honda Y, Mochizuki S, Machida K. *Clin Exp Hypertens* 2003; **25**: 183–9

BACKGROUND. Sleep apnoea causes fluctuations of the RR interval. In this investigation, the characteristics of sleep-related heart rate variability were studied in 13 heart failure patients with sleep apnoea. Heart rate variability occurred as a result of cyclical apnoea attacks between 0.005 and 0.03 Hz (apnoea band). The proportion of the apnoea band (percentage apnoea) increased with the number of apnoea episodes, and sleep apnoea was highly likely when the percentage apnoea was ≥80%. Low-flow oxygen administration effectively reduced apnoea frequency, and the apnoea-related heart rate variability also decreased.

INTERPRETATION. Instead of sending patients for full sleep studies, monitoring patients for apnoea-related heart rate variability can be useful for detecting and following sleep apnoea in patients with heart failure.

Comment

Oxymetry in association with nocturnal polysomnography is currently the 'gold standard' to diagnose sleep apnoea. However, full testing requires specialized equipment, is labour intensive, and may not be available as a tool to many practitioners. Nocturnal oxymetry alone has been used to document episodes of desaturation, and can be useful as a screening test in patients with and without heart failure. These investigators tested the utility of ambulatory ECG monitoring to detect alterations in heart rate variability that might be indicative of apnoeic episodes, and found a high predictive value in both the initial diagnosis as well as in the resolution of apnoeas following treatment with supplemental oxygen. While this could be useful as a screening tool, it should be noted that neither this technique nor nocturnal oxymetry alone can accurately detect the cause of the desaturation. Therefore, full sleep testing is indicated in patients with a high suspicion for sleep apnoea.

Enhanced ventilatory response to exercise in patients with chronic heart failure and central sleep apnea

Arzt M, Harth M, Luchner A, *et al. Circulation* 2003; **107**(15): 1998–2003

BACKGROUND. In patients with heart failure, CSA and an enhanced ventilatory response (VE/VCO$_2$ slope) to exercise are common, both of which alone indicate poor prognosis in chronic heart failure. Although augmented chemosensitivity to VCO$_2$ is thought to be one important underlying mechanism for both breathing disorders, it is unclear whether both breathing disorders are related closely in patients with heart failure. Twenty heart failure patients with clinically important CSA and ten heart failure patients without CSA were investigated. Exercise capacity (peak VO$_2$, determined by cardiopulmonary exercise testing) and LVEF were similar in both groups. The AHI was not correlated with either exercise capacity or LVEF. In contrast, the VE/VCO$_2$ slope was highly correlated with the AHI (P <0.001). The VE/VCO$_2$ slope was significantly increased in patients with CSA compared with those without CSA (29.7 vs 24.9; Fig. 9.4).

INTERPRETATION. The ventilatory response to exercise is significantly augmented in heart failure patients with CSA compared with those without CSA. In contrast to peak VO$_2$ and LVEF, the VE/VCO$_2$ slope is strongly related to the severity of CSA in patients with heart failure.

Comment

This study underscores that patients with heart failure and CSA exhibit augmented chemosensitivity to CO$_2$ as a common underlying pathophysiological mechanism. It is likely that this augmented sensitivity is what causes periods of apnoea in patients with CSA. Thus, administering increased inhaled CO$_2$, either by supplemental CO$_2$ or by increasing the dead space, may alleviate apnoeas in these patients. The corollary to this finding is that patients undergoing cardiopulmonary testing who show an exaggerated VE/VCO$_2$ slope may be those at risk of having CSA.

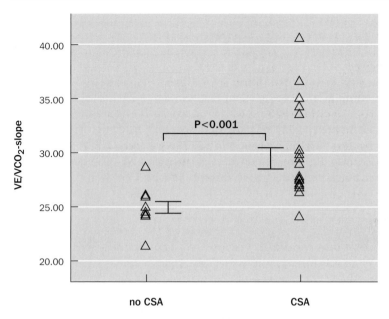

Fig. 9.4 Individual and mean values of the VE/VCO$_2$ slope of patients with heart failure, without and with central sleep apnoea. Source: Arzt *et al.* (2003).

Impact of sleep apnea on sympathetic nervous system activity in heart failure
Solin P, Kaye DM, Little PJ, Bergin P, Richardson M, Naughton MT. *Chest* 2003; **123**: 1119–26

BACKGROUND. Activation of the SNS is a hallmark of heart failure, and is exacerbated by sleep apnoea. However, the relative importance of CSA versus OSA to SNS activation is unknown. This was a prospective, controlled, observational trial in which the overnight urinary norepinephrine level (a measure of integrated overnight SNS activity) was measured in 15 healthy male volunteers, 15 male OSA patients who did not have heart failure, and 90 heart failure patients. Heart failure patients also had right heart pressure measurements. Compared with healthy individuals, the mean urinary norepinephrine level was significantly elevated in the OSA group and was even further elevated in the congestive heart failure group. Within the heart failure group, mean urinary norepinephrine levels were greatest in the heart failure–CSA group compared with the heart failure–OSA group and the congestive heart failure non-apnoea group (Fig. 9.5). Pulmonary capillary wedge pressure emerged as the best predictor of an elevated urinary norepinephrine level, whereas the AHI did not show a significant independent correlation to urinary norepinephrine level.

INTERPRETATION. Overnight SNS activity is significantly greater in heart failure patients than in OSA patients. Moreover, the haemodynamic severity of heart failure contributes to the elevated SNS activity in heart failure patients to a greater degree than apnoea-related hypoxaemia.

Comment

This study confirms previous observations that SNS activity is elevated in heart failure, and is further elevated in patients with sleep apnoea. It extends previous studies by showing that the presence of OSA alone does not result in additional activation of SNS activity, but that the presence of CSA in a patient with heart failure significantly increases SNS activity. This observation may help to explain why OSA does not additionally worsen prognosis in patients with heart failure, but CSA does.

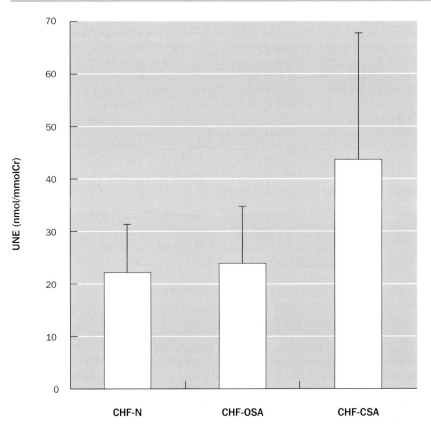

Fig. 9.5 Comparison of urinary norepinephrine (UNE) levels among patients with congestive heart failure (CHF) only (CHF-N), CHF with obstructive sleep apnoea (OSA), and CHF patients with central sleep apnoea (CSA). Source: Solin *et al.* (2003).

Raised sympathetic nerve activity in heart failure and central sleep apnea is due to heart failure severity

Mansfield D, Kaye DM, Brunner La Rocca H, Solin P, Esler MD, Naughton MT.
Circulation 2003; **107**(10): 1396–400

BACKGROUND. Patients with heart failure and CSA have elevated plasma norepinephrine levels compared with heart failure patients without apnoea. Patients with heart failure–CSA also demonstrate higher mean pulmonary artery pressure, which is suggestive of worse cardiac function. Whether CSA contributes to the chronic elevation of sympathetic nerve activity or is associated with more severe chronic heart failure remains unknown. In this investigation, awake total body and cardiac norepinephrine spillover were measured and related to measurements of cardiac haemodynamics and apnoea severity in 55 heart failure patients (21 with CSA, 19 with normal breathing, and 15 with OSA). The patients with heart failure and CSA had significantly higher total body norepinephrine spillover, cardiac norepinephrine spillover, and mean pulmonary artery pressure compared with heart failure patients with either OSA or no sleep apnoea. However, controlling for severity of heart failure resulted in no significant differences in norepinephrine kinetics among the three groups. Only the mean pulmonary artery pressure independently correlated with total body and cardiac norepinephrine spillover. Sleep apnoea severity bore no relationship to markers of sympathetic nerve activity.

INTERPRETATION. Total body and cardiac sympathetic nerve activity are elevated in heart failure patients with CSA compared with either those with heart failure alone or those with heart failure and OSA. SNS activity is related to heart failure and not apnoea severity.

Comment

The findings from this study show that the elevated levels of norepinephrine are due to increases in total body norepinephrine spillover in patients with heart failure and CSA. These investigators measured indices of the severity of heart failure and found that the higher levels of norepinephrine were more strongly associated with the severity of heart failure than the presence of CSA. This finding is somewhat at odds with previous studies showing not only strong correlations between the presence of CSA and elevated norepinephrine levels, but also that CSA episodes directly activate muscle sympathetic nerve activity (MSNA). Therefore, it is still not totally clear which is the 'chicken' and which is the 'egg'. Perhaps the only way to definitively answer this question will be a clinical trial demonstrating efficacy in reducing important endpoints in heart failure patients treated with specific therapy targeted to reduce CSA. A Toronto group is currently undertaking such a trial |**2**|.

Augmented sympathetic neural response to simulated obstructive apnoea in human heart failure

Bradley TD, Tkacova R, Hall MJ, Ando S, Floras JS. *Clin Sci* 2003; **104**: 231–8

BACKGROUND. In healthy subjects, simulated central apnoeas (breath holding) and obstructive apnoeas (Mueller manoeuvres) increase MSNA equally, due to the activation of chemoreceptors. In contrast, Mueller manoeuvres in patients with heart failure cause greater reductions in blood pressure than breath holds, possibly due to differential effects on arterial baroreceptor and chemoreceptor stimulation. In this investigation, the effects of these simulated apnoeas on MSNA were studied in control and heart failure patients. Breath holds evoked a progressive increase in MSNA in both groups, but had no effect on blood pressure. In healthy subjects, breath holds and Mueller manoeuvres caused equal peaks in sympathetic activity. In heart failure patients, Mueller manoeuvres caused a progressive decrease in blood pressure and greater increases in sympathetic activity than breath holds (Fig. 9.6).

INTERPRETATION. In patients with heart failure, simulated obstructive apnoea elicits greater increases in sympathetic activity than simulated central apnoea, due primarily to its additional hypotensive effect and deactivation of baroreceptors.

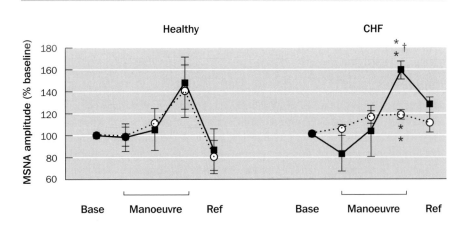

Fig. 9.6 Changes in muscle sympathetic nerve activity (MSNA) in response to simple breath holds (open circles) and Mueller manoeuvres (closed squares) in healthy subjects (left) and patients with heart failure (HF; right). Whereas in healthy subjects both breath holds and Mueller manoeuvres increased MSNA to the same degree, breath holds alone raised MSNA only to a small degree in HF, but was accentuated with Mueller manoeuvres. Source: Bradley *et al.* (2003).

Comment

This study confirmed previous findings of high levels of resting MSNA levels in heart failure. Despite this high resting level of MSNA, it was increased further by apnoea, and a simulated obstructive apnoea accentuated this increase in MSNA even more, but only in heart failure patients and not controls. It is difficult to reconcile this finding with those showing that norepinephrine levels in heart failure patients with OSA are similar to levels in heart failure patients with no OSA, but that the presence of CSA is associated with higher levels of norepinephrine. Perhaps one explanation is that in CSA the hypercapnoea phase replicates the mechanical effects of increasing negative intrathoracic pressure, therefore serving as 'functional OSA', in addition to being associated with more severe heart failure, accounting for the increased norepinephrine.

Treatment of sleep apnoea in patients with heart failure

Assisted ventilation for heart failure patients with Cheyne–Stokes respiration

Kohnlein T, Welte T, Tan LB, Elliott MW. *Eur Respir J* 2002; **20**: 934–41

BACKGROUND. Continuous positive airway pressure (CPAP) has been shown to be effective in reducing the episodes of apnoea in patients with both OSA and CSA. However, some patients do not tolerate CPAP. For these patients, bilevel ventilation has been proposed, but the relative effectiveness of one versus the other has not been tested in patients with heart failure. In this study, the effects of CPAP and bilevel ventilation were compared in patients with heart failure. Sixteen heart failure patients with LVEF ≥35% were identified, and the diagnosis of CSA was confirmed by polysomnography. All patients underwent treatment with both modes of assisted ventilation in a randomized, crossover manner.

INTERPRETATION. The AHI at baseline was 26.7 ± 10.7/h and was reduced significantly to approximately 7.0 by both modes of assisted ventilation, with no difference between the types of treatment. Improvements were also found in sleep quality, daytime fatigue, circulation time, and New York Heart Association functional class. It was concluded that both CPAP and bilevel ventilation improve CSA in patients with heart failure.

Comment

This was an unblinded, albeit randomized, study of two different treatment modalities for CSA–Cheyne–Stokes respiration. While only 16 patients were studied, they appeared to respond equally well to either CPAP or bilevel ventilation. As most of the data regarding improvement in cardiac function and reduction in norepinephrine levels are with CPAP, this should remain first-line therapy for patients with heart failure and CSA–Cheyne–Stokes respiration. However, for those patients unable to tolerate CPAP, bilevel ventilation appears to give a similar benefit. More data are needed to confirm that this approach leads to the clinical benefits seen with CPAP in addition to a reduction in apnoeas.

The effect of theophylline on sleep-disordered breathing in patients with stable chronic congestive heart failure

Hu K, Li Q, Yang J, Hu S, Chen X. *Chin Med J (Engl)* 2003; **116**: 1711–16

BACKGROUND. Theophylline has been used in a variety of disorders of respiration due to its effects on the lungs (bronchodilator), diaphragm (improved contractility), and central nervous system (central respiratory stimulation). As a weak phosphodiesterase inhibitor, it also has mild effects on cardiac output. These effects might also be beneficial in heart failure patients with sleep apnoea, although any potential therapeutic benefits may be limited by gastrointestinal and central nervous system toxicity, as well as adverse effects on sleep quality. In this study, the effect of short-term oral theophylline therapy on periodic breathing in stable heart failure patients was investigated.

INTERPRETATION. In 13 patients with documented sleep-disordered breathing, theophylline (average dose 4.3 mg/kg for 5–7 days) decreased the AHI from 43 ± 16 to 21 ± 13 ($P<0.001$) and the number of episodes of central apnoea–hypopnoea/h from 32 ± 10 to 10 ± 8 ($P<0.001$). The percentage of total sleep time during which arterial oxyhaemoglobin saturation was less than 90% was also reduced from 23 ± 24 to $9 \pm 9\%$ ($P<0.05$), as was the number of arousals/h (from 37 ± 21 to 19 ± 21, $P<0.05$). There were no significant differences in the characteristics of sleep or obstructive AHI before and after theophylline treatment.

Comment

In heart failure patients with CSA, short-term oral theophylline administration improved indices of sleep-disordered breathing without significant adverse effects. Whether these short-term improvements can be sustained chronically in patients with heart failure is not known, especially with the increasing complexity of pharmacological regimens in these patients and the potential for toxicity, given the relatively narrow therapeutic window of this medication. Also, the long-term effects of theophylline administration on heart failure outcomes remain unknown. Therefore, this therapy should not be used until long-term data become available.

The effect of successful heart transplant treatment of heart failure on central sleep apnea

Mansfield DR, Solin P, Roebuck T, Bergin P, Kaye DM, Naughton MT. *Chest* 2003; **124**: 1675–81

BACKGROUND. The most abrupt 'cure' for heart failure is cardiac replacement via transplantation. Short-term studies of the effects of cardiac transplantation on sleep-disordered breathing have shown varying results. In this study, the impact of heart transplant on SNS activity and CSA severity in patients with congestive heart failure was determined.

INTERPRETATION. In this prospective trial, 22 heart failure patients were studied with polysomnography before and after cardiac transplantation. In 13 patients with CSA, the AHI fell from 28 ± 15 to 7 ± 6/h (*P* <0.001), and the urine norepinephrine concentration fell from 48 ± 31 to 6 ± 4.8 nmol/mmol creatinine (*P* <0.001) at 13.2 ± 8.3 months following heart transplantation. Transplantation relieved the CSA in seven of 13 patients, but three patients had persistent CSA and four patients acquired OSA following transplant. None of nine heart failure patients without sleep-disordered breathing developed either CSA or OSA after transplantation.

Comment

These investigators confirmed and extended findings from previous studies showing significant improvement in sleep-disordered breathing following cardiac replacement therapy, associated with normalization of cardiac function and decreased indices of sympathetic activation. However, abnormalities of sleep-disordered breathing can persist in some patients. This suggests that while abnormalities of sleep are tightly correlated with advanced heart failure, the driving mechanisms may be independent of heart failure, at least in some patients who have both disorders.

Cardiovascular effects of continuous positive airway pressure in patients with heart failure and obstructive sleep apnea

Kaneko Y, Floras JS, Usui K, *et al. N Engl J Med* 2003; **348**: 1233–41

BACKGROUND. Small, non-randomized studies have suggested that in patients with heart failure who have OSA, CPAP therapy not only improved sleep architecture, but also can lead to improvements in left ventricular function and heart failure status. This was a randomized study of CPAP in 24 heart failure patients shown to have OSA in which a number of sleep- and cardiac-related parameters were measured before and 1 month following either CPAP or no CPAP.

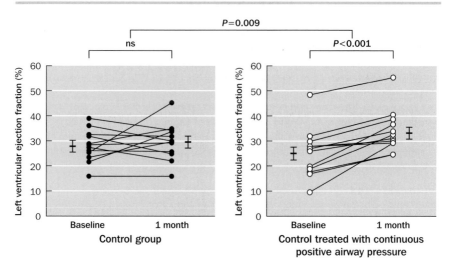

Fig. 9.7 Effect of 1-month CPAP therapy on ejection fraction in patients with HF and OSA (right) vs controls (no CPAP, left). Source: Kaneko *et al.* (2003).

INTERPRETATION. CPAP was effective in reducing sleep-disordered breathing, heart rate, left ventricular end-systolic dimension, and increasing LVEF (Fig. 9.7).

Comment

This study importantly extends previous observational studies in patients with heart failure and OSA to a clinical trial in patients randomized to either CPAP or continued medical therapy alone. While β blockers were used in only about 50% of the patients, and therefore the patients might not have been optimized medically, the effectiveness of CPAP in improving both sleep-associated pathology as well as parameters of left ventricular function is clear. This supports the concept that OSA contributes significantly to worsening heart failure, and that treatment aimed at correcting the OSA improves cardiac function. Whether CPAP would decrease mortality in heart failure remains to be shown.

Cardiorespiratory effects of added dead space in patients with heart failure and central sleep apnea

Khayat RN, Xie A, Patel AK, Kaminski A, Skatrud JB. *Chest* 2003; **123**: 1551–60

BACKGROUND. Inhaled CO_2 has been shown to stabilize the breathing pattern of patients with CSA. Added dead space as a form of supplemental CO_2 has been effective in eliminating idiopathic CSA. In this study, the respiratory and cardiovascular effects of added dead space were investigated in eight patients with heart failure and CSA. The dead space consisted of a facemask attached to a cylinder of adjustable volume. During the nocturnal study, patients slept with and without the addition of dead space to the mask. During sleep, the addition of dead space increased the end-tidal CO_2, reduced apnoeic episodes, decreased the number of arousals, and increased the mean arterial oxygen saturation (Fig. 9.8).

INTERPRETATION. The addition of dead space to spontaneously breathing heart failure patients stabilized CSA and improved sleep quality in patients with congestive heart failure without significant acute adverse effects on cardiovascular function.

Comment

As hyperventilation probably plays an important role in the development of CSA in heart failure, previous studies have used inhalation of low levels of CO_2 as a potential treatment, and have demonstrated a marked reduction in the frequency of apnoeas. However, applying inhaled CO_2 to patients with heart failure seems limited, in part because of the difficulty with the acceptance of this therapy to physicians and patients. These investigators used a more 'physiological' approach in heart failure patients with CSA by applying a mask that simply increased the dead space, thereby resulting in increased delivery of CO_2. The marked resolution of apnoeas is a promising alternative or replacement to CPAP or supplemental oxygen in the treatment of CSA in heart failure. Whether this will become an accepted approach to the treatment of CSA in heart failure remains to be determined.

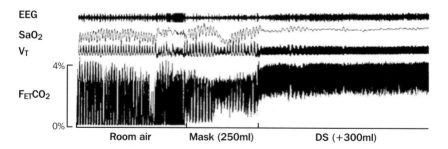

Fig. 9.8 Continuous recording from a nocturnal polygraph of room air and dead space breathing. The first portion shows a segment of room air breathing followed by a segment of breathing through a face mask with 250 ml of dead space, then an additional 300 ml of dead space was added to the mask. The segment with added dead space shows resolution of the fluctuations in mean arterial oxygen saturation and tidal volume (V_T), indicating a decrease in arousals, oxygen desaturations, and apnoeas. Source: Khayat *et al.* (2003).

Conclusion

Abnormalities of sleep-disordered breathing are highly prevalent in patients with heart failure. Whereas formerly it was not clear whether this correlation was important in terms of progression of the disease, accumulating evidence points to a significant role of sleep apnoea in the progression of left ventricular dysfunction and worsening heart failure. This appears to be mediated through furthering the sympathoexcitatory state of heart failure. Currently, therapy to alleviate OSA is indicated to relieve symptoms attributable to sleep apnoea, although there is less consensus with respect to CSA in heart failure, especially as good medical treatment of heart failure can alleviate the severity of both heart failure and CSA. While it is tempting to speculate that CPAP and related therapies will improve outcome in patients with heart failure, proof of this concept awaits the results of large-scale, prospectively designed, clinical trials.

References

1. Cheyne JA. A case of apoplexy in which the fleshy part of the heart was converted into fat. *Dublin Hospital Rep* 1818; 2: 216–23.
2. Bradley TD, Logan AG, Floras JS; CANPAP Investigators. Rationale and design of the Canadian Continuous Positive Airway Pressure Trial for Congestive Heart Failure patients with Central Sleep Apnea—CANPAP. *Can J Cardiol* 2001; 17(6): 677–84.

10

Exercise testing and training in heart failure

STEVEN KETEYIAN, ILEANA PIÑA, MATT SAVAL

Introduction

Chronic heart failure remains a clinical disorder with increasing cost, incidence and prevalence. As a result, new drug, surgical and device therapies continue to be investigated.

Some 15 years ago, initial reports began to appear addressing the role of exercise testing and training in the assessment and treatment of patients with chronic heart failure. Preliminary investigations showed that measured peak oxygen uptake (VO_2) or the ability of the body to transport and utilize oxygen, played a powerful role in predicting 3-year survival. Additionally, regular modest exercise improved both exercise tolerance and quality of life.

Through the 1990s, evidence continued to mount relative to the value of exercise testing and training in this patient population. Presently, based on dozens of database and prospective trials, we know that peak VO_2 measured during exercise testing remains an important marker for survival. However, more work is required relative to whether it should be used as a discrete indicator or a continuous variable that is part of a multicomponent model [1]. Additionally, much of the original work involving exercise testing was completed in patients not on angiotensin-converting enzyme (ACE) inhibitor or β-adrenergic blockade therapy.

Whether peak VO_2, chronotropic incompetence or other exercise testing markers such as VE–VCO_2 slope (ratio of rate of change for minute ventilation versus rate of change for CO_2 production) remain independent and strong predictors of survival among patients with heart failure taking ACE inhibitor or β-adrenergic blockade therapy remains to be determined. Recent work is conflicting relative to the use of peak VO_2 in these patients. Specifically, although Peterson *et al.* (see below) suggest that treatment with adrenergic blockade therapy does not change the predictive power of peak VO_2 in patients with heart failure, Pohwani *et al.* [2] disagree, indicating that peak VO_2 as a criterion to list patients for cardiac transplantation is no longer valid. Future studies analysing clinical databases are needed relative to delineating the role of measured peak VO_2. Perhaps a different VO_2 cut-off point or exercise marker will be identified that can be used clinically to help guide risk stratification or need for transplant.

In addition to exercise testing, the role of exercise training has been extensively investigated over the past 15 years, to the extent that we know that exercise tolerance is improved 15–35%, quality of life is enhanced, no further worsening of left ventricular function appears likely and many of the physiological and histochemical abnormalities that occur in conjunction with the disorder are partially reversed with training. Some of those histochemical changes include improvement in mitochondria density, changes in skeletal muscle fibre types and increases in capillary density. In addition, exercise training appears to be safe and free of major complications.

All of these beneficial findings related to exercise training should nonetheless be defined as surrogates. Should peak VO_2 improve with exercise training, there is no guarantee that it will translate to improvements in survival, in spite of the powerful predictive value of peak VO_2. The literature on heart failure is replete with instances of improvements in exercise function which have not translated to improvements in survival. Typical examples are flosequinan, pimobendan, and hydralazine nitrate versus ACE inhibitor. All these agents improved exercise function but were either neutral on mortality or actually increased mortality.

At present, definitive, large trial exercise training evidence does not exist for safety and clinical outcomes such as deaths and hospitalizations. Numerous smaller trials suggest that it is safe, and one trial has shown improved clinical outcomes such as hospitalizations and deaths [3]. (Most of these trials have been small and single centre and, thus, these important findings need to be confirmed in a large randomized, controlled trial which would include a broad-based group of patients including the elderly and women, as well as diverse racial groups.)

Fortunately, such a trial is presently underway. Heart Failure–A Controlled Trial Investigating Outcomes of Exercise Training (HF-ACTION) is a multisite trial study which proposes to enrol 3000 patients to usual care or usual care plus supervised and then home-based exercise training. The study is planned to continue into 2006 and is scheduled to report its findings in 2007. The primary end-points are combined all-cause mortality and all-cause hospitalization. With strong penetration of β blockers and ACE inhibitors, this trial will be applicable to accepted current clinical care. The inclusion of academic medical centres as well as smaller community practices will make the findings applicable to a general population of heart failure patients. Most patients enrolled into HF-ACTION are on β-adrenergic blockade therapy, so the generalizability of this trial to other patients with New York Heart Association class II–IV heart failure due to systolic dysfunction will be intact.

Exercise training

Antiremodeling effect of long-term exercise training in patients with stable chronic heart failure

Giannuzzi P, Temporelli PL, Corra U, Tavazzi L, for the ELVD-CHF Study Group.
Circulation 2003; **108**: 554–9

BACKGROUND. To examine the effects of exercise training on left ventricle remodelling in patients with chronic heart failure, 90 patients were randomized to a 6-month exercise training group or usual care. In this multicentre trial, a resting echocardiogram, cardiopulmonary exercise test and other measures were performed at entry and at 6 months. Exercise training consisted of three to five supervised sessions per week, each for 30 min on a cycle ergometer. Intensity was set at 60% of peak VO_2. In addition, the subjects were asked to walk briskly each day at home for 30 min.

INTERPRETATION. After 6 months, left ventricular end-diastolic volume decreased 5% and left ventricular end-systolic volume decreased 9% in the exercise training group (Table 10.1). Among the controls, left ventricular end-diastolic volume increased 6% and left ventricular end-systolic volume increased 7% at 6 months. The changes over time between the groups for both measures were significant. Additionally, left ventricular ejection fraction (LVEF) was significantly increased after training in the exercise group compared with controls. Significant improvements at follow-up testing were also reported for peak VO_2 (19%), 6-min walking distance (20%) and quality of life among exercise-trained patients but not controls. The authors concluded that moderate exercise training has no detrimental effect on left ventricular volumes and function; rather it attenuates abnormal remodelling.

Comment

In 1989, Jugdutt *et al.* |**4**|, using a very small sample of patients suffering a large anterior myocardial infarction with left ventricular dysfunction, showed worsening of left ventricular function and greater remodelling in an exercise-trained group of patients versus those receiving usual care alone. However, since then numerous trials

Table 10.1 LV function and remodelling

	Exercise training group ($n = 45$)		Control group ($n = 44$)	
	Baseline	**6 months**	**Baseline**	**6 months**
EDV, ml/m^2	142 ± 26	135 ± 26*	147 ± 41	156 ± 42*†
ESV, ml/m^2	107 ± 24	97 ± 24*	110 ± 34	118 ± 34*‡
EF, %	25 ± 4	29 ± 4*	25 ± 4	25 ± 5‡

EDV, end-diastolic volume; ESV, end-systolic volume; EF, ejection fraction. Data are mean ± SD.
*P <0.01, time effect within group; †P <0.001, interaction; ‡P <0.01, interaction.
Source: Giannuzzi *et al.* (2003).

using more conventional training methods have demonstrated no exercise training-related worsening of left ventricular function |5|.

Using an exercise regimen involving moderate-intensity training (i.e. 60%), a central finding from this trial was that not only was exercise training free of any further worsening of left ventricular function, it attenuated (and slightly improved upon) the remodelling that was observed in the control group. Unfortunately, the scope of this trial only allows us to speculate about the possible mechanisms responsible for the differences observed in left ventricular function between the two study groups. The possible mechanisms involved might include lower heart rate and blood pressure responses during submaximal exercise leading to less left ventricular wall tension; improved skeletal and cardiac muscle vasculature and endothelial function resulting in a further reduction in total systemic peripheral resistance and improved blood flow or perfusion; and an exercise training reduction in the pro-inflammatory cytokines.

It is important to point out that in this study only 40% of patients were taking ACE inhibitors and only 10% were receiving β-adrenergic blockade. Clearly, the use of these agents has increased markedly and as both have been shown to favourably impact left ventricular function and remodelling, the specific aim addressed in this paper needs to be reassessed in a group of patients where >90% are taking an ACE inhibitor or angiotensin receptor blocker and >60% are taking a β-adrenergic blocker.

Exercise training for heart failure patients improves respiratory muscle endurance, exercise tolerance, breathlessness, and quality of life

McConnell T, Mandak J, Sykes J, Fesniak H, Dasgupta H. *J Cardiopulm Rehabil* 2003; **23**: 10–16

BACKGROUND. The purpose of this study was to evaluate if exercise training resulted in an increased respiratory muscle function that in turn contributed to an increased exercise tolerance, decreased perceived breathlessness, and improved quality of life. Maximal sustainable ventilatory capacity, submaximal and peak exercise responses (VO$_2$, cardiac output via CO$_2$ rebreathing), perceived breathlessness, and quality of life were measured in 24 patients (New York Heart Association class III, 24% ejection fraction (EF)) before and after 12 weeks of exercise training. The training included treadmill walking, stationary leg ergometry, combined arm and leg ergometry, and rowing at 70–85% of maximum heart rate, followed by two sets of eight to ten repetitions of upper extremity resistance training exercises. The training sessions lasted 1 h, three times per week.

INTERPRETATION. Peak VO$_2$ and maximal sustainable ventilatory capacity increased after training (1377 vs 1488 ml/min; $P = 0.01$; 45 vs 52 l/min; $P < 0.001$, respectively). After 12 weeks, no changes were observed for peak heart rate or for stroke volume while exercising at 25 watts. Maximal ventilatory capacity contributed to a larger proportion of the variability for peak VO$_2$ at study completion ($r^2 = 0.57$ post vs 0.42 pre). Perceived breathlessness was reduced ($P < 0.05$) and quality of life was increased ($P < 0.05$).

Respiratory muscle function endurance improved with exercise training, contributing to increased exercise capacity, decreased breathlessness, and decreased perception of breathlessness.

Comment

A common complaint in patients with heart failure is dyspnoea during exertion. For many patients, this feeling of laboured breathing leads to a self-imposed restriction of physical activity, which then leads to an even further decrease in exercise capacity. In this trial involving New York Heart Association class III patients with heart failure, the authors further partition the mechanisms responsible for the improved exercise capacity that occurs in patients who undergo regular exercise.

Specifically, we know that although the primary and initial abnormality involves the heart and this alone can diminish their exercise capacity, other factors develop over time to attenuate the exercise tolerance as well. These other factors include reduced respiratory muscle function, histochemical abnormalities of the skeletal muscle |6|, loss of muscle strength and endurance |7|, and decreased nutrient blood flow to metabolically active skeletal muscles due to endothelial dysfunction |8| and over-activation of the sympathetic nervous system |5|.

In contrast, numerous trials have shown that regular exercise partially reverses many of the above-mentioned abnormalities |9|. This study provides further evidence that an exercise training-induced improvement in respiratory muscle endurance contributes, in part, to the improved peak exercise capacity that occurs in these patients, even when no apparent change is observed in central transport (i.e. cardiac output).

Although the authors did not assess what mechanism(s) specifically acts to improve respiratory muscle function, one can speculate that several may be involved. These might include improved oxygenation, decreased diaphragmatic work and improved function within the respiratory muscles themselves.

It is important to point out that there are several limitations associated with this trial, two of which are the small sample size and the absence of a control group. However, their work does help us better describe the important role that respiratory muscle function plays with regards to impacting exercise intolerance, and its plasticity when you exercise train patients with heart failure with the intent of improving exercise capacity.

The effects of exercise training on sympathetic neural activation in advanced heart failure

Roveda F, Middlekauff H, Rondon M, *et al. J Am Coll Cardiol* 2003; **42**(5): 854–60

BACKGROUND. In this study, the authors tested the hypothesis that exercise training reduces resting sympathetic neural activation in patients with chronic heart failure. Sixteen New York Heart Association class II–III patients were randomized to either an

exercise training ($n = 7$) or sedentary control ($n = 9$) group. Another group of subjects free of coronary heart disease who also underwent exercise training served as a normal control group ($n = 8$). Four months of exercise training included three 60-min sessions per week, at heart rates up to 10% below the respiratory compensation point. Muscle sympathetic nerve activity (MSNA) was recorded directly from the peroneal nerve using microneurography, and forearm blood flow was measured using venous plethysmography.

INTERPRETATION. MSNA among the group of all patients with heart failure was greater at baseline when compared with normal controls. MSNA decreased after exercise training in heart failure patients (60 vs 38 bursts/100 heartbeats), with the mean reduction (~46%) being significantly ($P <0.05$) greater than that observed in either the sedentary heart failure group (2%) or the trained normal controls (7%) (Fig. 10.1). After training, resting MSNA in patients with heart failure was not significantly different than that in the trained normal controls. Peak VO$_2$ increased (39%) and forearm blood flow increased (76%) in the exercise-trained patients, both of which represented significant changes when compared with the no exercise group of patients with heart failure. In summary, exercise training among heart failure patients resulted in dramatic reductions in directly recorded resting sympathetic nerve activity.

Comment

This trial provides important information that contributes to our understanding of how exercise training can favourably attenuate or reverse one of the many systemic or non-cardiac abnormalities that develop in patients with heart failure. To date, most of our data concerning the effects of exercise training on autonomic dysfunction have come from an indirect assessment using plasma catecholamines, norepinephrine spill-over or heart rate variability analyses. Using a direct measure of sympathetic neural traffic via contemporary technology and accepted methods, the authors showed that sympathetic nerve traffic (bursts/min) was reduced some 70%—approaching that observed in controls who were free of heart failure.

The authors suggested that the change in central sympathetic outflow may have led to the decrease in forearm vascular resistance and improved forearm blood flow, as measured by venous occlusion plethysmography. Although not measured during exercise, any reduction in sympathetic activity that contributed to an improved nutrient blood flow in the metabolically active skeletal muscles has the potential to improve exercise capacity. Also, such a change would further the improvement that has been observed in endothelial function, which has been shown to occur not only locally within metabolically active skeletal muscles but systemically as well |10|.

Taken in aggregate, it is likely that both the improvement in central sympathetic outflow to, and improved endothelial function within, the vascular responsible for nourishing metabolically active skeletal muscles delays the local activation of the group IV afferent chemoreceptors-receptors that are activated when muscle ischaemia leads to the release of muscle metabolites (e.g. lactic acid).

(a)

MSNA (bursts/min)

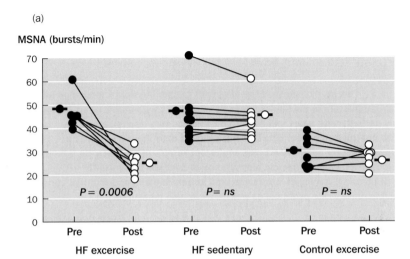

(b)

MSNA (bursts/100 heart beats)

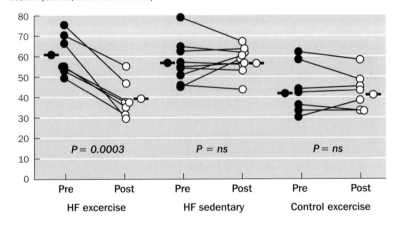

Fig. 10.1 Muscle sympathetic nerve activity (MSNA) pre/post excercise/sedentary periods quantified as bursts/min (a) and bursts/100 heart beats (b). Post-exercise training MSNA levels compared with pre-training MSNA levels in heart failure patients are uniformly and markedly reduced and are no longer higher than normal controls; MSNA remained unchanged in the heart failure sedentary group and the normal control exercise group. Source: Roveda *et al.* (2003).

Anti-inflammatory effects of exercise training in the skeletal muscle of patients with chronic heart failure

Gielen S, Adams V, Möbius-Winkler S, *et al. J Am Coll Cardiol* 2003; **42**(5): 861–8

BACKGROUND. This study assessed the effects of regular physical exercise on local inflammatory parameters in the skeletal muscle of patients with stable heart failure. Twenty male patients with heart failure were randomized to a training group (*n* = 10) or a no exercise control group (*n* = 10). Training included daily 20-min sessions of stationary leg ergometry near a heart rate equivalent to 70% of peak VO_2 for 6 months. Serum and local (obtained via muscle biopsy) tumour necrosis factor-α (TNF-α), interleukin (IL)-6 and IL-1β levels were measured at baseline and at 6 months. Local tissue inducible nitric oxide synthase expression was also measured.

INTERPRETATION. Peak VO_2 increased 29% in the training group ($P <0.001$ versus control). Serum TNF-α, IL-6 and IL-1β were unchanged after training. However, local skeletal muscle tissue TNF-α decreased ($P <0.05$ for change with training versus control), IL-6 decreased ($P <0.05$ versus baseline) and IL-1β decreased ($P = 0.02$ for change with training versus control) (Fig. 10.2). Inducible nitric oxide synthase expression also decreased 52% ($P = 0.007$ versus control). Exercise training significantly reduced the local expression of TNF-α, IL-1β, IL-6 and inducible nitric oxide synthase in the skeletal muscle of chronic heart failure patients. These local anti-inflammatory effects of exercise may attenuate the catabolic wasting process associated with the progression of chronic heart failure.

Comment

An ever-increasing number of investigations are examining problems other than central function in patients with the heart failure. This suggests that although the disorder begins with an initial insult to the heart, it becomes a progressive systemic disorder over time, involving the autonomic, skeletal muscle and humoral systems as well. Abnormalities associated with the skeletal muscle include muscle size, strength, endurance, histology and chemistry |5|.

This trial showed that despite mild to no elevation of the inflammatory markers TNF-α, IL-6 and IL-1β in serum, the local expressions of these cytokines were all increased. This information is potentially important because it offers one possible mechanism by which damage to the heart leads to abnormalities within the skeletal muscles. It is possible that as these agents are released in response to the disease and disease progression, they influence muscle function and exercise capacity.

However, exercise training is known to alter skeletal muscle parameters favourably and each of the inflammatory markers assessed in this trial was favourably altered with training as well. Future work is needed to identify whether the exercise-induced favourable changes in tissue inflammatory markers are directly linked with training-related improvements in muscle strength, endurance and histochemistry.

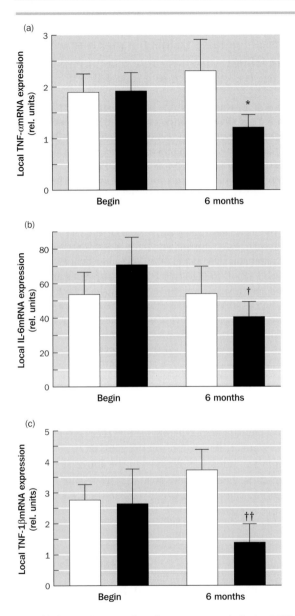

Fig. 10.2 Local expression of tumour necrosis factor (TNF)-α (a) interleukin (IL)-6 (b), and IL-1-β (c) in skeletal muscle biopsies of patients in the training group (black bars) and the control group (open bars) at study baseline and after six months. *P <0.05 for change at six months from baseline in training versus control group; †P <0.05 versus respective baseline at six months; ††P <0.05 versus control group at six months. mRNA, messenger ribonucleic acid. Source: Gielen et al. (2003).

Differential effects of exercise training in men and women with chronic heart failure

Keteyian S, Duscha B, Brawner C, *et al. Am Heart J* 2003; **145**: 912–18

BACKGROUND. The purpose of this study was to describe and compare the effects of exercise training on exercise capacity and skeletal muscle histochemistry in men and women with chronic heart failure. Fifteen patients (ten males) completed a 14–24-week training programme. Training included walking, leg and arm ergometry, and rowing at 60–80% of heart rate reserve three times per week for 14–24 weeks. Peak VO$_2$, myosin heavy chain, capillary density, and selected metabolic enzymes were assessed before and after training.

INTERPRETATION. Peak VO$_2$ increased 14% (P <0.05). However, most of this improvement was observed in men versus women (20 vs 2%; P <0.01). Myosin heavy chain I before training content was lower in men than women (33 vs 50%; P <0.05) and myosin heavy chain I was improved with training in men to 46% (increased 38%; P <0.05) versus no change in women (decreased 3%; P <0.82; Table 10.2). No significant changes in capillary density or muscle enzyme activity were observed in the group as a whole or in men and women separately. Improvements in peak exercise capacity may be more pronounced in men than women. The differential response of VO$_2$ to training paralleled that observed between men and women for changes in myosin heavy chain I isoforms.

Comment

The response of skeletal muscle to exercise training in patients with heart failure remains somewhat variable. Although several trials have shown an improvement in skeletal muscle histology (capillary density, fibre type, myosin heavy chain isoform) and chemistry (mitochondrial enzymes) with cardiorespiratory |**11,12**| or resistance |**13**| training, other studies have not |**14**|. Interestingly, most of the above-cited trials involved men. Therefore, the preliminary observations made in this trial of exercise

Table 10.2 Response of relative myosin heavy chain content to 14 to 24 weeks of exercise training

	All		Men (*n* = 10)		Women (*n* = 5)	
	Baseline	**Change**	**Baseline**	**Change**	**Baseline**	**Change**
MHC-I (%)	38.5 ± 3.3	8.0 ± 4.2	33.0 ± 3.0*	12.6 ± 5.2†	49.6 ± 5.5	−1.3 ± 5.5
MHC-IIa (%)	35.8 ± 2.2	−6.1 ± 3.5	36.6 ± 3.2	−9.7 ± 4.7	34.2 ± 1.9	1.3 ± 2.3
MHC-IIX	25.1 ± 3.4	−1.3 ± 3.5	29.6 ± 3.6*	−2.1 ± 4.9	16.0 ± 5.4	0.3 ± 4.2

Values presented as mean ± SE. MHC, myosin heavy chain.
*P <0.05, men versus women at baseline.
†P <0.05, change compared to baseline.
Source: Keteyian *et al.* (2003).

training-induced changes in exercise capacity and skeletal muscle in men, but not women, may suggest a possible gender-specific response.

Specifically, the increase in peak VO_2 was almost fully attributable to the change observed in men; albeit different from prior reports showing that peak VO_2 can be improved in women with heart failure as well. Additionally, it was only the male subjects in this trial who showed a significant shift in the relative content of myosin heavy chain I isoforms, from 33% before training to 46% after training. Data such as this are intriguing and might suggest that skeletal muscle abnormalities that are not attributable to deconditioning develop in men with heart failure, whereas abnormalities of the same magnitude do not develop in women. Clearly, further research is needed to fully explore this issue for any possible gender-specific differences. It is important to point out that the sample size in this trial, both for men and certainly for women, was quite small. Therefore, the results should only be viewed as preliminary.

Strength/endurance training versus endurance training in congestive heart failure

Delagardelle C, Feiereisen P, Autier P, Shita R, Krecke R, Beissel J. *Med Sci Sports Ex* 2002; **34**(12): 1868–72

BACKGROUND. The aim of this investigation was to compare the effects of endurance training alone (ET group) with combined endurance and strength training (CT group) on haemodynamic and strength parameters in patients with heart failure. Twenty males were randomized into the ET group ($n = 10$) or CT group ($n = 10$). The ET group performed 40 min of interval cycle ergometry (20 min at 50% peak VO_2, 20 min at 75% peak VO_2) three times per week for 40 sessions. The CT group performed 20 min of the same interval cycling followed by 20 min of strength training. Left ventricular function, peak VO_2, lactate, and muscle strength were assessed before and after 40 sessions.

INTERPRETATION. In the ET group, functional class (–23%), work capacity (10%), peak torque (3%) and muscular endurance (9%) were improved. However, peak lactate and peak VO_2 remained unchanged, while EF was decreased and end-diastolic diameter increased. In the CT group, functional class (–22%), work capacity (16%), peak torque (7%), muscular endurance (9%), peak lactate (25%) and peak VO_2 (8%) were all improved. EF increased, whereas end-diastolic diameter decreased. Although endurance training alone showed favourable results, for patients with stable heart failure a greater overall benefit in cardiorespiratory endurance and muscle function may be achieved using a combined programme of strength training and endurance training.

Comment

A limitation of this randomized trial was its small ($n = 20$) sample size. However, despite this shortcoming, it was the first trial to properly assess to what extent, if any, improvements in muscle strength lead to additional improvements in peak VO_2. This was accomplished because two exercise groups were studied, one receiving cardiorespiratory training only and the other receiving both cardiorespiratory and resistance training.

Several groups have shown that skeletal muscle endurance and strength are related to the observed exercise intolerance or reduced peak VO_2 that is characteristic of patients with heart failure |5|. This paper showed that the greater increase in exercise capacity among patients in the CT group was due to improvements in muscle strength. Surprisingly, no meaningful increase in peak VO_2 was observed with aerobic training, which is contrary to what has been observed in well over 20 other trials to date |9|.

The resistance training protocol described in this trial appeared sufficient to stimulate muscle adaptation and should take <30 min to complete. Three sets of ten repetitions (3 s of concentric and 3 s of eccentric movement per repetition) with 1 min of rest between sets was well tolerated. The prescribed workload for resistance training was reasonably set at 60% of one repetition maximum. However, further work is needed to help to identify the optimal dose of resistance training.

Exercise testing

Contribution of peak respiratory exchange ratio to peak VO_2 prognostic reliability in patients with chronic heart failure and severely reduced exercise capacity

Mezzani A, Corrà U, Bosimini E, Giordano A, Giannuzzi P. *Am Heart J* 2003; **145**: 1102–7

BACKGROUND. The purpose of this study was to evaluate the influence of peak respiratory exchange ratio (pRER) on peak VO_2 prognostic reliability in patients with chronic heart failure. Cardiopulmonary exercise testing was performed in 570 patients with chronic heart failure, 193 of whom had a peak VO_2 >10 but ≤14 ml/kg/min, and 80 of whom had a peak VO_2 ≤10 ml/kg/min. Exercise tests were performed in a symptom-limited manner, on a stationary cycle ergometer and using a ramp protocol that increased the work rate by 10 watts/min. Volitional effort or physiological stress was stratified based on pRER at cut-off points of 1.00, 1.05, 1.10 and ≥1.15.

INTERPRETATION. Overall use of ACE inhibitors and β-adrenergic blockade therapy was 93 and 42%, respectively. Seventy-eight events (72 deaths, six heart transplants) occurred during a mean follow-up period of 19.6 ± 14 months. The 2-year survival rate was 69% in patients with a peak VO_2 ≤10 ml/kg/min and 83% in patients with a peak VO_2 >10 but ≤14 ml/kg/min (P <0.0001). Within the group with a peak VO_2 ≤10 ml/kg/min and a pRER >1.15, the 2-year survival rate was 52%, and this pRER was the only independent predictor of the composite end-point (P = 0.03). Within the group of subjects with a peak VO_2 ≤10 ml/kg/min and a pRER <1.15, the survival rate was 83%. Patients with heart failure and a peak VO_2 <10 ml/kg/min should be encouraged to achieve a pRER of 1.15 to ensure the reliability of peak VO_2 as a prognostic measure.

Comment

This paper addressed the topic of the sensitivity of pRER relative to its ability to help assess prognostic reliability in patients with heart failure and a peak VO_2 ≤10 ml/kg/min. Clearly, this is important given the fact that information shared with a patient relative to prognosis and the need for cardiac transplant must be based on accurate information.

For those centres performing and using peak VO_2 to help guide treatment strategies, they must be sure that a true peak effort is achieved, as determined by a pRER ≥1.15. The failure or inability to accomplish this may actually diminish the predictive accuracy of peak VO_2. Specifically, patients who achieve a peak VO_2 ≤10 ml/kg/min and achieve a pRER <1.15 may have results that are suspect relative to prognostic ability and risk stratification. Therefore, and given the generally recognized safety of exercise testing in patients with New York Heart Association class II–III heart failure, testing personnel should be encouraged to motivate patients to achieve the greatest possible level of physiological stress. Doing so will help to ensure that a true peak VO_2 is achieved, one that can accurately help guide and differentiate prognosis and clinical decision making.

The authors correctly pointed out that pRER is associated with inter-individual variation. Therefore, the cut-off for pRER of ≥1.15 may not represent the same level of metabolic stress for everyone. However, based on the findings of this trial, achieving a pRER above or below 1.15 does discriminate survival in patients with a peak VO_2 ≤10 ml/kg/min. This suggests that clinical decisions should be made with caution in patients who achieve this level of exercise capacity but do so with less physiological stress, as measured by pRER.

Combining low-intensity and maximal exercise test results improves prognostic prediction in chronic heart failure

Rickli H, Kiowski W, Brehm M, *et al. J Am Coll Cardiol* 2003; **42**: 116–22

BACKGROUND. To investigate the combined advantages of maximal- and low-intensity exercise testing in predicting prognosis in chronic heart failure using a single exercise test (two-step protocol), a cardiopulmonary or metabolic treadmill exercise test was performed in 202 heart failure patients. VO_2 kinetics were defined as oxygen deficit (ΔVO_2 × time [rest to steady state] – ΣVO_2 [rest to steady state]) and mean response time (oxygen deficit/ΔVO_2). The mean follow-up was 873 ± 628 days. The primary end-point was cardiac mortality and the need for heart transplantation.

INTERPRETATION. Fifty-nine events (44 deaths, 15 transplants) occurred. A mean response time >50 s was the most powerful predictor of the primary end-point (hazard ratio [HR] 4.44), followed by a maximal VO_2 that was <50% of predicted (HR 3.50), and a resting systolic blood pressure <105 mmHg (HR 2.49; all P <0.01). Sixty-four per cent (130 patients) had one or none of the above risk predictors, with a 1-year event rate of 3%. Patients with two risk predictors (n = 45 [22%]) had a 1-year event rate of 33%.

Twenty-seven patients (13%) had all three risk predictors, with a 1-year event rate of 59%. A combination of low- and maximal-intensity exercise testing improved prognosis assessment in patients with heart failure.

Comment

Over the past decade, much research has focused on identifying variables that could be used to better determine prognosis in patients with heart failure. Much of this research has involved a variety of variables obtained during cardiopulmonary exercise testing. This trial provides yet another piece of important information, in that a multicomponent analysis may better predict future risk or prognosis versus peak VO_2 alone. This concept is consistent with the work of Myers *et al.* [1], who also suggested the utility of a multicomponent model.

However, a shortcoming of this paper and any others that also promote a multi-component model involving gas exchange is that it may not be available to the general cardiologist caring for patients with heart failure. Specifically, ordering a gas exchange test to acquire peak VO_2 or other cardiopulmonary parameters can be a challenge in the community-based setting, where the equipment or staff to perform these tests may not exist. All of this makes the use of cardiopulmonary testing for the simple acquisition of peak VO_2, let alone a multicomponent model requiring several metabolic variables and advanced interpretation, even less attractive.

As a result, one area of research that has not been well investigated is whether office-based measures could serve as a surrogate for peak VO_2 and the determination of prognosis. Bittner *et al.* [15] have shown that the 6-min walk is related to prognosis. However, whether this approach can be improved upon remains open for investigation.

Finally, it is important to re-emphasize that the information in this paper is significant and worth repeating for confirmation. The abnormal kinetics of gas exchange are well known in these patients and the model presented takes this into account, suggesting that the logic is sound and related to the underlying disease. Finally, the generalizability of this trial to other cardiac transplant/advanced heart failure centres that typically do have the trained staff and necessary equipment to measure gas exchange is quite good, in that 99% of patients were taking an ACE inhibitor or an angiotensin II receptor blocker. Likewise, 45% of patients were receiving β-adrenergic blockade therapy.

Effect of erythropoietin on exercise capacity in patients with moderate to severe chronic heart failure

Mancini D, Katz S, Lang C, LaManca J, Hudaihed A, Androne A. *Circulation* 2003; **107**: 294–9

BACKGROUND. The effect of erythropoietin on exercise performance in anaemic patients with heart failure was evaluated. Twenty-six anaemic patients were randomized

Table 10.3 Maximal and submaximal exercise capacity at baseline and end of study

	Control				EPO			
	Baseline		End		Baseline		End	
	Rest	Exercise	Rest	Exercise	Rest	Exercise	Rest	Exercise
Heart rate, bpm	77 ± 9	100 ± 19	81 ± 11	102 ± 22	76 ± 9	106 ± 14	73 ± 7	102 ± 13
Blood pressure, mmHg	88 ± 8	96 ± 9	81 ± 8	90 ± 10	87 ± 8	94 ± 12	87 ± 8	94 ± 15
Respiratory quotient	0.83 ± 0.04	1.14 ± 0.11	0.88 ± 0.07	1.10 ± 0.11	0.84 ± 0.06	1.13 ± 0.08	0.85 ± 0.07	1.10 ± 0.08
VO_2, ml/kg/min		10.0 ± 1.9		9.5 ± 1.6		11.0 ± 1.8		12.7 ± 2.8*
VO_2 AT, ml/kg/min		8.2 ± 1.2		7.1 ± 0.8		7.5 ± 1.1		8.7 ± 1.9*
Exercise duration, s		542 ± 115		459 ± 172		590 ± 107		657 ± 119†
6-minute walk distance, ft		929 ± 356		1052 ± 403		1187 ± 279		1328 ± 254*

VO_2 AT, oxygen consumption at anaerobic threshold.
*$P < 0.05$ rest vs exercise; †$P < 0.004$ rest vs exercise.
Source: Mancini et al. (2003).

to receive erythropoietin or placebo for 3 months. Measured variables in both groups at baseline and 3 months included haemoglobin, haematocrit, plasma volume, peak VO$_2$, exercise duration, 6-min walk, muscle aerobic metabolism, and forearm vasodilatory function.

INTERPRETATION. In the erythropoietin group, haemoglobin increased from 11.0 to 14.3 g/dl (P <0.05), whereas peak VO$_2$ increased from 11.0 to 12.7 ml/min/kg (P <0.05) and exercise duration increased from 590 to 657 s (P <0.05) (Table 10.3). No significant changes were observed in the control group. For both groups there was no change in resting and hyperaemic forearm vascular resistance or muscle oxidative capacity. The use of erythropoietin was well tolerated, with no thrombotic or hypertensive events. Erythropoietin significantly enhanced exercise capacity in anaemic patients with heart failure. This improvement in exercise capacity was due to increased oxygen delivery that resulted from an increased haemoglobin concentration.

Comment

Patients with heart failure are frequently anaemic, due, in part, to a variety of direct and indirect disease-related factors. At the same time, patients with heart failure often complain of exercise intolerance, with the majority of the investigations to date focusing on central haemodynamic and peripheral abnormalities. Given the known effect of correcting anaemia on improving exercise intolerance in patients with other chronic diseases, this study represents the logical next step relative to addressing whether correcting anaemia in patients with heart failure would similarly lead to an improved exercise capacity.

In fact, 3 months of erythropoietin therapy in patients with heart failure and anaemia at baseline improved haemoglobin ~30% and peak VO$_2$ ~15%. Similar changes were not observed among patients randomized to usual care. Given the absence of improvements in muscle or endothelial function with erythropoietin, the increase in exercise capacity appears to be due to an increased oxygen delivery that results from the increased haemoglobin concentration. The fact that the increase was more likely due to increases in haemoglobin and not an increase in central cardiac function was supported by the absence of any increase in peak heart rate with erythropoietin therapy. An increase in peak heart with exercise training often occurs in patients with heart failure, and can account for up to 40–50% of the observed increase in VO$_2$ |**16**|. At least one trial is currently underway reproducing the benefits of anaemia therapy in improving exercise capacity in patients with heart failure. Another trial is being planned to determine whether the strategy of treating anaemia with a erythropoietin congener affects mortality.

The effect of β-adrenergic blockers on the prognostic value of peak exercise oxygen uptake in patients with heart failure

Peterson L, Schechtman K, Ewald G, *et al. J Heart Lung Transplant* 2003; **22**: 70–7

BACKGROUND. The aim of this study was to determine the effect of β-adrenergic blockade on the prognostic value of peak VO_2 relative to deaths, heart transplants, and event-free survival days in 369 patients (170 patients not on β blockers) with heart failure. The patients were divided into those taking β blockers and those not taking them. The patients included in this study were referred for assessment between October 1993 and December 2000. All patients underwent symptom-limited exercise treadmill tests with gas exchange.

INTERPRETATION. The median follow-up was 1.6 years and peak VO_2 trended towards being an independent predictor of event-free survival ($P = 0.055$). At all levels of peak VO_2 the event rate was lower in the group taking β blockers. In both patients taking and not taking β blockers, a peak VO_2 of >14 ml/kg/min was associated with a 1-year event rate of approximately half that of a VO_2 ≤ 14 ml/kg/min (Fig. 10.3).

Comment

The timely importance of this paper and other similar papers |**2,17**| should not be overlooked. Given the improving and still increasing use of β blockers in patients with heart failure and the increasing reliance on using peak VO_2 to help establish risk and the need for cardiac transplantation, much work is needed to determine whether this measure remains an important and simple marker of survival and, if so, whether the same cut-off point of 14 ml/kg/min remains. Lund *et al.* |**17**| reported no survival differences in analyses performed with patients divided at a threshold of 10 ml/kg/min. Similar to the work of Pohwani *et al.* |**2**|, this paper also showed that patients treated with β blockers have an improved survival versus similar patients not on β blocker therapy.

An obvious limitation of this trial, and other trials that rely on an observational database, is that it was not conducted in a randomized, controlled manner. Similarities and differences in outcomes might be attributed to differences in patient characteristics at baseline or selection bias rather than the measure of interest or treatment being assessed. Additionally, the follow-up period was relatively short, which means that future trials should address event rates at 3 years or more.

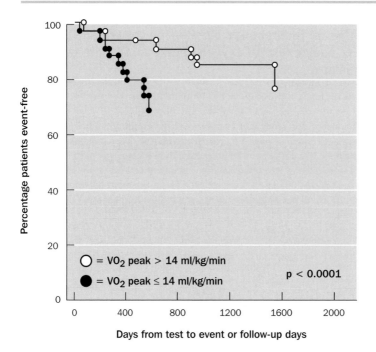

Fig. 10.3 Event-free survival as a function of VO_2 peak in patients on β-blockers. Source: Peterson *et al.* (2003).

Prognostic significance of exercise plasma noradrenaline levels for cardiac death in patients with mild heart failure

Kinugawa T, Ogino K, Osaki S, *et al. Circ J* 2002; **66**(3): 261–6

BACKGROUND. The aim of this study was to determine whether exercise plasma noradrenaline levels could predict cardiac death in patients with mild heart failure, in whom plasma noradrenaline levels were only minimally elevated. One hundred and forty-two patients and 26 age-matched normal subjects performed treadmill exercise testing with serial measurement of plasma noradrenaline.

INTERPRETATION. Twenty-seven cardiac deaths occurred during a median follow-up of 9.6 years among patients. Univariate hazard analysis showed several significant prognostic markers including left ventricular end-systolic dimension ($P < 0.001$), age ($P < 0.01$), peak exercise heart rate ($P < 0.01$), exercise plasma noradrenaline level ($P < 0.01$), and LVEF ($P < 0.001$). Multivariate analysis identified exercise plasma noradrenaline level as the most powerful prognostic marker ($P < 0.001$), followed by left ventricular end-systolic dimension and peak exercise heart rate. Exercise plasma noradrenaline levels can provide prognostic information in patients with mild heart failure, which suggests an important link between an exercise-induced activation of the sympathetic nervous system activity and prognosis.

Comment

The important and, at times, deleterious activation of the sympathetic nervous system in patients with heart failure has been defined |9|. The onset of heart failure activates the sympathetic nervous system and both direct and indirect markers of this heightened state, such as increased plasma noradrenaline at rest, represent a predictor of long-term survival. It is also well known that heart failure treatment strategies such as ACE inhibitors and β-adrenergic blockade favourably attenuate this sympathetic over-activation, providing one explanation of how these agents exert their beneficial influence on survival.

This study is unique for several reasons. First, it involved a 'less sick' group of patients with heart failure, presenting with New York Heart Association class I–II status. Secondly, it was conducted over almost 10 years. Their finding that the magnitude of the exercise-induced increase in plasma noradrenaline is related to survival extends what we know about sympathetic activity at rest in patients with more advanced heart failure. Specifically, we now know that an exercise-induced over-activation of the sympathetic nervous system, even in patients with relatively mild heart failure, is an unfavourable risk factor.

Clinically, preliminary work such as this addressing survival, especially given that it was completed over almost 10 years, forces us to begin paying more attention to these 'less sick' patients. As this group represents a large segment of all patients with heart failure, long-term research assessing various assessment and treatment strategies appears warranted.

Effects of cold exposure on submaximal exercise performance and adrenergic activation in patients with congestive heart failure and the effects of beta-adrenergic blockade (carvedilol or metoprolol)

Blanchet M, Ducharme A, Racine N, *et al. Am J Cardiol* 2003; **92**: 548–53

BACKGROUND. The aim of this study was to investigate the impact of cold exposure on submaximal exercise capacity, systemic adrenergic drive, and the effects of long-term β-adrenergic blockade on these parameters. Thirty-three patients with heart failure were randomized to receive metoprolol or carvedilol for 6 months. Observations were compared with twelve age-matched healthy subjects. Maximal exercise testing with gas exchange was performed, and endurance capacity was measured using two constant-load exercise tests performed randomly at 20 and –8°C.

INTERPRETATION. In response to cold exposure, healthy volunteers increased submaximal exercise time by 20% (*P* <0.05), whereas heart failure patients showed a 21% decrease (*P* <0.05). However, in patients with heart failure, β blockers increased submaximal exercise time at both temperatures ($P < 0.05$). Norepinephrine increased to a greater extent at 4 min of exercise and exhaustion (at $-8°C$) only in heart failure patients. β-adrenergic blockade caused no significant decrease in norepinephrine levels. β blocker therapy with either metoprolol or carvedilol significantly increased submaximal exercise time and attenuated the impact of cold exposure on functional capacity.

Comment

Patients with moderate and advanced heart failure typically complain of dyspnoea and fatigue with exertion—symptoms that commonly mark the exercise intolerance that develops in these patients. This study identified that the already abnormal exercise capacity of these patients is only worsened with cold exposure.

Although this study did provide an interesting look at the mechanisms that might account for the cold-induced decrease in exercise tolerance in patients with heart failure (e.g. increased heart rate and increased after load due to sympathetic activation), what is possibly even more relevant is the fact that β blocker therapy attenuated the cold-induced reduction in exercise capacity. Given that β blocker therapy now approaches 60% in patients with heart failure, its use should help those patients routinely exposed to cold temperatures due to their place of residence or work-related duties.

Conclusion

Although the above research and, for that matter, most of the exercise and heart failure research over the last 15 years have advanced the use of exercise testing and training in the assessment and routine care of patients with stable heart failure, these accomplishments may someday pale when compared with potential findings yet to be revealed over the next 5 to 7 years. Therefore, we believe that it is important to focus our summary on the many questions that remain. At the top of the list is assessing the effect of regular exercise on all-cause and cardiac mortality and hospitalizations. Additionally, trials are also needed relative to the application of exercise training in various subpopulations.

Specifically, if favourable, will the biological, economic, clinical and psychological effects of exercise training apply equally regardless of age, gender, race, severity of illness, failure and aetiology of illness? Concerning the latter, we know that patients with an ischaemic cardiomyopathy often have a poorer prognosis when compared with those with a non-ischaemic cardiomyopathy. Does exercise provide similar benefits regardless of aetiology of illness, or does exercise need to be more narrowly applied? Likewise, similar questions should be answered for men versus women, those with diabetes versus those free of diabetes, and younger versus older patients.

Although we would like to think that current research has most of the answers to these questions, the truth of the matter is that this is not the case. Fortunately, the HF-ACTION trial is now underway, which will report its findings in 2007. In addition to this trial, however, work is also needed relative to several specific exercise-related investigations. For example, the proper dose of both aerobic and resistance training exercise needs further investigation. Also, exercise, regardless of the population involved, is a difficult behaviour to maintain relative to long-term compliance. If HF-ACTION finds that long-term exercise improves clinical outcome, then additional and complementary research must address how best to achieve compliance—so that its therapeutic benefits are, in fact, derived.

The key here is not simply to wait for the results of the HF-ACTION trial to be reported. In this interim period of time much can be accomplished concerning not only how exercise might act to improve symptoms and exercise capacity, but how we can apply it using a dose that is safe and favours long-term compliance. Even if the HF-ACTION trial shows no improvement in all-cause mortality or hospitalizations with training, as long as exercise is shown to be safe it will probably still be recommended for selected patients because of its well-established effect on improving exercise capacity and symptoms.

Concerning the use of exercise testing, as the background medical therapy continues to evolve so should the nature and type of data derived from exercise testing. In fact, much emphasis is currently being placed on looking at other cardiopulmonary measures, not just peak VO_2, to predict survival. A point to remember, however, is that any evaluation method that is explored should keep the concept of generalizability in mind. Clearly, for the practising cardiologist we need to investigate assessment options that are realistic and accessible, and do so using patient groups that are similar to those they care for each day.

Finally, it would be remiss if we did not point out that nearly all of the research conducted to date has involved patients with heart failure due to systolic dysfunction. Given that many patients with diastolic heart failure complain of similar symptoms, is not research needed relative to defining the role of exercise testing and training in these patients as well? As stated previously, the next 5 years will be quite exciting.

References

1. Myers J, Gullestad L, Vagelos R, Do D, Bellin D, Ross H, Fowler M. Cardiopulmonary exercise testing and prognosis in severe heart failure: 14 mls/kg/min revisited. *Am Heart J* 2000; **139**: 78–84.
2. Pohwani AL, Murali S, Mathier MM, Tokarczyk T, Kormos RL, McNamara DM, MacGowan GA. Impact of b-blocker therapy on functional capacity of criteria for heart transplant listing. *J Heart Lung Transplant* 2003; **22**: 78–86.
3. Belardinelli R, Georgiou D, Purcaro A. Randomized, controlled trial of long-term moderate exercise training in chronic heart failure. *Circulation* 1999; **99**: 1173–82.

4. Jugdutt BI, Michorowski BL, Kappagoda CT. Exercise training after anterior Q wave myocardial infarction: importance of regional left ventricular function and topography. *J Am Coll Cardiol* 1988; **12**: 362–72.

5. Afzal A, Brawner C, Keteyian S. Exercise training in heart failure. *Prog Cardiovasc Dis* 1998; **41**: 175–90.

6. Sullivan MJ, Green HJ, Higginbotham FR. Exercise training in patients with severe left ventricular dysfunction. *Circulation* 1988; **78**: 506–15.

7. Minotti JR, Christoph I, Ika R, Weiner MW, Wells L, Massie BM. Impaired skeletal muscle function in patients with congestive heart failure. *J Clin Invest* 1991; **88**: 2077–82.

8. Hambrecht R, Fiehn E, Weigl C, Gielen S, Hamann C, Kaiser R, Yu J, Adams V, Niebauer J, Schuler G. Regular physical exercise corrects endothelial dysfunction and improves exercise capacity in patients with chronic heart failure. *Circulation* 1998; **98**; 2709–15.

9. Keteyian SJ, Spring TJ. Chronic heart failure. In: Ehrman J, Gordon P, Visich P, Keteyian SJ (eds). *Clinical Exercise Physiology*. Champaign, Illinois: Human Kinetics, 2003; pp 261–80.

10. Linke A, Schoene N, Gielen S, Hofer J, Erbs S, Schuler G, Hambrecht R. Endothelial dysfunction in patients with chronic heart failure: systemic effects of lower-limb exercise training. *J Am Coll Cardiol* 2001; **37**: 392–7.

11. Hambrecht R, Niebauer J, Fiehn E, Kalberer B, Offner B, Hauer K, Riede U, Schlierf G, Kubler W, Schuler G. Physical training in patients with stable chronic heart failure: effects on cardiorespiratory fitness and ultrastructural abnormalities of leg muscles. *J Am Coll Cardiol* 1995; **25**: 1239–49.

12. Hambrecht R, Fiehn E, Yu J, Niebauer J, Weigl C, Hilbrich L, Adams V, Riede U, Schuler G. Effects of endurance training on mitochondrial ultrastructure and fiber type distribution in skeletal muscle of patients with chronic heart failure. *J Am Coll Cardiol* 1997; **29**: 1067–73.

13. Pu CT, Johnson MT, Forman DE, Hausdorff JM, Roubenoff R, Foldvari M, Fielding RA, Singh MA. Randomized trial of progressive resistance training to counteract the myopathy of chronic heart failure. *J Appl Physiol* 2001; **90**: 2341–50.

14. Kiilavuori K, Naveri H, Salmi T, Harkonen M. The effect of physical training on skeletal muscle in patients with chronic heart failure. *Eur J Heart Failure* 2000; **2**: 53–63.

15. Bittner V, Weiner DH, Yusuf S, Rogers WJ, McIntyre KM, Bangdiwala SI, Kronenberg MW, Kostis JB, Kohn RM, Guillotte M, *et al.* for the SOLVD Investigators. Prediction of mortality and morbidity with a 6-minute walk test in patients with left ventricular dysfunction. *JAMA* 1993; **270**: 1702–7.

16. Keteyian SJ, Brawner CA, Schairer JR, Levine TB, Levine AB, Rogers FJ, Goldstein S. Effects of exercise training on chronotropic incompetence in patients with heart failure. *Am Heart J* 1999; **138**: 233–40.

17. Lund LH, Aaronson KD, Mancini DM. Predicting survival in ambulatory patients with severe heart failure on beta-blocker therapy. *Am J Cardiol* 2003; **92**: 1350–4.

11

Future of cardiac rehabilitation in Spain for patients with heart failure

RICARDO SERRA-GRIMA

In the last 5 years, cardiac rehabilitation services directed to heart failure patients with an ischaemic aetiology have developed at a slow and uneven pace. During that time, the number of cardiac rehabilitation programmes in Spain has increased. The majority of cardiologists have accepted that exercise training for patients with heart failure can have significant benefits and is efficacious. Yet, recommending exercise therapy in conjunction with other measures of secondary prevention is not being carried out in all patients once discharged from hospital. Therefore, there are still many patients in whom an appropriate exercise programme has never been recommended or prescribed. Rehabilitation programmes have not applied the tenets of training across all patient types, including those with ischaemic cardiomyopathies, often due to economic restraints and the lack of available physical space in many hospitals. Nonetheless, there are other factors that could, in the future, affect the cardiac rehabilitation of patients with heart failure due to an ischaemic aetiology.

Heart failure guidelines developed by the Spanish Society of Cardiology include exercise training among the basic recommendations for patients with heart failure. In general, cardiologists agree, to a large degree, that these recommendations are based on evidence that exercise training generally benefits this patient population. An increase in functional capacity as measured objectively, in addition to the subjective improvement in quality of life, are the two most solid reasons to recommend that cardiac rehabilitation services be prescribed to patients with heart failure, once a clinical assessment has been completed. However, notwithstanding the good intentions of the physician, the lack of physical space, personnel and technical equipment makes it difficult to accomplish the goals of the guidelines.

It is time for a community-based effort to add guidelines and to form advisory groups composed of cardiologists, rehabilitation and physical therapists, to resolve these issues which prevent turning a theoretical benefit into a reality. We are hopeful that the mortality and morbidity trials that are ongoing in the USA will contribute further to our knowledge base and lead to a better application of rehabilitation services to the greatest number of patients.

As mentioned above, economic factors have not only limited the expansion of rehabilitation services to countries with a socialized financial system of medical care, but have also impacted on the private sector. Spain currently has a socialized health system for the entire population. However, the private insurance sector is rapidly growing. In addition, there has been a movement towards decentralization of health services in order to allow each region (similar to the states in the USA) to disburse health according to its own priorities or needs. This movement has further affected the uniformity of rehabilitation services throughout Spain and most definitely has impacted on the heart failure population. Consequently, guidelines, although accepted in theory, are not applied in practice.

Solutions to our current problems include: (a) assigning sufficient funds, (b) providing technical equipment and (c) training personnel who can carry out the training programmes. In Spain, cardiology fellows do not rotate through cardiac rehabilitation programmes, but are more interested in imaging and invasive techniques. Functional capacity assessment by cardiopulmonary testing should be part of the standard training programme along with all other technical interventions, whether invasive or non-invasive. If exposed to it during training, more cardiologists would be better informed about exercise in heart failure and would take those practices to the community. This expanded training would in large part help to solve our current problem. Similarly, neither nurses nor physical therapists are routinely trained in cardiac rehabilitation and yet these are the individuals needed to administer the programmes of exercise training and secondary prevention.

It may be of value to involve sports medicine specialists who are very interested in exercise physiology and functional capacity assessment. These individuals do train in exercise programmes with wide applications across many disease states. Their involvement in exercise training of the ever-growing heart failure population may be an intermediate and temporary solution to bringing the benefits of exercise training to patients with this syndrome. Specialists in sports medicine currently supervise patients with heart failure who are referred by cardiologists for post-hospitalization cardiac rehabilitation programmes. For several years, residents in sports medicine programmes from the School of Medicine of Barcelona have rotated through the exercise laboratory and cardiac rehabilitation programme at St Paul Hospital. This is an elective rotation lasting a minimum of 6 months. My colleagues and I hope that this trend continues with increased emphasis on activity training for patients with heart failure. In parallel, exercise training in heart failure patients should be an integral part of the training of nurses and physical therapists. Of note, physical therapists are well versed on the negative effects of a sedentary lifestyle and on the consequences of immobilization.

In conclusion, cardiac rehabilitation in heart failure patients is in its infancy in Spain, although the wealth of information on its benefits is solid in the literature. Supervised exercise training is gradually being extended to those who suffer from heart failure along with the application of current evidenced-based medical therapy.

A guarantee for the future expansion of these programmes will only occur with adequate financial resources, better-trained personnel and coordination among cardiologists who are charged with its recommendation and exercise prescription.

12

Women and heart failure: a failure of trials?

ILEANA PIÑA

Introduction

Cardiovascular disease is the leading cause of death in women, responsible for more deaths each year than all other causes combined. Because medical therapy has improved survival, more women are living with the chronic syndrome known as heart failure. As illustrated by the Framingham data, the incidence of heart failure declined in women during the decades from 1950 to 1999, as did mortality. However, of the patients diagnosed in the 1990s, 50% had died by 5 years. Almost half the patients in the USA with heart failure are women. Among persons older than 70 years, the incidence of heart failure in women is higher than in men. Therefore, women are just as capable as men of developing heart failure. In spite of these facts, medical therapy has been tested primarily in men. Nonetheless, the same medical therapy is applied to both genders with little knowledge of the differences that may exist. This chapter will briefly review some of the differences in prevalence, clinical presentation and mortality between men and women with heart failure.

To better understand the incidence, prevalence and risk factors for heart failure in women, several sets of data need to be examined: epidemiological databanks, registries derived from trials or procedures, health plans, large clinical trials or heart failure speciality clinics. Some of these information sources, in fact, will seem at first to be contradictory.

Epidemiological data, such as the Framingham cohort, describe the growing prevalence of heart failure in women in parallel with increasing age, with the greatest increase occurring after 80 years of age. The increase in heart failure with age is similar in men. More recently, investigators from the Framingham study have reported a decline in the incidence of heart failure in women, but not in men. Reviewing the periods from 1950 to 1969, 1970 to 1979, 1980 to 1989 and 1990 to 1999, the 30-day mortality in women dropped from 18 to 10%, with mortality at 28, 28, 27 and 24%, respectively, for those time periods.

The American Heart Association and the Center for Vital Statistics report that approximately 2 440 000 women in the USA have heart failure and are alive today. A common misconception is that women have less myocardial infarctions (MIs) than men and may fare better in the post-MI period. In fact, however, 46% of women who are victims of MI will develop heart failure within 6 years, compared with 22% of men.

If one were to examine the clinical trials, one would be led to believe that the number of women with heart failure is small. Clinical trials of pharmacotherapy have enrolled only an average of 20% women. Health plans, however, such as the Henry Ford Health System, report that in over 4 million covered lives, 57% are women and that in 29 686 patients with heart failure, 53% are women. The women are older than the men and 54% are African–American. These figures undoubtedly include women with heart failure and preserved systolic function. The mortality of the women in the Henry Ford Health System is significantly better than in the men, but the statistics do not differentiate aetiology.

Published clinical trials, including those with reported improved survival, have performed poorly in the recruitment of women. This small number of women may reflect the high penetration of patients with ischaemia and the exclusion, thus far, of patients with preserved systolic function. The Candesartan in Heart Failure—Assessment of Reduction in Mortality and Morbidity (CHARM) trial has now prospectively enrolled patients with heart failure due to preserved systolic function and compared candesartan with placebo. In this study, the women comprised 40% of the population. Other studies of this important patient group with heart failure are in progress.

In the registry of the Studies of Left Ventricular Dysfunction (SOLVD), the women were older than their male counterparts and were more likely to have hypertension and less ischaemic heart disease, but had an equivalent depression of systolic function. Valvular disease was twice as common in the women. The event rates followed in the registry are worrisome, however, with women having a higher total mortality, explained by a higher overall cardiac mortality of 22% compared with 17% in men. The combined observations of death and/or hospitalization were also higher in women.

Heart failure speciality clinics provide perhaps a more realistic view of patients referred to these centres, which are dedicated to the care of heart failure patients. As published by Adams *et al.* (1996), the women in their speciality clinic were more likely to be African–American with higher ejection fractions (EFs) than the men. The women were also more likely to have oedema and 40% were New York Heart Association class IV compared with 25% of the men. In contrast, the men were more likely to have ischaemic heart disease and to have undergone bypass surgery with worse ventricular function than the women. Although at first glance the women had a better survival, when assigned to aetiology, both the men and the women had a similar mortality if ischaemia was the aetiological factor in the heart failure. This observation was also noted in the Beta Blocker Evaluation of Survival Trial (BEST). Although the number of women in clinical therapeutic trials has been small, the results have been extrapolated to the heart failure population of both genders. A close look at SOLVD will show that death and/or hospitalizations were similar in men and women, but the women seemed to benefit less from enalapril than the men.

This observation is best explained by a lesser benefit on first heart failure hospitalization and new or worsening heart failure. The benefits to mortality appear to be as positive.

β blockers have now taken their place next to the angiotensin-converting enzyme (ACE) inhibitors in the prevention of death and hospitalizations. The Metoprolol CR/XL Randomized Intervention Trial (MERIT) has published an analysis of the women included in this randomized trial comparing metoprolol CR/XL with placebo in class II–IV heart failure. The women demonstrated significant reductions in all-cause and heart failure-cause hospitalizations. In the women with severe heart failure, the reductions in hospitalizations were even more striking. Total mortality was lower in the women when compared with the men, after adjustment for differences in baseline variables. The benefits of drug versus placebo in the women were statistically significant. When the three important β blocker trials are summarized, the benefits to women favour the β blockers, although the confidence intervals are larger due to the smaller number of female subjects. Therefore, at this time, women with heart failure should receive both ACE inhibitors and β blockers for the prevention of hospitalizations and death. The Randomized Aldactone Evaluation Study (RALES) trials of spironolactone versus placebo in patients with severe heart failure, which showed improvements in survival, did not analyse the women separately and, therefore, no other comments can be made about this therapeutic agent and its specific benefits to women with heart failure.

Aetiology of heart failure

The University of North Carolina database has been in existence since 1984 and provides valuable information on the relationship between gender, aetiology and survival in patients with symptomatic heart failure. A study of 557 patients (380 men and 177 women) with symptomatic heart failure, predominantly non-ischaemic in origin (68%), and severe left ventricular dysfunction with a mean left ventricular ejection fraction (LVEF) of 25%, revealed a better survival in women compared with men when heart failure was due to a non-ischaemic cause. The mean follow-up period was 2.4 years and the relative risk of death for men 2.36 ($P <0.001$). The risk of death was similar for the subset of men and women with ischaemic heart disease as the primary cause of heart failure. Although baseline LVEF was higher in women than in men with non-ischaemic heart failure, the mortality in women remained lower after adjustment for this variable.

Gender and cardiac physiology

A growing body of basic and clinical data points to fundamental gender-related differences in the nature and extent of myocardial hypertrophy and adaptation, which might account for the survival advantage for women. Early studies of spontaneously hypertensive rats suggested that the adverse influence of hypertrophy on cardiac function was greater in male than female rats. Gender differences in the up-regulation of left ventricular ACE activity during pressure-overload hypertrophy have been reported. Importantly, gender has been found to influence the nature of left ventricular adaptation in patients with aortic stenosis dilatation and hypertrophy. A similar situation exists with regard to hypertension, with women more likely to have left ventricular hypertrophy.

Treatment of established heart failure: ACE inhibitors

Early meta-analysis of ACE inhibitor trials found significant reductions in mortality and the combined end-point of all-cause mortality and hospitalizations for heart failure for men only. The apparent lack of benefit for women in this analysis probably reflects the small number of women (1991) in these trials. A recently reported meta-analysis of the long-term ACE inhibitor trials in patients with a low EF found no significant heterogeneity of effects by gender. This meta-analysis incorporated data on 12 763 patients followed for an average of 35 months.

Treatment of established heart failure: β blockers

The Cardiac Insufficiency Bisoprolol Study (CIBIS II) was the first large-scale randomized, double-blind, placebo-controlled European study to show a reduction in all-cause mortality rates with the addition of the β1 selective antagonist bisoprolol to standard treatment with ACE inhibitors and diuretics. Out of 2647 patients with New York Heart Association class III–IV heart failure and an LVEF of less than or equal to 35%, 515 were women. As noted and consistent with other trials, the women were older than the men at the time of enrolment and had a higher New York Heart Association Class, with 21% of the women in Class IV compared with 16% of the men. Despite signs of more advanced symptoms, the women enjoyed a better survival after an average follow-up of 1.3 years. The rates of sudden death, fatal MI, unknown cause of death and all-cause hospital admissions did not differ between the men and women.

MERIT-HF was a randomized, placebo-controlled study of metoprolol controlled-release/extended-release in 3991 patients with New York Heart Association Class II–IV heart failure due to left ventricular systolic dysfunction, of which 898 were women (23% of the population). The two primary outcome events were total mortality and the combined end-point of all-cause mortality or all-cause hospitalization (time to first event). Compared with the men, the women were older, were more likely to have New York Heart Association Class III and IV, and had similar LVEFs.

The women also had a higher prevalence of hypertension and diabetes mellitus and a lower prevalence of ischaemic heart disease and prior MI.

Overall, treatment with extended-release metoprolol led to a 21% decrease in the combined end-point of all-cause hospitalization and all-cause mortality in women, but did not lead to a significant reduction in mortality when viewed as a separate end-point, perhaps due to the limited percentage of women. Another explanation for the lack of mortality benefit in women was the fact that there was a limited number of deaths in the women (totalling 64). There was a 29% decrease in cardiovascular hospitalizations, and a 42% decrease in hospitalization due to worsening heart failure. In the subset of women with severe heart failure, there was a 44% reduction in the combined end-point, a 57% reduction in cardiovascular hospitalization and a 72% reduction in hospitalization due to worsening heart failure. In contrast to women, actively treated men had a significant but less robust reduction in all-cause hospitalization rates. A significant reduction in all-cause mortality was seen with actively treated men.

A pooling of mortality results from three recent large β blocker trials (MERIT-HF, CIBIS II and COPERNICUS), providing the statistical power of a large sample size of more than 8900 patients, showed very similar survival benefits in women and men treated with β blockers.

Treatment of established heart failure: other vasodilators

ACE inhibitors are recommended in all patients with reduced left ventricular systolic function, regardless of the absence, presence or severity of symptoms. However, a significant number of people develop intolerable side effects from these medications, limiting their use. Alternative vasodilator medications for patients who are intolerant of ACE inhibitors include the non-specific vasodilating combination of hydralazine and isosorbide (as studied in the V-HeFT I trials) and angiotensin II receptor blockers, which have been more extensively studied. The V-HeFT trials, conducted in the Veterans Administration hospitals, included no women. A trial of African–Americans, A HeFT was recently stopped prematurely due to benefits of the combination of hydralazine and nitrates in addition to ACE inhibitors and β blockers in a population with moderate to severe heart failure symptoms. The results of this trial are eagerly awaited.

The Val-HeFT trial studied the angiotensin receptor blocker valsartan versus placebo in combination with background therapy including digoxin, diuretics and β blockers in 5010 patients (20% of whom were women) with Class II–IV heart failure due to left ventricular systolic dysfunction. Although overall mortality was similar in the two groups, there was a 13.2% reduction in the combined end-point of morbidity and mortality, defined as mortality plus the incidence of cardiac arrest with successful resuscitation, hospitalization for heart failure requiring intravenous inotropic or vasodilator therapy. The significance was noted in hospitalizations and not in mortality. A similar benefit was seen in women and men.

The CHARM trial compared the angiotensin receptor blocker candesartan with either ACE inhibitor or placebo in three distinct heart failure patient populations: those with reduced LVEF either receiving or intolerant of ACE inhibition and those with clinical heart failure despite a preserved LVEF. This trial enrolled 7601 patients. While women represented 32% of total enrolment, they comprised 40% of the subset with heart failure despite preserved left ventricular systolic function. The women with heart failure in this trial were older than the men (mean age 68 vs 65 years), more likely to have a hypertensive aetiology for their heart failure (21 vs 9%) and less likely to be treated with β blockers (57 vs 52%). At baseline, women were also found to have more symptoms and clinical evidence of systemic and pulmonary vascular congestion despite a higher LVEF (43 vs 37%). In the CHARM-added arm, a reduction in the combined end-point of cardiovascular death or heart failure hospitalization of 15% was observed. To date, the results in the women have not been published separately. In the group of patients who were ACE intolerant, the reduction in the primary end-point was 23% ($P = 0.0004$).

The Eplerenone Post-acute Myocardial Infarction Heart Failure Efficacy and Survival Study (EPHESUS) randomized 6632 patients who had suffered an MI resulting in an EF of less than 40% or symptoms of heart failure to eplerenone versus placebo. The trial population included approximately 29% women. All-cause mortality was reduced by 15%. A subgroup analysis of men and women showed similar benefits of eplerenone in this population. It should be noted that the population of EPHESUS was not one of chronic heart failure. Whether the trial results can be extrapolated to the chronic heart failure population is purely speculative.

Clinical trials versus clinical practice

Although women have represented, on average, only 20% of patients enrolled in large trials of heart failure, they represent a substantially larger percentage of heart failure patients seen clinically, in either general or speciality clinics, in either the inpatient or outpatient setting. It is also becoming clear that many older women with heart failure have preserved systolic function and comprise as much as 40% of hospital admissions for decompensated heart failure. Nonetheless, to date, there is no reason to exclude women from the heart failure therapy applicable to men, i.e. ACE inhibitors and β blockers. Clinicians, however, should have a high index of suspicion when diagnosing and treating women who exhibit signs and symptoms of heart failure. The presentation may be more advanced, but the therapeutic benefits of drug therapy appear to be consistent. Should the aetiology of heart failure not be clear, it is imperative to rule out or rule in coronary artery disease, given that the prognosis of women may in fact be worse than men with a similar disease burden. It is hoped that future trials will prospectively enrol more women in accordance with the reality of the population and that prospective analyses will be planned for women. To do anything less would be a disservice to the female heart failure population.

Further reading

1. Levy D, Kenchaiah S, Larson MG, Benjamin EJ, Kupka MJ, Ho KK, Murabito JM, Vasan RS. Long-term trends in the incidence of and survival with heart failure. *N Engl J Med* 2002; **347**: 1397–402.

2. Luchi RJ, Taffet GE, Teasdale TA. Congestive heart failure in the elderly. *J Am Geriatr Soc* 1991; **39**(8): 810–25.

3. Senni M, Tribouilloy CM, Rodeheffer RJ, Jacobsen SJ, Evans JM, Bailey KR, Redfield MM. Congestive heart failure in the community: trends in incidence and survival in a 10-year period. *Arch Intern Med* 1999; **159**(1): 29–34.

4. American Heart Association. *Heart Disease and Stroke Statistics—2003*. Dallas: American Heart Association, 2002.

5. McCullough PA, Philbin EF, Spertus JA, Kaatz S, Sandberg KR, Weaver WD. Confirmation of a heart failure epidemic: findings from the Resource Utilization Among Congestive Heart Failure (REACH) study. *J Am Coll Cardiol* 2002; **39**(1): 60–9.

6. Yusuf S, Pfeffer MA, Swedberg K, Granger CB, Held P, McMurray JJ, Michelson EL, Olofsson B, Ostergren J; CHARM Investigators and Committees. Effects of candesartan in patients with chronic heart failure and preserved left-ventricular ejection fraction: the CHARM-Preserved Trial. *Lancet* 2003; **362**(9386): 777–81.

7. Bourassa MG, Gurne O, Bangdiwala SI, Ghali JK, Young JB, Rousseau M, Johnstone DE, Yusuf S. Natural history and patterns of current practice in heart failure. The Studies of Left Ventricular Dysfunction (SOLVD) Investigators. *Am J Cardiol* 1993; **22**(4 Suppl A): 14A–19A.

8. Adams KF Jr, Dunlap SH, Sueta CA, Clarke SW, Patterson JH, Blauwet MB, Jensen LR, Tomasko L, Koch G. Relation between gender, etiology and survival in patients with symptomatic heart failure. *J Am Coll Cardiol* 1996; **28**: 1781–8.

9. Ghali JK, Krause-Steinrauf HJ, Adams KF Jr, Khan SS, Rosenberg YD, Yancy CW, Young JB, Goldman S, Peberdy MA, Lindenfeld J. Gender differences in advanced heart failure: insights from the BEST study. *J Am Coll Cardiol* 2003; **42**: 2128–34.

10. Pina IL. A better survival for women with heart failure? It's not so simple... *J Am Coll Cardiol* 2003; **42**(12): 2135–8.

11. Limacher MC, Yusuf S. Gender differences in presentation, morbidity and mortality in the Studies of Left Ventricular Dysfunction (SOLVD): a preliminary report. In: Wenger NK, Speroff L, Packard B (eds). *Cardiovascular Health and Disease in Women*. Greenwich, CT: Le Jacq Communications, 1993; pp 345–8.

12. The SOLVD Investigators. Effect of enalapril on survival in patients with reduced left-ventricular ejection fractions and congestive heart failure. *N Engl J Med* 1991; **325**: 293–302.

13. Johnstone D, Limacher M, Rousseau M, Liang CS, Ekelund L, Herman M, Stewart D, Guillotte M, Bjerken G, Gaasch W, *et al.* Clinical characteristics of patients in Studies of Left Ventricular Dysfunction (SOLVD). *Am J Cardiol* 1992; **70**: 894–900.

14. Hjalmarson A, Goldstein S, Fagerberg B, Wedel H, Waagstein F, Kjekshus J, Wikstrand J, El Allaf D, Vitovec J, Aldershvile J, Halinen M, Dietz R, Neuhaus KL, Janosi A, Thorgeirsson G, Dunselman PH, Gullestad L, Kuch J, Herlitz J, Rickenbacher P, Ball S, Gottlieb S, Deedwania P. Effects of controlled-release metoprolol on total mortality, hospitalizations, and well-being in patients with heart failure: the Metoprolol CR/XL Randomized Intervention Trial in congestive heart failure (MERIT-HF). MERIT-HF Study Group. *JAMA* 2000; **283**: 1295–302.

15. Ghali JK, Pina IL, Gottlieb SS, Deedwania PC, Wikstrand JC. Metoprolol CR/XL in female patients with heart failure: analysis of the experience in Metoprolol Extended-release Randomized Intervention Trial in Heart Failure (MERIT-HF). *Circulation* 2002; **105**(13): 1585–91.

16. Shekelle PG, Rich MW, Morton SC, Atkinson CS, Tu W, Maglione M, Rhodes S, Barrett M, Fonarow GC, Greenberg B, Heidenreich PA, Knabel T, Konstam MA, Steimle A, Warner Stevenson L. Efficacy of angiotensin-converting enzyme inhibitors and beta-blockers in the management of left ventricular systolic dysfunction according to race, gender, and diabetic status: a meta-analysis of major clinical trials. *J Am Coll Cardiol* 2003; **41**: 1529–38.

17. Pitt B, Zannad F, Remme WF, Cody R, Castaigne A, Perez A, Palensky J, Wittes J. The effect of spironolactone on morbidity and mortality in patients with severe heart failure. Randomized Aldactone Evaluation Study Investigators. *N Engl J Med* 1999; **341**: 709–17.

18. Jessup M, Pina IL. Is it important to examine gender differences in the epidemiology and outcome of severe heart failure? *J Thorac Cardiovasc Surg* 2004; **127**(5): 1247–52.

19. Pfeffer JM, Pfeffer MA, Fletcher P, Fishbein MC, Braunwald E. Favorable effects of therapy on cardiac performance in spontaneously hypertensive rats. *Am J Physiol* 1982; **242**(5): H776–84.

20. Lorell BH. Cardiac renin-angiotensin system: role in development of pressure-overload hypertrophy. *Can J Cardiol* 1995; **11**(Suppl F): 7F–12F.

21. Carroll JD, Carroll EP, Feldman T, Ward DM, Lang RM, McGaughey D, Karp RB. Sex-associated differences in left ventricular function in aortic stenosis of the elderly. *Circulation* 1992; **86**(4): 1099–107.

22. Devereux RB, Pickering TG, Alderman MH, Chien S, Borer JS, Laragh JH. Left ventricular hypertrophy in hypertension: prevalence and relationship to pathophysiologic variables. *Hypertension* 1987; **9**(2 Pt 2): II53–II60.

23. Garg R, Yusuf S. Overview of randomized trials of angiotensin-converting enzyme inhibitors on mortality and morbidity in patients with heart failure; Collaborative Group on ACE Inhibitor Trials. *JAMA* 1995; **273**(18): 1450–6.

24. Flather MD, Yusuf S, Kober L, Pfeffer M, Hall A, Murray G, Torp-Pedersen C, Ball S, Pogue J, Moye L, Braunwald E. Long-term ACE-inhibitor therapy in patients with heart failure or left-ventricular dysfunction: a systematic overview of data from individual patients; ACE-Inhibitor Myocardial Infarction Collaborative Group. *Lancet* 2000; **355**(9215): 1575–81.

25. The Cardiac Insufficiency Bisoprolol Study II (CIBIS-II): a randomised trial. *Lancet* 1999; **353**: 9–13.

26. Simon T, Mary-Krause M, Funck-Brentano C, Jaillon P. Sex differences in the prognosis of congestive heart failure: results from the Cardiac Insufficiency Bisoprolol Study (CIBIS II). *Circulation* 2001; **103**(3): 375–80.

27. Packer M, Fowler MB, Roecker EB, Coats AJ, Katus HA, Krum H, Mohacsi P, Rouleau JL, Tendera M, Staiger C, Holcslaw TL, Amann-Zalan I, DeMets DL; Carvedilol Prospective Randomized Cumulative Survival (COPERNICUS) Study Group. Effect of carvedilol on the morbidity of patients with severe chronic heart failure: results of the Carvedilol Prospective Randomized Cumulative Survival (COPERNICUS) study. *Circulation* 2002; **106**: 2194–9.

28. Cohn JN, Archibald DG, Ziesche S, Franciosa JA, Harston WE, Tristani FE, Dunkman WB, Jacobs W, Francis GS, Flohr KH, *et al.* Effect of vasodilator therapy on mortality in chronic congestive heart failure: results of a Veterans Administration Cooperative Study. *N Engl J Med* 1986; **314**: 1547–52.

29. Cohn JN, Johnson G, Ziesche S, Cobb F, Francis G, Tristani F, Smith R, Dunkman WB, Loeb H, Wong M, *et al.* A comparison of enalapril with hydralazine–isosorbide dinitrate in the treatment of chronic congestive heart failure. *N Engl J Med* 1991; **325**: 303–10.

30. Cohn JN, Tognoni G. A randomized trial of the angiotensin-receptor blocker valsartan in chronic heart failure. *N Engl J Med* 2001; **345**(23): 1667–75.

31. Pfeffer MA, Swedberg K, Granger CB, Held P, McMurray JJ, Michelson EL, Olofsson B, Ostergren J, Yusuf S, Pocock S; CHARM Investigators and Committees. Effects of candesartan on mortality and morbidity in patients with chronic heart failure: the CHARM-Overall programme. *Lancet* 2003; **362**(9386): 759–66.

32. McMurray J, Ostergren J, Pfeffer M, Swedberg K, Granger C, Yusuf S, Held P, Michelson E, Olofsson B; CHARM Committees and Investigators. Clinical features and contemporary management of patients with low and preserved ejection fraction heart failure: baseline characteristics of patients in the Candesartan in Heart Failure-Assessment of Reduction in Mortality and Morbidity (CHARM) programme. *Eur J Heart Fail* 2003; **5**: 261–70.

33. McMurray JJ, Ostergren J, Swedberg K, Granger CB, Held P, Michelson EL, Olofsson B, Yusuf S, Pfeffer MA; CHARM Investigators and Committees. Effects of candesartan in patients with chronic heart failure and reduced left-ventricular systolic function taking angiotensin-converting-enzyme inhibitors: the CHARM-Added trial. *Lancet* 2003; **362**(9386): 767–71.

34. Pitt B, Williams G, Remme W, Martinez F, Lopez-Sendon J, Zannad F, Neaton J, Roniker B, Hurley S, Burns D, Bittman R, Kleiman J. The EPHESUS trial: eplerenone in patients with heart failure due to systolic dysfunction complicating acute myocardial infarction; Eplerenone Post-AMI Heart Failure Efficacy and Survival Study. *Cardiovasc Drugs Ther* 2001; **15**(1): 79–87.

The following article is reproduced with kind permission of the *Journal of the American College of Cardiology*

A better survival for women with heart failure? It's not so simple...

PIÑA IL. *J Am Coll Cardiol* 2003; **42**(12): 2135–8

The value of experience is not in seeing much, but in seeing wisely—William Osler |**1**|

Good news! The incidence of heart failure in women has dropped by one-third from the 1950s through the 1990s although it has remained unchanged in men over the same time period |**2**|. This decline may be due in part to the availability of anti-hypertensive medications and the increased recognition among physicians of elevated blood pressure levels, given that hypertension predominates in women as a risk factor for heart failure. Another possible explanation is the decrease in the incidence of rheumatic heart disease after the 1970s in the US, which had affected more women than men |**3–5**|.

More good news! The 30-day mortality rate among women dropped from 18% in the 1950 to 1969 decades to 11% in 1990 to 1999. Moreover, the 1- and 5-year mortality in women also declined in the years 1950 to 1999 from 28% to 24% and from 57% to 45%, respectively |**2**|. Therefore, women have an overall better survival than men with heart failure.

However, that is where the good news ends. In women diagnosed with heart failure in the Framingham cohort from 1990 to 1999, approximately 50% had died by 5 years despite an improvement in survival rates from 1950 to 1999 |**2**|. These improvements in survival rates are undoubtedly due to the advances made in heart failure therapy over the last 30 years.

Heart failure presentation in women

Information about heart failure in women can be acquired from registries, from large group data (insurers/health plans), from statistical data of large organizations, or from clinical trials such as the Beta Blocker Evaluation of Survival Trial (BEST) about which Ghali *et al.* |**6**| report in this same issue of *J Am Coll Cardiol*. If we were only to review clinical trials, however, the number of women would appear to barely reach one-third of all heart failure patients |**7–23**| (Table 1). Yet in registries, health plans, and national statistics, such as the American Heart Association Statistics, the number of women with heart failure approaches one-half of all diagnosed patients |**24**|. Rather than speculate on the reasons for the under-representation of women in trials, there is a lot to be learned from these same clinical trials.

Discrepancies between the presentation of men and women with heart failure are worth noting |25|. Women with heart failure present at an older age and have a lower prevalence of ischaemic heart disease and previous MI than men and are more likely to have systemic hypertension |26|. When controlling for ischaemic disease, women are less likely to have undergone coronary bypass surgery. When suffering an MI, women are more likely than men to develop heart failure |26,27|. More women than men with heart failure also have diabetes as an additional comorbidity |28|. In addition, diabetic women have two to four times the cardiovascular mortality than women without diabetes |24|.

On presentation, women with heart failure are more symptomatic than men with a greater degree of oedema, a third heart sound, murmurs, and more noticeable jugular venous distension |29|. In addition, health-related quality of life is low in women who are admitted with heart failure when compared with men and has a smaller improvement over the hospitalization |30|. When controlling for New York Heart Association functional class, women have a greater impairment in daily living activities, which usually require low level effort and, therefore, are less functional than men |31|.

In the US, hospitalization rates for heart failure have increased from 377 000 in 1979 to 962 000 in 1999 |24|. When hospitalized for heart failure, women have a longer length of stay, leading to higher costs, less involvement by cardiology specialists,

Table 1 Women in heart failure trials

Study	Number of patients	Number of Women in	Percentage of women in
V-HeFT-I |7|	0	0	0
V-HeFT-II |8|	0	0	0
CONSENSUS-I |9|	253	75	30
SOLVD-T |10|	2569	504	23
SOLVD-P |11|	4228	476	31
ELITE-I |12|	722	240	31
ELITE-II |13|	3152	966	30
MERIT-HF |14|	3991	451	23
CIBIS II |15|	2647	515	20
COPERNICUS |16|	2287	465	28
Val HEFT |17|	5010	1002	20
RALES |18|	1663	446	27
SAVE |19|	2231	390	28
TRACE |20|	1749	501	22
CHARM |21|	7599	243	32
SCD HeFT |22|	2521	580	23
DIG |23|	6800	1520	22.4
TOTAL	**47 422**	**10 907**	**23**

and a higher inpatient mortality |**32**|. In the Studies of Left Ventricular Dysfunction (SOLVD) trials, female gender was one of the factors associated with hospitalization for heart failure and 1-year mortality |**28,33**|.

Heart failure therapy in women

Given the discrepancies of presentation, burden of disease, aetiology, and hospitalizations between men and women, it is necessary to assess the benefits of medical therapy and its impact on disease progression and mortality. Although heart failure trials have under-represented women, they do provide important data, in subgroup analysis, which should help clinicians recommend therapy to their female patient population.

Angiotensin-converting enzyme (ACE) inhibitors

Preliminary analysis of the SOLVD data suggested that women had a lesser benefit from the ACE inhibitor, enalapril, than the men in the treatment arm of the trial |**34**|. A recent meta-analysis of ACE inhibitors in both treatment and prevention trials reported that women did benefit from ACE inhibition in treatment trials, although the benefits were attenuated |**35**|. However, a significant mortality benefit from ACE inhibitors in prevention trials was not noted for women. The differences, however, did not reach statistical significance and may be attributable to the small number of women in the trials. Although ACE inhibitors should be the standard of care for heart failure patients, fewer women may be receiving these agents in practice. In the Metoprolol Extended-release Randomized Intervention Trial in Heart Failure (MERIT-HF), fewer women were receiving an ACE inhibitor at entry in the trial than their male counterparts (MERIT-HF women). This difference was not observed in the BEST trial |**36**|.

β blockers

β blockers have become important therapeutic agents in patients with heart failure who are on ACE inhibitors. Although the number of women in the large β blocker trials with carvedilol or metoprolol succcinate (extended release) has been limited, the benefits have been definitive in mortality reduction and equal for both men and women |**36,37**|.

Digoxin

In the Digitalis Investigation Group trials, digoxin failed to show an improvement in overall survival but did result in a reduction in hospitalization rates when compared with placebo |**23**|. However, a recent *post hoc* analysis of the data showed that women may have an increased risk of death with digoxin and a smaller improvement in hospitalization rate |**38**|. This difference could be due to a smaller body mass in women and, therefore, a higher comparable blood level of digoxin |**39**|.

The BEST trial

Ghali *et al.* |6| describe the female cohort in the BEST trial. Features of the women in BEST are consistent with those of other reports, such as a higher EF, lower prevalence of atrial fibrillation, and a lower presence of ischaemic disease. As in the parent trial, the women in the bucindolol group did not have an improvement in survival when compared with placebo. The crude mortality in women was overall lower when compared with the men. Nonetheless, those women with ischaemic disease did not enjoy the same survival benefits over men as those with non-ischaemic disease. The investigators should be congratulated in going beyond the simple mortality rates and examining in more detail the women with ischaemic disease. Taken separately, women with an ischaemic aetiology for heart failure had a different course, with a 2.5-fold increase in the risk of death compared with a 1.5-fold increase in men. Ghali *et al.* |6| offer various hypotheses for this mortality difference. The answer is not clear but should stimulate more research into gender differences in heart failure. Adams *et al.* |40| had already reported that the mortality was similar for men and women when heart failure was due to ischaemic disease and that the mortality benefit for women was only in the dilated cardiomyopathy group. Their data, however, were derived from a heart failure clinic experience where selection bias due to referrals could exist. The current findings in the BEST trial confirm the observations of Adams *et al.* |40| in a larger number of women enrolled in a multicentre, randomized, double-blind trial.

What does the future hold?

With the continuing increase in the prevalence of obesity |41|, the already high prevalence of smoking among women, the prevalence of hypertension in women, and an ever-increasing number of diabetics in the US (33% increase in men and women from 1990 to 1998) |24|, the number of women with ischaemic disease will only continue to grow. Today, cardiovascular disease claims the lives of more women than men, and the gap is widening even further (Fig. 1). Clinicians cannot afford to be less aggressive in prescribing medical therapy to their women patients with heart failure when compared with men. Furthermore, we can no longer be complacent in attempting to stem the tide by using measures of prevention, although efforts in this arena have been traditionally focused on men. These primary prevention measures need to be implemented in women as well. Extensive national campaigns, for example, the American Heart Association 'Women's Heart Day', need to be supported by local communities. Other such measures could include the dissemination of the Seventh Report of the Joint National Committee on Prevention, Detection, Evaluation, and Treatment of High Blood Pressure |42| to the female lay public, programmes that address weight reduction coupled with information on exercise and targeting of these programmes to women groups, and community-based smoking cessation programmes, among others. The advocates for dissemination of breast cancer awareness have been highly successful in spreading their message. Should we not do the same?

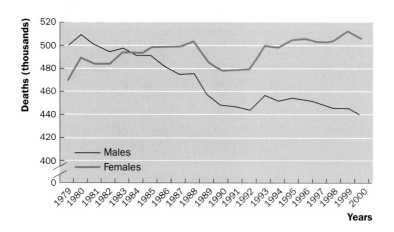

Fig. 1 Cardiovascular disease mortality trends for males and females, United States 1979–2000.

References

1. Osler W. Army surgeon. Philadelphia, 1894.
2. Levy D, Kenchaiah S, Larson MG, Benjamin EJ, Kupka MJ, Ho KK, Murabito JM, Vasan RS. Long-term trends in the incidence of and survival with heart failure. *N Engl J Med* 2002; **347**: 1397–402.
3. Kannel WB. Epidemiological aspects of heart failure. *Cardiol Clin* 1989; 7: 1–9.
4. Schaffer WL, Galloway JM, Roman MJ, Palmieri V, Liu JE, Lee ET, Best LG, Fabsitz RR, Howard BV, Devereux RB. Prevalence and correlates of rheumatic heart disease in American Indians (the Strong Heart Study). *Am J Cardiol* 2003; **91**: 1379–82.
5. Soler-Soler J, Galve E. Worldwide perspective of valve disease. *Heart* 2000; **83**: 721–5.
6. Ghali JK, Krause-Steinrauf HJ, Adams KF Jr, Khan SS, Rosenberg YD, Yancy CW, Young JB, Goldman S, Peberdy MA, Lindenfeld J. Gender differences in advanced heart failure: insights from the BEST study. *J Am Coll Cardiol* 2003; **42**: 2128–34.
7. Cohn JN, Archibald DG, Ziesche S, Franciosa JA, Harston WE, Tristani FE, Dunkman WB, Jacobs W, Francis GS, Flohr KH, *et al*. Effect of vasodilator therapy on mortality in chronic congestive heart failure: results of a Veterans Administration Cooperative Study. *N Engl J Med* 1986; **314**: 1547–52.

8. Cohn JN, Johnson G, Ziesche S, Cobb F, Francis G, Tristani F, Smith R, Dunkman WB, Loeb H, Wong M, *et al.* A comparison of enalapril with hydralazine–isosorbide dinitrate in the treatment of chronic congestive heart failure. *N Engl J Med* 1991; **325**: 303–10.

9. The CONSENSUS Trial Study Group. Effects of enalapril on mortality in severe congestive heart failure. Results of the Cooperative North Scandinavian Enalapril Survival Study (CONSENSUS). *N Engl J Med* 1987; **316**: 1429–35.

10. The SOLVD Investigators. Effect of enalapril on survival in patients with reduced left ventricular ejection fractions and congestive heart failure. *N Engl J Med* 1991; **325**: 293–302.

11. The SOLVD Investigators. Effect of enalapril on mortality and the development of heart failure in asymptomatic patients with reduced left ventricular ejection fractions. *N Engl J Med* 1992; **327**: 685–91.

12. Pitt B, Segal R, Martinez FA, Meurers G, Cowley AJ, Thomas I, Deedwania PC, Ney DE, Snavely DB, Chang PI. Randomised trial of losartan versus captopril in patients over 65 with heart failure (Evaluation of Losartan in the Elderly Study, ELITE). *Lancet* 1997; **349**: 747–52.

13. Pitt B, Poole-Wilson PA, Segal R, Martinez FA, Dickstein K, Camm AJ, Konstam MA, Riegger G, Klinger GH, Neaton J, Sharma D, Thiyagarajan B. Effect of losartan compared with captopril on mortality in patients with symptomatic heart failure: randomised trial—the Losartan Heart Failure Survival Study ELITE II. *Lancet* 2000; **355**: 1582–7.

14. Hjalmarson A, Goldstein S, Fagerberg B, Wedel H, Waagstein F, Kjekshus J, Wikstrand J, El Allaf D, Vitovec J, Aldershvile J, Halinen M, Dietz R, Neuhaus KL, Janosi A, Thorgeirsson G, Dunselman PH, Gullestad L, Kuch J, Herlitz J, Rickenbacher P, Ball S, Gottlieb S, Deedwania P. Effects of controlled-release metoprolol on total mortality, hospitalizations, and well-being in patients with heart failure: the Metoprolol CR/XL Randomized Intervention Trial in congestive heart failure (MERIT-HF). MERIT-HF Study Group. *JAMA* 2000; **283**: 1295–302.

15. The Cardiac Insufficiency Bisoprolol Study II (CIBIS-II): a randomised trial. *Lancet* 1999; **353**: 9–13.

16. Packer M, Fowler MB, Roecker EB, Coats AJ, Katus HA, Krum H, Mohacsi P, Rouleau JL, Tendera M, Staiger C, Holcslaw TL, Amann-Zalan I, DeMets DL; Carvedilol Prospective Randomized Cumulative Survival (COPERNICUS) Study Group. Effect of carvedilol on the morbidity of patients with severe chronic heart failure: results of the Carvedilol Prospective Randomized Cumulative Survival (COPERNICUS) study. *Circulation* 2002; **106**: 2194–9.

17. Cohn JN, Tognoni G; Valsartan Heart Failure Trial Investigators. A randomized trial of the angiotensin-receptor blocker valsartan in chronic heart failure. *N Engl J Med* 2001; **345**: 1667–75.

18. Pitt B, Zannad F, Remme WF, Cody R, Castaigne A, Perez A, Palensky J, Wittes J. The effect of spironolactone on morbidity and mortality in patients with severe heart failure. Randomized Aldactone Evaluation Study Investigators. *N Engl J Med* 1999; **341**: 709–17.

19. Pfeffer MA, Braunwald E, Moye LA, Basta L, Brown EJ Jr, Cuddy TE, Davis BR, Geltman EM, Goldman S, Flaker GC, *et al*; the SAVE investigators. Effect of captopril on mortality and morbidity in patients with left ventricular dysfunction after myocardial infarction; results of the Survival And Ventricular Enlargement trial. *N Engl J Med* 1992; **327**: 669–77.

20. The TRACE Study Group. The Trandolapril Cardiac Evaluation (TRACE) study: rationale, design, and baseline characteristics of the screened population. *Am J Cardiol* 1994; **73**: 44C–50C.

21. McMurray J, Ostergren J, Pfeffer M, Swedberg K, Granger C, Yusuf S, Held P, Michelson E, Olofsson B; CHARM Committees and Investigators. Clinical features and contemporary management of patients with low and preserved ejection fraction heart failure: baseline characteristics of patients in the Candesartan in Heart Failure-Assessment of Reduction in Mortality and Morbidity (CHARM) programme. *Eur J Heart Fail* 2003; **5**: 261–70.

22. Klein H, Auricchio A, Reek S, Geller C. New primary prevention trials of sudden cardiac death in patients with left ventricular dysfunction: SCD-HeFT and MADIT-II. *Am J Cardiol* 1999; **83**: 91D–7D.

23. The Digitalis Investigation Group. The effect of digoxin on mortality and morbidity in patients with heart failure. *N Engl J Med* 1997; **336**: 525–33.

24. American Heart Association. *Heart Disease and Stroke Statistics—2003*. Dallas: American Heart Association, 2002.

25. Petrie MC, Dawson NF, Murdoch DR, Davie AP, McMurray JJ. Failure of women's hearts. *Circulation* 1999; **99**: 2334–41.

26. Tofler GH, Stone PH, Muller JE, Willich SN, Davis VG, Poole WK, Strauss HW, Willerson JT, Jaffe AS, Robertson T, *et al.* Effects of gender and race on prognosis after myocardial infarction: adverse prognosis for women, particularly black women. *J Am Coll Cardiol* 1987; **9**: 473–82.

27. Kimmelstiel C, Goldberg RJ. Congestive heart failure in women: focus on heart failure due to coronary artery disease and diabetes. *Cardiology* 1990; 77(Suppl 2): 71–9.

28. Bangdiwala SI, Weiner DH, Bourassa MG, Friesinger GC, Ghali JK, Yusuf S. Studies of Left Ventricular Dysfunction (SOLVD) registry: rationale, design, methods and description of baseline characteristics. *Am J Cardiol* 1992; **70**: 347–53.

29. Johnstone D, Limacher M, Rousseau M, Liang CS, Ekelund L, Herman M, Stewart D, Guillotte M, Bjerken G, Gaasch W, *et al.* Clinical characteristics of patients in Studies of Left Ventricular Dysfunction (SOLVD). *Am J Cardiol* 1992; **70**: 894–900.

30. Chin MH, Goldman L. Gender differences in 1-year survival and quality of life among patients admitted with congestive heart failure. *Med Care* 1998; **36**: 1033–46.

31. Riedinger MS, Dracup KA, Brecht ML, Padilla G, Sarna L, Ganz PA. Quality of life in patients with heart failure: do gender differences exist? *Heart Lung* 2001; **30**: 105–16.

32. Philbin EF, Disalvo TG. Influence of race and gender on care process, resource use, and hospital-based outcomes in congestive heart failure. *Am J Cardiol* 1998; **82**: 76–81.

33. Bourassa MG, Gurne O, Bangdiwala SI, Ghali JK, Young JB, Rousseau M, Johnstone DE, Yusuf S. Natural history and patterns of current practice in heart failure. The Studies of Left Ventricular Dysfunction (SOLVD) Investigators. *Am J Cardiol* 1993; **22**(4 Suppl A): 14A–19A.

34. Limacher MC, Yusuf S. Gender differences in presentation, morbidity and mortality in the Studies of Left Ventricular Dysfunction (SOLVD): a preliminary report. In: Wenger NK, Speroff L, Packard B (eds). *Cardiovascular Health and Disease in Women*. Greenwich, CT: Le Jacq Communications, 1993; pp 345–8.

35. Shekelle PG, Rich MW, Morton SC, Atkinson CS, Tu W, Maglione M, Rhodes S, Barrett M, Fonarow GC, Greenberg B, Heidenreich PA, Knabel T, Konstam MA, Steimle A, Warner Stevenson L: Efficacy of angiotensin-converting enzyme inhibitors and beta-blockers in the management of left ventricular systolic dysfunction according to race, gender, and diabetic status: a meta-analysis of major clinical trials. *J Am Coll Cardiol* 2003; **41**: 1529–38.

36. Ghali JK, Piña IL, Gottlieb SS, Deedwania PC, Wikstrand JC; MERIT-HF Study Group. Metoprolol CR/XL in female patients with heart failure: analysis of the experience in Metoprolol Extended-release Randomized Intervention Trial in Heart Failure (MERIT-HF). *Circulation* 2002; **105**: 1585–91.

37. Packer M, Bristow MR, Cohn JN, Colucci WS, Fowler MB, Gilbert EM, Shusterman NH. The effect of carvedilol on morbidity and mortality in patients with chronic heart failure. US Carvedilol Heart Failure Study Group. *N Engl J Med* 1996; **334**: 1349–55.

38. Rathore SS, Wang Y, Krumholz HM. Sex-based differences in the effect of digoxin for the treatment of heart failure. *N Engl J Med* 2002; **347**: 1403–11.

39. Eichhorn EJ, Cheorghiade M. Digozin—new perspective on an old drug. *N Engl J Med* 2002; **347**: 1394–5.

40. Adams KF Jr, Dunlap SH, Sueta CA, Clarke SW, Patterson JH, Blauwet MB, Jensen LR, Tomasko L, Koch G. Relation between gender, etiology and survival in patients with symptomatic heart failure. *J Am Coll Cardiol* 1996; **28**: 1781–8.

41. Steinberger J, Daniels SR. Obesity, insulin resistance, diabetes, and cardiovascular risk in children: an American Heart Association scientific statement from the Atherosclerosis, Hypertension, and Obesity in the Young Committee (Council on Cardiovascular Disease in the Young) and the Diabetes Committee (Council on Nutrition, Physical Activity, and Metabolism). *Circulation* 2003; **107**: 1448–53.

42. Chobanian AV, Bakris GL, Black HR, Cushman WC, Green LA, Izzo JL Jr, Jones DW, Materson BJ, Oparil S, Wright JT Jr, Roccella EJ; National Heart, Lung, and Blood Institute Joint National Committee on Prevention, Detection, Evaluation, and Treatment of High Blood Pressure; National High Blood Pressure Education Program Coordinating Committee. The Seventh Report of the Joint National Committee on Prevention, Detection, Evaluation, and Treatment of High Blood Pressure: the JNC 7 report. *JAMA* 2003; **289**: 2560–72.

The following article is reproduced with kind permission of the Journal of Thoracic and Cardiovascular Surgery

Is it important to examine gender differences in the epidemiology and outcome of severe heart failure?

JESSUP M, PIÑA IL. *J Thorac Cardiovasc Surg* 2004; **127**(5): 1247–52

Introduction

Nearly five million Americans have heart failure today, with an incidence approaching ten per 1000 population in persons above 65 years of age; approximately 50% of these cases are in women (see Fig. 1). In 2000, 62.3% of all heart failure mortalities occurred among women; 20% of those died within 1 year of their diagnosis and less than 15% of women survive more than 8–12 years after diagnosis |**1**|. These results notwithstanding, the Framingham study recently noted that the age-adjusted rates of heart failure are higher among men, with no significant change in this rate over a 50-year period |**2**|. Among women, the incidence of heart failure has declined by 31–40% in the decades following 1950.

Heart failure is the reason for at least 20% of all hospital admissions in persons above age 65 and, over the past decade, hospitalizations for heart failure have increased by 159%. Women who have been hospitalized with heart failure have less improvement in physical health status and perceive their quality of care to be lower than their male cohorts |**3**|. Of the thousands of patients disabled from heart failure within 6 years of their diagnosis, 46% are adult women as compared to only 22% of men. In 1997, an estimated $5501 was spent for every hospital-discharge diagnosis of heart failure, and another $1742 per month was required to care for each patient after discharge. Gender has been shown to be an important determinant of hospital length of stay, hospital charges and mortality during hospitalization |**4**|.

The above statistics, and countless other graphs, studies and reports chronicle two very important issues: (1) the syndrome of heart failure has reached epidemic proportions in the United States and throughout the world, and (2) the disease appears to have different characteristics in men and women. It is reasonable to postulate that an elucidation of these sex-specific differences might suggest novel approaches to the prevention of this serious disorder. Moreover, additional insights into gender-specific pathophysiologic mechanisms that lead to heart failure might be used to

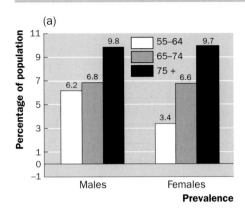

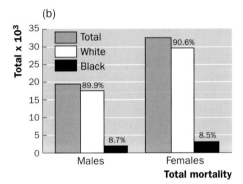

Fig. 1 Prevalence and mortality of heart failure by gender. (a) Prevalence of heart failure in the United States, 1988–1994, by age group and gender. (b) Mortality: 51 546 total deaths, including Hispanics, in 2000; 37.6% of deaths were male and 62.4% were female |5|.

develop unique therapies for this relentlessly lethal disease. This review, then, should be regarded as more than a politically expedient exercise, but as one part of the larger battle to fight the syndrome of heart failure in all its forms. We would also like to acknowledge the newer literature on this subject since the outstanding review of Petrie and colleagues was published in 1999 |6|.

Epidemiology

Elderly patients in the United States represent an increasing proportion of patients with heart failure. There is the general ageing of the population, a progressive increase in the age of onset of heart failure and improved treatment of other cardiovascular diseases, such as hypertension and MI, to account for these figures |7|. Although the overall prevalence of heart failure is similar in men and women, there is a striking impact of age on the prevalence of the disease. Men have a much higher prevalence of heart failure under the age of 75 years, while women surpass the male prevalence over age 75. Importantly, these elderly, female patients are much more likely to have heart failure with preserved systolic function |**8–11**| or 'diastolic heart failure' than their younger cohorts |**7,12**|.

Over the past 50 years, the incidence of heart failure has declined among women but not among men |**2**|. What could account for this differing gender trend? Treatment of hypertension reduces the incidence of heart failure by about 50% and important advances have occurred in the awareness, treatment, and control of high blood pressure during this time period |**13,14**|. The risk of heart failure imparted by hypertension is greater for women than for men; the population attributable risk effect of hypertension was 59% in women and only 39% in men in an earlier Framingham report |**15**|. Increasing use of antihypertensive medications has led to a decline in the prevalence of high blood pressure and may have affected the incidence of heart failure in women, more so than in men. In men, the greater incidence of heart failure is partly explained by the greater prevalence and incidence of arteriosclerosis and coronary artery disease. Some data also suggest a sex difference in the cardiac response to increased afterload or hypertension, as discussed subsequently.

Ventricular arrhythmias are thought to be secondary to a dispersion of normal conduction through non-homogeneous myocardial tissue, promoting repetitive ventricular rhythms. The rate of sudden cardiac death among persons with heart failure is six to nine times that seen in the general population |**16**|, and is more common in men than women |**17**|. One study suggested that women who present with sudden cardiac death are less likely to have a prior history of heart disease than men, 37% versus 56%. More recent data revealed that women who suffer a cardiac arrest are less likely than men to have ventricular fibrillation as an initial rhythm |**18**|. Albert and colleagues prospectively followed a cohort of 121 701 women aged 30–55 years at baseline, and identified 244 cases of sudden cardiac death between 1976 and 1998 |**19**|. Although the risk of sudden death increased markedly as the women grew older, the percentage of cardiac deaths that were sudden decreased with age. Most (69%) women who suffered a sudden cardiac death had no history of cardiac disease before their death, but almost all (94%) of the women who died reported at least one coronary risk factor. Smoking, hypertension and diabetes conferred a significantly elevated risk of sudden death, similar to men.

Mortality from heart failure

There has been considerable scrutiny of a possible survival advantage of women once they develop heart failure, in contrast to men. Two large epidemiological studies, Framingham |**20**| and NHANES-1 |**21**|, both reported an improved survival for women, despite a greater average age in the female cohorts. In contrast, the SOLVD investigators noted a worse outlook, with a 1-year mortality rate of 22% in women and a 17% rate in the men of the study |22|. All patients in SOLVD had a formal measurement of LVEF; entry into the large epidemiological studies was on the basis of symptoms without an assessment of LVEF. Thus it is probable that the women followed in the earlier studies had a higher incidence of diastolic heart failure, as compared to SOLVD, and may account for their survival advantage. Data from the Italian Network CHF Registry, where patients were enrolled on the basis of signs and symptoms, reported a similar 1-year mortality in men and women |23|. However, the women of the cohort were significantly older, had a worse functional class, and exhibited a higher heart rate and systolic blood pressure, with more atrial fibrillation but less ventricular tachycardia. In this study also, women were more likely to have preserved left ventricular function than the men.

It appears that the underlying aetiology of heart failure in women, in general, is different than men, and these baseline risk factors, outside the development of heart failure, may have an important impact on prognosis. Diabetes, for example, is a stronger risk factor for heart failure in women than men, especially in younger women |24|. In a Framingham report, increased wall thickness and left ventricular mass were found in women but not in men with diabetes mellitus |25|. Moreover, left ventricular mass and wall thickness increases with worsening glucose intolerance, an effect that is also more striking in women |26|. Thus, if one were to examine a given population of patients with heart failure, the women in the group would more likely be older, have diabetes and hypertension. Age, hypertension and diabetes are powerful determinants of prognosis in other cardiovascular disorders, such as in patients after MI or cardiac surgery, and women frequently do less well because of these additional risk factors. Why is it that women with the same comorbid conditions and heart failure fare better than their male counterparts?

Mortality outcomes become even more muddled as the large, randomized, clinical trials are examined with regard to this issue. As mentioned earlier, women survived less frequently in SOLVD, a study of patients with left ventricular systolic dysfunction |22|. In the FIRST study, involving patients with far-advanced systolic dysfunction and refractory symptoms, only women without ischaemic heart disease had a better prognosis compared to men |27|. However, in two large trials studying patients with systolic dysfunction and symptomatic heart failure, MERIT-HF |28| and CIBIS-II |29|, women had a significantly improved survival even after adjustment for baseline differences, including β blocker treatment and ischaemic aetiology. The mechanisms that determine an enhanced survival for women with heart failure require elucidation.

Pathophysiology

Numerous studies have shown that the clinical manifestations and prognosis in women with ischaemic heart disease differ significantly from those of men. In spite of having preserved left ventricular systolic function more often than men, women have more symptoms of heart failure |30–32|. Mendes and colleagues sought to understand more completely the relationship between sex and left ventricular pressure and volume in patients referred for cardiac catheterization |33|. Women comprised 35% of the 1667 patients undergoing catheterization; they had a higher prevalence of hypertension (41% in women, 31% in men), diabetes (18% in women, 12% in men) and heart failure (13% in women, 10% in men). At the time of the procedure, women had a higher LVEF, 61% compared to the men's 56%, but had less three vessel coronary disease. In a multivariate analysis, female sex remained an independent predictor of heart failure. Left ventricular end-diastolic volume index was smaller in women despite similar left ventricular end-diastolic pressure. When patients were stratified according to left ventricular end-diastolic pressure, women had a significantly smaller end-diastolic volume. The authors suggested that the response of the left ventricle to the pressure-overload state, such as seen in hypertension, might be modified by sex. The pressure–volume relationship noted in the study by Mendes *et al.* accounts for the diastolic abnormalities seen so often in women with heart failure, and explains the degree of symptoms despite a preserved LVEF.

Other pathophysiologic differences exist in patients with heart failure that appear to be sex determined. Aronson *et al.* examined heart rate variability in patients with non-ischaemic heart failure and found that women have attenuated sympathetic activation and an attenuated parasympathetic withdrawal |34|. Current understanding about the critical role of the sympathetic nervous system in the progression of heart failure suggests that the above findings might be advantageous. Likewise, investigators have shown that myocyte necrosis and apoptosis are significantly reduced in women with heart failure, despite a longer duration of disease compared to the men in the study populations |35|. There is also considerable data to conclude that gender and sex hormones affect the components of the renin–angiotensin system by a number of mechanisms |36|.

Fig. 2 depicts a possible schema of the pathophysiologic response to a myocardial injury in men and women, derived in part from the above and other studies. The clinical observation that women present with symptoms of heart failure later in life, with more concentric left ventricular hypertrophy, might be explained by a gender-specific tendency that confers an improved survival in many instances. Recent reports suggest that the gender response to post-infarction injury favours women in that they develop less hypertrophy, a pattern quite different than that observed in non-ischaemic cardiomyopathy |37|.

Management of heart failure

Our ability to discern whether women respond to pharmacotherapy for heart failure in a meaningfully dissimilar manner from men has been impaired by the failure to enrol adequate numbers of women into many of the heart failure trials, as shown in Table 1 |38|. To be fair, this low enrolment rate is probably due, in part, to a greater proportion of diastolic heart failure in women, making them ineligible for the trials outlined in Table 1 |39|.

Gender-related survival rates

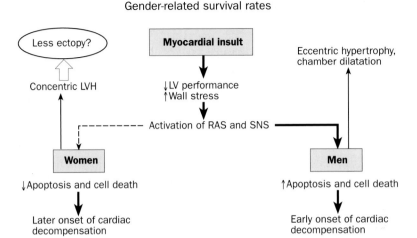

Possible pathophysiologic mechanisms

Fig. 2 Gender-related survival rates and how they may be influenced by different pathophysiologic mechanisms in men and women. LV, left ventricle; LVH, left ventricular hypertrophy; RAS, renin–angiotensin system; SNS, sympathetic nervous system.

Women may receive less optimal care for a variety of reasons. Harjai *et al.* showed that, even after adjusting for age, race, coronary artery disease and LVEF, there was a higher utilization of combination therapy by cardiologists in male versus female patients |40|. Improvements in peak exercise capacity may be more pronounced in men than in women with heart failure after exercise training, and yet women are referred less often to cardiac rehabilitation |41|. In addition, the skeletal muscle abnormalities described in the legs of male patients with heart failure are not as pronounced in women |42|. Women suffered more side effects in the SOLVD trial |43|. Most important, however, is the lack of definitive, randomized trials in patients with diastolic heart failure, a group of patients who are predominantly women |44|. Some of the differences between men and women at baseline when enrolled in clinical trials are shown in Table 1. Note the greater degree of hypertension and diabetes in women |22,27–29,45,46|.

In summary, there is mounting evidence that there are important sex differences in the phenotype of heart failure as we understand it currently. Women appear to have an overall improved outlook once they become symptomatic with heart failure. The mechanisms behind this advantage are worthy of further exploration.

Table 1 Differences in heart failure: women to men compared

	SOLVD[22,45]	FIRST[27]	MERIT[28]	CIBIS-II[29]	Heart failure clinic[46]
N (% women)	6271 (26)	471 (24)	898 (22.5)	2647 (19)	557 (32%)
Age	Older	Older	Older	Older	Younger
Ischaemia	Less	Less	Less	Less	Less
EF	Same	Same	Same	Same	Higher
Diabetes	More	Same	More	More	More
Hypertension	More	More	More	More	More
HR	Higher	Higher	Higher	Same	–
Race	?AA	?AA	–	–	?AA
Mortality	Higher	Lower in IDC	Lower	Lower in non-IDC	Lower in non-IDC

References

1. American Heart Association. *2001 Heart and Stroke Statistical Update*. Dallas: American Heart Association, 2000.

2. Levy D, Kenchaiah S, Larson MG, Benjamin EJ, Kupka MJ, Ho KK, Murabito JM, Vasan RS. Long-term trends in the incidence of and survival with heart failure [comment]. *N Engl J Med* 2002; **347**: 1397–402.

3. Chin MH, Goldman L. Gender differences in 1-year survival and quality of life among patients admitted with congestive heart failure. *Medical Care* 1998; **36**: 1033–46.

4. Philbin EF, DiSalvo TG. Influence of race and gender on care process, resource use, and outcomes in congestive heart failure. *Am J Cardiol* 1998; **82**: 76–81.

5. American Heart Association. *Heart Disease and Stroke Statistics—2003*. Dallas; American Heart Association, 2002.

6. Petrie MC, Dawson NF, Murdoch DR, Davie AP, McMurray JJV. Failure of women's hearts. *Circulation* 1999; **99**: 2334–41.

7. Gottdiener JS, Arnold AM, Aurigemma GP, Polak JF, Tracy RP, Kitzman DW, Gardin JM, Rutledge JE, Boineau RC. Predictors of congestive heart failure in the elderly: the Cardio-vascular Health Study. *J Am Coll Cardiol* 2000; **35**: 1628–37.

8. Redfield MM, Jacobsen SJ, Burnett JC Jr, Mahoney DW, Bailey KR, Rodeheffer RJ. Burden of systolic and diastolic ventricular dysfunction in the community: appreciating the scope of the heart failure epidemic. *JAMA* 2003; **289**: 194–202.

9. Vasan R, Levy D. Defining diastolic heart failure. A call for standardized diagnostic criteria. *Circulation* 2000; **101**: 2118–21.

10. Zile MR, Brutsaert DL. New concepts in diastolic dysfunction and diastolic heart failure: part II: causal mechanisms and treatment. *Circulation* 2002; **105**: 1503–8.

11. Zile MR, Brutsaert DL. New concepts in diastolic dysfunction and diastolic heart failure: part I: diagnosis, prognosis, and measurements of diastolic function. *Circulation* 2002; **105**: 1387–93.

12. Masoudi FA, Havranek EP, Smith G, Fish RH, Steiner JF, Ordin DL, Krumholz HM. Gender, age, and heart failure with preserved left ventricular systolic function [comment]. *J Am Coll Cardiol* 2003; **41**: 217–23.

13. Dahlof B, Lindholm LH, Hansson L, Schersten B, Ekbom T, Wester PO. Morbidity and mortality in the Swedish Trial in Old Patients with Hypertension (STOP-Hypertension) [comment]. *Lancet* 1991; **338**: 1281–5.

14. SHEP Cooperative Research Group. Prevention of stroke by antihypertensive drug treatment in older persons with isolated systolic hypertension. Final results of the Systolic Hypertension in the Elderly Program (SHEP). *JAMA* 1991; **265**: 3255–64.

15. Levy D, Larson MG, Vasan RS, Kannel WB, Ho KKL. The progression from hypertension to heart failure. *J Am Coll Cardiol* 1996; **275**: 1557–62.

16. Stevenson WG, Stevenson LW. Prevention of sudden death in heart failure. *J Cardiovasc Electrophysiol* 2001; **12**: 112–14.

17. Kannel WB, Wilson PW, D'Agostino RB, Cobb J. Sudden coronary death in women. *Am Heart J* 1998; **136**: 205–12.

18. Kim C, Fahrenbruch CE, Cobb LA, Eisenberg MS. Out-of-hospital cardiac arrest in men and women. *Circulation* 2001; **104**: 2699–703.

19. Albert CM, Chae CU, Grodstein F, Rose LM, Rexrode KM, Ruskin JN, Stampfer MJ, Manson JE. Prospective study of sudden cardiac death among women in the United States [comment]. *Circulation* 2003; **107**: 2096–101.

20. Ho K, Anderson K, Kannel W, Grossman W, Levy D. Survival after the onset of congestive heart failure in Framingham Heart Study subjects. *Circulation* 1993; **88**: 107–15.

21. Schocken DD, Arrieta MI, Leaverton PE, Ross EA. Prevalence and mortality rate of congestive heart failure in the United States. *J Am Coll Cardiol* 1992; **20**: 301–6.

22. Bourassa MG, Gurne O, Bangdiwala SI, Ghali JK, Young JB, Rousseau, M, Johnstone DE, Yusuf S. Natural history and patterns of current practice in heart failure. The Studies of Left Ventricular Dysfunction (SOLVD) Investigators. *J Am Coll Cardiol* 1993; **22**: 14A–19A.

23. Opasich C, Tavazzi L, Lucci D, Gorini M, Albanese MC, Cacciatore G, Maggioni AP. Comparison of one-year outcome in women versus men with chronic congestive heart failure. *Am J Cardiol* 2000; **86**: 353–7.

24. Wenger NK. Women, heart failure, and heart failure therapy. *Circulation* 2002; **105**: 1526–8.

25. Galderisi M, Anderson KM, Wilson PWF, Levy D. Echocardiographic evidence for the existence of a distinst diabetic cardiomyopathy (The Framingham Heart Study). *Am J Cardiol* 1991; **68**: 85–9.

26. Rutter MK, Parise H, Benjamin EJ, Levy D, Larson MG, Meigs JB, Nesto RW, Wilson PW, Vasan RS. Impact of glucose intolerance and insulin resistance on cardiac structure and function: sex-related differences in the Framingham Heart Study. *Circulation* 2003; **107**: 448–54.

27. Adams KF Jr, Sueta CA, Gheorghiade M, O'Connor CM, Schwartz TA, Koch GG, Uretsky B, Swedberg K, McKenna W, Soler-Soler J, Califf RM. Gender differences in survival in advanced heart failure. Insights from the FIRST study. *Circulation* 1999; **99**: 1816–21.

28. Ghali JK, Pina IL, Gottlieb SS, Deedwania PC, Wikstrand JC, The M-HFSG. Metoprolol CR/XL in female patients with heart failure: analysis of the experience in Metoprolol Extended-release Randomized Intervention Trial in Heart Failure (MERIT-HF). *Circulation* 2002; **105**: 1585–91.

29. Simon T, Mary-Krause M, Funck-Brentano C, Jaillon P. Sex differences in the prognosis of congestive heart failure: results from the Cardiac Insufficiency Bisoprolol Study (CIBIS II). *Circulation* 2001; **103**: 375–80.

30. Fisher LD, Kennedy JW, Davis KB, Maynard C, Fritz JK, Kaiser G, Myers WO. Association of sex, physical size, and operative mortality after coronary artery bypass in the Coronary Artery Surgery Study (CASS). *J Thorac Cardiovasc Surg* 1982; **84**: 334–41.

31. Kennedy JW, Kaiser GC, Fisher LD, Fritz JK, Myers W, Mudd JG, Ryan TJ. Clinical and angiographic predictors of operative mortality from the collaborative study in coronary artery surgery (CASS). *Circulation* 1981; **63**: 793–802.

32. Jacobs AK, Kelsey SF, Brooks MM, Faxon DP, Chaitman BR, Bittner V, Mock MB, Weiner BH, Dean L, Winston C, Drew L, Sopko G. Better outcome for women compared with men undergoing coronary revascularization: a report from the bypass angioplasty revascularization investigation (BARI) [comment]. *Circulation* 1998; **98**: 1279–85.

33. Mendes LA, Davidoff R, Cupples LA, Ryan TJ, Jacobs AK. Congestive heart failure in patients with coronary artery disease: the gender paradox. *Am Heart J* 1997; **134**: 207–12.

34. Aronson D, Burger AJ. Gender-related differences in modulation of heart rate in patients with congestive heart failure. *J Cardiovasc Electrophysiol* 2000; **11**: 1071–7.

35. Guerra S, Leri A, Wang X, Finato N, Di Loreto C, Beltrami CA, Kajstura J, Anversa P. Myocyte death in the failing human heart is gender dependent [comment]. *Circ Res* 1999; **85**: 856–66.

36. Fischer M, Baessler A, Schunkert H. Renin angiotensin system and gender differences in the cardiovascular system. *Cardiovasc Res* 2002; **53**: 672–7.

37. Crabbe DL, Dipla K, Ambati S, Zafeiridis A, Gaughan JP, Houser SR, Margulies KB. Gender differences in post-infarction hypertrophy in end-stage failing hearts. *J Am Coll Cardiol* 2003; **41**: 300–6.

38. Harris D, Douglas PS. Enrollment of women in cardiovascular clinical trials funded by the National Heart, Lung, and Blood Institute. *N Engl J Med* 2000; **343**: 475–80.

39. Jessup M. The less familiar face of heart failure [comment]. *J Am Coll Cardiol* 2003; **41**: 224–6.

40. Harjai KJ, Nunez E, Stewart Humphrey J, Turgut T, Shah M, Newman J. Does gender bias exist in the medical management of heart failure? *Int J Cardiol* 2000; **75**: 65–9.

41. Keteyian SJ, Duscha BD, Brawner CA, Green HJ, Marks CR, Schachat FH, Annex BH, Kraus WE. Differential effects of exercise training in men and women with chronic heart failure. *Am Heart J* 2003; **145**: 912–18.

42. Duscha BD, Annex BH, Green HJ, Pippen AM, Kraus WE. Deconditioning fails to explain peripheral skeletal muscle alterations in men with chronic heart failure. *J Am Coll Cardiol* 2002; **39**: 1170–4.

43. Kostis JB, Shelton BJ, Yusuf S, Weiss MB, Capone RJ, Pepine CJ, Gosselin G, Delahaye F, Probstfield JL, Cahill L. Tolerability of enalapril initiation by patients with left ventricular dysfunction: results of the medication challenge phase of the Studies of Left Ventricular Dysfunction. *Am Heart J* 1994; **128**: 358–64.

44. Tandon S, Hankins SR, Le Jemtel TH. Clinical profile of chronic heart failure in elderly women [comment]. *Am J Geriatr Cardiol* 2002; **11**: 318–23.

45. Johnstone D, Limacher M, Rousseau M, Liang CS, Ekelund L, Herman M, Stewart D, Guillotte M, Bjerken G, Gaasch W, *et al.* Clinical characteristics of patients in Studies of Left Ventricular Dysfunction (SOLVD). *Am J Cardiol.* 1992; **70**: 894–900.

46. Adams KF Jr, Dunlap SH, Sueta CA, Clarke SW, Patterson JH, Blauwet MB, Jensen LR, Tomasko L, Koch G. Relation between gender, etiology and survival in patients with symptomatic heart failure. *J Am Coll Cardiol* 1996; **28**: 1781–8.

13

Pulmonary hypertension: an increasingly common challenge for clinicians

EUGENIA NATALE, ILEANA PIÑA

Introduction

The pulmonary circulation is one of the determinants of right ventricular afterload, therefore determining its output. Although the right ventricle can accommodate large increases in systemic venous return without a rise in pulmonary artery pressures, acute increases in pulmonary vascular tone can result in right ventricular failure. As therapy for heart failure has improved, the survival of patients with this syndrome has also improved. In addition, given the increased use of defibrillators, the incidence of sudden death will drop and, thus, more patients will develop the haemodynamic consequences of advanced pump failure. One of the manifestations of advanced pump failure is secondary pulmonary hypertension. Furthermore, as ventricular dilatation ensues, mitral regurgitation can increase, due to dilatation of the mitral annulus. This additional retrograde flow adds burden to the already compromised pulmonary circulation.

Pulmonary hypertension can develop insidiously in a patient who has been stable, thereby gradually developing increasing right ventricular failure leading to peripheral oedema and ascites. This type of presentation is often resistant to increases in diuretics and, in an effort to eliminate volume, the patient can become pre-renal and develop azotaemia with increases in creatinine. A careful physical examination will often reveal an elevated pulmonary component of the second heart sound (P2) and concomitant tricuspid regurgitation. This clinical presentation should prompt a review of a previous echocardiogram or provoke a new echocardiogram. Careful Doppler assessment will identify pulmonary hypertension fairly accurately.

In patients being considered for cardiac transplantation, it is important to establish the levels of pulmonary pressures and to make every attempt to lower them, if elevated.

Pulmonary hypertension will detect patients at high risk of adverse outcomes after heart transplantation [1]. Secondary pulmonary hypertension places a newly transplanted heart at risk of acute right ventricular failure. Therefore, in transplant programmes, every effort is made to identify and treat pulmonary hypertension aggressively. Should there prove to be no reversibility, patients can be turned down for transplantation.

Over the past few years there has been an enormous advance in the comprehension of the mechanisms involved in the pathophysiology of end-stage heart failure. In spite of this progress, some issues still need to be resolved. The current evidence suggests that there is no reliable haemodynamic threshold beyond which right ventricular failure is certain to occur, nor are there values below which right ventricular failure is always avoidable. Regarding this issue, there are two important questions to answer about a patient who has chronic heart failure: (a) does a particular patient have pulmonary hypertension? (b) If so, is it reversible or not?

Pathophysiology of pulmonary hypertension in heart failure

The endothelium, probably the body's largest organ, is the core of vasomotor tone. Endothelin, which is one of the most potent vasoconstrictors known, plays an important role in the regulation of vascular tone |**2**|. The endothelin family includes three isopeptides: ET-1, ET-2 and ET-3, and studies have shown that at least two different types of receptor exist: selective (ETa) and non-selective (ETb). ETa has a high affinity for ET-1 and ET-2 and is located on the vascular smooth muscle cells responsible for vasoconstriction. ETb is found primarily on vascular endothelial cells and mediates vasodilatation via the release of nitric oxide and prostacyclin. Studies in both experimental models and patients suggest that nitric oxide-dependent pulmonary vasodilatation is impaired in heart failure |**3,4**|.

Dysfunctional endothelial cells play a critical role in the initiation and progression of pulmonary hypertension. In secondary pulmonary hypertension, local factors such as increased levels of vasoconstrictors (impaired nitric oxide availability and increased endothelin expression) and enhanced shear stress are the triggers in endothelial cell proliferation, leading to the plexiform lesions, which are histologically indistinguishable from those in primary pulmonary hypertension |**5**|. Due to these changes, pulmonary vascular resistance (PVR) is frequently elevated. This elevation may be reversible (dysregulation of vascular smooth muscle tone) or irreversible (structural remodelling) |**6**|.

In patients with rheumatic valvular disease, for example, there is a positive correlation between the pre-operative plasma ET-1 level and pulmonary haemodynamic variables (pulmonary artery pressure, pulmonary capillary wedge pressure and PVR), which strongly implies that ET-1 might be involved in the pathological process of secondary pulmonary hypertension |**7**|. Plasma ET-1 levels predict mortality in chronic heart failure |**8**|. The development of endothelin receptor antagonists (bosentan, sitaxsentan) has provided important information about the role of ET-1 in the pathophysiology of heart failure. ET-1 antagonists improve haemodynamics, ameliorate left ventricular remodelling and improve survival in animal models of heart failure. Unfortunately, the recent trials with endothelin antagonists have not shown reductions in mortality. This may be due to a patient mix of the less ill to those with more advanced disease. A current programme of clinical trials with another endothelin antagonist, tezosentan, is ongoing |**9**|. In patients with chronic heart failure, the renin–angiotensin system activity is greatly activated, with volume overload as a result and elevation of pulmonary pressures. Therapy in these patients using angiotensin-converting enzyme (ACE) inhibitors, β blockers and other vasodilators reduces PVR in the long term. It has also been shown that neurohormonal activation rapidly decreases after short-term therapy tailored to decrease elevated filling pressures and systemic vascular resistance |**10**|.

Diagnosing pulmonary hypertension

Pulmonary hypertension is classically defined as pulmonary artery systolic pressure greater than 30 mmHg or as mean pulmonary artery pressure equal to or greater than 19 mmHg. The first step in evaluating the patient is to establish the existence of pulmonary hypertension. The diagnosis can be defined with a simple, non-invasive and cost-effective study such as Doppler echocardiography |**11**|, but to be more accurate, the diagnosis is usually defined by cardiac catheterization, obtaining the following measurements: pulmonary artery pressures, PVR, transpulmonary gradient. The transpulmonary gradient (pulmonary artery mean pressure–wedge pressure), which is defined as the mean arterial pressure minus the pulmonary capillary wedge pressure, may be a better predictor of outcome than PVR alone, as cardiac output is not needed for its measurement. In addition, a transpulmonary gradient greater than 15 mmHg correlates with 6- and 12-month mortality after orthotopic heart transplantation |**9**|.

Pulmonary hypertension in heart failure patients may reflect structural remodelling of the arterioles (abnormalities of elastic fibres, medial hypertrophy, intimal fibrosis), resulting in vascular stiffness and reduced vasodilator responsiveness. Pulmonary hypertension attributable to these structural changes is referred to as fixed or irreversible as it is not rapidly responsive to reversal with pharmacological manoeuvres. However, in most patients, the major component is likely to reverse with vasodilators, due to the central role played by the endothelium in the control of pulmonary vascular tone. The time elapsed between the onset of the passive increase in pulmonary venous pressure and its correct treatment is critical for these patients (the importance of aggressive therapy of fluid overload) |**12**|.

Multiple agents are available to attempt to prove reversibility. These include: oxygen (100%), nitrates, sodium nitroprusside, adenosine, prostacyclin, inhaled nitric oxide, nesiritide.

Treatment

The standard therapy for heart failure (ACE inhibitors, β blockers and most vaso-dilators) reduces PVR. In patients with elevated pulmonary pressures, the renin–angiotensin system is activated, with consequent sodium and water retention, as angiotensin-II is a potent pulmonary vasoconstrictor. Acute hypoxic pulmonary vasoconstriction is significantly attenuated by lisinopril. This is probably related to the effect of lisinopril in suppressing plasma levels of angiotensin-II |13| and therefore reducing PVR.

Medical therapy in the arena of pulmonary hypertension has been disappointing thus far. For example, the long-term administration of prostacyclin (PGI2/epoprostenol) improves haemodynamic parameters, symptoms and survival in patients with primary pulmonary hypertension, but it increases mortality in patients with heart failure despite haemodynamic benefits |14|. Montalescot *et al.* |15| tried to find an explanation for these negative results and found that, in patients with end-stage heart failure and pulmonary hypertension, PGI2 improved pulmonary haemo-dynamics with a 47% reduction in PVR and a doubling of pulmonary compliance. However, they also found that at therapeutic doses, endothelin exerts a significant positive inotropic effect. This positive inotropic effect may explain the increased mortality rate observed with the long-term use of PGI2 in this type of patient |16|.

Studies of endothelin antagonisits in heart failure have thus far been disappoint-ing, but studies with tezosentan continue in the form of the Randomized Intravenous Tezosentan Study (RITZ) |17|. The acute intravenous |18| and short-term oral |19| administration of bosentan, a non-selective (ETa/ETb) receptor antagonist, caused systemic and pulmonary vasodilatation in patients with severe heart failure. There-fore, it is not recommended in this type of patient |20|. Bosentan is currently used with caution for primary pulmonary hypertension.

Therefore, although the mechanisms of secondary pulmonary hypertension in chronic heart failure implicate endothelin, blocking endothelin receptors has not improved outcomes as could be expected.

References

1. Chen JM, Michler RE. The problem of pulmonary hypertension and the potential recipi-ent. In: Cooper DKC (ed). *The Transplant and Replacement of Thoracic Organs*. Hingham, MA: Kluwer, 1997; pp 177–84.
2. Lerman A, Burnett JC Jr. Intact and altered endothelium in regulation of vasomotion. *Circulation* 1992; **86**(6 Suppl): III12–19.

3. Porter TR, Taylor DO, Cycan A, Fields J, Bagley CW, Pandian NG, Mohanty PK. Endothelium-dependent pulmonary artery responses in chronic heart failure: influence of pulmonary hypertension. *J Am Coll Cardiol* 1993; **22**: 1418–24.

4. Cooper CJ, Jevnikar FW, Walsh T, Dickinson J, Mouhaffel A, Selwyn AP. The influence of basal nitric oxide activity on pulmonary vascular resistance in patients with congestive heart failure. *Am J Cardiol* 1998; **82**: 609–14.

5. Tuder RM, Cool CD, Yeager M, Taraseviciene-Stewart L, Bull TM, Voelkel NF. The pathobiology of pulmonary hypertension. Endothelium. *Clin Chest Med* 2001; **22**(3): 405–18.

6. Moraes DL, Colucci WS, Givert MM. Secondary pulmonary hypertension in chronic heart failure: the role of endothelium in pathophysiology and management. *Circulation* 2000; **102**(14): 1718–23.

7. Zhu ZG, Wang MS, Jiang ZB, Jiang Z, Xu AX, Ren CY, Shi MX. The dynamic change of plasma endothelin-1 during the perioperative period in patients with rheumatic valvular disease and secondary pulmonary hypertension. *J Thorac Cardiovasc Surg* 1994; **108**(5): 960–8.

8. Hulsmann M, Stanek B, Frey B, Sturm B, Putz D, Kos T, Berger R, Woloszczuk W, Putz D, Kos T, Berger R, Woloszczuk W, Maurer G, Pacher R. Value of cardiopulmonary exercise testing and big endothelin plasma levels to predict short-term prognosis of patients with chronic heart failure. *J Am Coll Cardiol* 1998; **32**: 1695–700.

9. Ooi H, Colucci WS, Givertz MM. Endothelin mediates increased pulmonary vascular tone in patients with heart failure: demonstration by direct intrapulmonary infusion of sitaxsentan. *Circulation* 2002; **106**(13): 1618–21.

10. Johnson W, Omland T, Hall C, Lucas C, Myking OL, Collins C, Pfeffer M, Rouleau JL, Stevenson LW. Neurohormonal activation rapidly decreases after intravenous therapy with diuretics and vasodilators for class IV heart failure. *J Am Coll Cardiol* 2002; **39**(10): 1623–9.

11. Abramson SV, Burke JF, Kelly JJ Jr, Kitchen JG 3rd, Dougherty MJ, Yih DF, McGeehin FC 3rd, Shuck JW, Phiambolis TP. Pulmonary hypertension predicts mortality and morbidity in patients with dilated cardiomyopathy. *Ann Intern Med* 1992; **116**: 888–95.

12. Steimle AE, Stevenson LW, Chelimsky-Fallick C, Fonarow GC, Hamilton MA, Moriguchi JD, Kartashov A, Tillisch JH. Sustained hemodynamic efficacy of therapy tailored to reduce filling pressures in survivors with advanced heart failure. *Circulation* 1997; **96**: 1165–72.

13. Cargill RI, Lipworth BJ. Lisinopril attenuates acute hypoxic pulmonary vasoconstriction in humans. *Chest* 1996; **109**: 424–9.

14. Califf RM, Adams KF, McKenna WJ, Gheorghiade M, Uretsky B, McNulty SE, Darius H, Schulman K, Zannad F, Handberg-Thurmond E, Harrell FE, Wheeler W, Soler-Soler J, Swedberg K. A randomized controlled trial of epoprosterenol therapy for severe congestive heart failure: the Flolan International Randomized Survival Trial (FIRST). *Am Heart J* 1997; **134**: 44–54.

15. Montalescot G, Drobinski G, Meurin P, Maclouf J, Sotirov I, Philippe F, Choussat R, Morin E, Thomas D. Effects of prostacyclin on the pulmonary vascular tone and cardiac contractility in patients with pulmonary hypertension secondary to end-stage heart failure. *Am J Cardiol* 1998; **82**(6): 749–55.

16. Kramer BK, Nishida M, Kelly RA, Smith TW. Endothelins: myocardial actions of a new class of cytokines. *Circulation* 1992; **85**: 350–6.

17. O'Connor CM, Gattis WA, Adams KF Jr, Hasselblad V, Chandler B, Frey A, Kobrin I, Rainisio M, Shah MR, Teerlink J, Gheorghiade M, Randomized Intravenous TeZosentan Study-4 Investigators. Tezosentan in patients with acute heart failure and acute coronary syndromes: results of the Randomized Intravenous TeZosentan Study (RITZ-4). *J Am Coll Cardiol* 2003; **41**(9): 1452–7.

18. Kiowski W, Sutsch G, Hunziker P, Muller P, Kim J, Oechslin E, Schmitt R, Jones R, Bertel O. Evidence for endothelin-1-mediated vasoconstriction in severe chronic heart failure. *Lancet* 1995; **346**: 732–6.

19. Sutsch G, Kiowski W, Yan X-W, Hunziker P, Christen S, Strobel W, Kim JH, Rickenbacher P, Bertel O. Short-term oral endothelin-receptor antagonist therapy in conventionally treated patients with symptomatic severe chronic heart failure. *Circulation* 1998; **98**: 2262–8.

20. Kalra PR, Moon JC, Coats AJ. Do results of the ENABLE (Endothelin Antagonist Bosentan for Lowering Cardiac Events in Heart Failure) study spell the end for non-selective endothelin antagonism in heart failure? *Int J Cardiol* 2002; **85**(2–3): 195–7.

Part IV

The future

14

Devices in heart failure: new approaches

MANDEEP MEHRA

Introduction

Therapy targeted towards neurohormonal aberrations in heart failure has served us well. In this regard, the strategy of using angiotensin-converting enzyme (ACE) inhibitors in concert with β-adrenergic blockade has demonstrated clinically important improvements in outcomes for patients with heart failure [1]. As investigators have sought to evaluate other incremental neurohormonal targets in further improving outcomes, it has become evident that a ceiling effect might exist in the serial exploitation of the neurohormonal model [2]. Thus, cytokine antagonism, endothelin receptor blockade and centrally acting sympatholytics (moxonidine) have demonstrated worse outcomes, while vasopeptidase inhibitors (omapatrilat) that enhance circulating natriuretic peptides have shown little additional benefits. Even angiotensin receptor blockers (ARBs) have shown divergent effects in the setting of β-adrenergic blockade, with one trial suggesting adverse outcomes (using valsartan) and another pointing to modest improvement (using candesartan) [3,4]. Only aldosterone antagonists have suggested a glimmer of hope, with a putative effect on sudden death reduction in the setting of post-myocardial infarction heart failure [5] (Fig. 14.1).

This emerging dilemma has led to the proposition that therapeutic targets beyond the neurohormonal model must be entertained if we are to derive ongoing incremental improvements in outcomes in heart failure. These specific strategies include modulation of myocardial metabolic substrate utilization, alleviation of myocardial ischaemia, and relief of arrhythmic burden. Other novel areas of investigation relate to identifying and treating sleep disordered breathing, amelioration of anaemia and renal dysfunction, and resynchronization of contraction as well as the use of other antiremodelling strategies such as mechanical ventricular assistance and passive restraint devices [2].

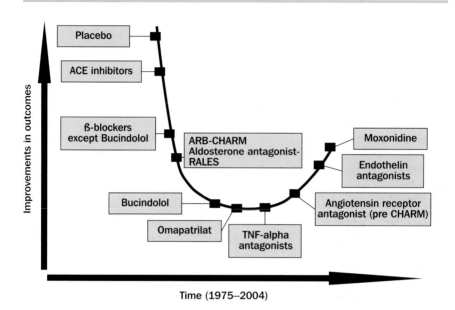

Fig. 14.1 A schema depicting a possible ceiling effect to the incremental targeting of the neurohormonal model. This exemplifies the need to investigate targets beyond the traditional concept of neurohormonal antagonism, thereby making the case for device therapy in the treatment of heart failure. Source: adapted from Mehra *et al.* (2003) |**2**|.

Cardiac resynchronization therapy

The concept of cardiac resynchronization therapy that seeks to harmonize ventricular contractility by decreasing areas of focal asynchrony is widely gaining clinical acceptance. Several recent clinical trials have provided support for the usefulness of cardiac resynchronization therapy using biventricular pacing |**6**|. Recent randomized clinical trials of cardiac resynchronization therapy have suggested that the application of this treatment modality in severe systolic heart failure despite optimal drug therapy yields benefits that result in improved functional capacity, reversal of adverse ventricular remodelling, and decreased hospitalizations. Indeed, a recent meta-analysis of these trials has even suggested decreased deaths from progressive heart failure as a consequence of cardiac resynchronization.

Cardiac resynchronization in chronic heart failure

Abraham WT, Fisher WG, Smith AL, *et al*. MIRACLE Study Group. *N Engl J Med* 2002; **346**(24): 1845–53

BACKGROUND. These investigators conducted a double-blind trial to evaluate cardiac resynchronization therapy in 453 patients with moderate to severe symptoms of heart failure associated with an ejection fraction (EF) of 35% or less and a QRS interval of 130 ms or more. The patients were randomly assigned to a cardiac resynchronization group (228 patients) or to a control group (225 patients) for 6 months, while conventional therapy for heart failure was maintained. As compared with the control group, patients assigned to cardiac resynchronization experienced an improvement in the distance walked in 6 min (+39 vs +10 m; *P* = 0.005), functional class (*P* <0.001), quality of life (–18.0 vs –9.0 points; *P* = 0.001), time on the treadmill during exercise testing (+81 vs +19 s; *P* = 0.001), and EF (+4.6 vs –0.2%; *P* <0.001). In addition, fewer patients in the group assigned to cardiac resynchronization than control patients required hospitalization (8 vs 15%) or intravenous medications (7 vs 15%) for the treatment of heart failure (*P* <0.05 for both comparisons). Implantation of the device was unsuccessful in 8% of patients and was complicated by refractory hypotension, bradycardia, or asystole in four patients (two of whom died) and by perforation of the coronary sinus requiring pericardiocentesis in two others.

INTERPRETATION. Cardiac resynchronization resulted in significant clinical improvement in patients who had moderate to severe heart failure and an intraventricular conduction delay.

Comment

This study was rigorously conducted and was constructed to maintain blinding in the heart failure specialist. One of the difficulties in translating this data to the 'real world' setting lies in the fact that this trial randomized patients only after pacemaker implantation was deemed successful (92% of patients). This study also brought to

Table 14.1 Problems and uncertainties with cardiac resynchronization therapy

QRS width fails to define site and magnitude of ventricular dys-synchrony
Electrical and mechanical dys-synchrony are not consistent, as 'normal' QRS width can also be associated with dys-synchrony
Failure to define the location and magnitude of mechanical dys-synchrony leads to a 'hit or miss' approach with a high non-responder rate
Uncertain if patients with atrial fibrillation benefit from resynchronization therapy
Risk–benefit ratio may be narrow: New York Heart Association class II might be 'too well' for cardiac resynchronization therapy or class IV might be 'too sick'
Unclear when cardiac resynchronization therapy should be performed alone or in conjunction with an implantable cardioverter defibrillator
Technical learning curve, cost and potential morbidity are substantial
Longevity of benefit not completely established

Source: Abraham *et al.* (2002).

light the importance of the placebo response that occurs in patients with heart failure who undergo device implantation. Once the placebo effect is adjusted for, only 30% of the study patients actually appeared to benefit primarily as a result of the device effect. This low response rate points out that there are several unknowns with cardiac resynchronization therapy and much needs to be understood with regards to appropriate patient selection by detecting mechanical dys-synchrony, optimal location of lead placement and correcting mechanical ventricular dys-synchrony by the pacing technique |6| (Table 14.1).

Cardiac resynchronization and death from progressive heart failure: a meta-analysis of randomized controlled trials

Bradley DJ, Bradley EA, Baughman KL, *et al. JAMA* 2003; **289**(6): 730–40

BACKGROUND. Progressive heart failure is the most common mechanism of death among patients with advanced heart failure. The objective of this meta-analysis was to determine whether cardiac resynchronization reduces mortality from progressive heart failure. Eligible studies were randomized controlled trials of cardiac resynchronization for the treatment of chronic symptomatic left ventricular dysfunction. Eligible studies reported death, hospitalization for heart failure, or ventricular arrhythmia as outcomes. Of the 6883 potentially relevant reports initially identified, eleven reports of four randomized trials with 1634 total patients were included in the meta-analysis. Pooled data from the four selected studies showed that cardiac resynchronization reduced death from progressive heart failure by 51% relative to controls (odds ratio [OR] 0.49; 95% confidence interval [CI] 0.25–0.93). Progressive heart failure mortality was 1.7% for cardiac resynchronization patients and 3.5% for controls. Cardiac resynchronization also reduced heart failure hospitalization by 29% (OR 0.71; 95% CI 0.53–0.96) and showed a trend towards reducing all-cause mortality (OR 0.77; 95% CI 0.51–1.18). Cardiac resynchronization was not associated with a statistically significant effect on non-heart failure mortality (OR 1.15; 95% CI 0.65–2.02). Among patients with implantable cardioverter defibrillators (ICDs), cardiac resynchronization had no clear impact on ventricular tachycardia or ventricular fibrillation (OR 0.92; 95% CI 0.67–1.27).

INTERPRETATION. Cardiac resynchronization reduced mortality from progressive heart failure in patients with symptomatic left ventricular dysfunction. This finding suggests that cardiac resynchronization may have a substantial impact on the most common mechanism of death among patients with advanced heart failure.

Comment

Caution must be exercised in interpreting the results of meta-analyses that seek to separate the mode of death in heart failure trials. Much controversy exists in adjudicating the mode of death in the context of clinical trials, and investigators agree that distinguishing between different modes of death is not always crystal clear. Furthermore, this review lumped together trials in which patients received either pacemakers alone or in combination with implantable defibrillators. The natural history and prognosis of these different patient groups might not be similar. Also, when assessing treatments that have the capacity to be harmful, all-cause mortality is the appropriate end-point that deserves to be examined. In this regard it is vital to point out that all-cause mortality was not demonstrated to improve using cardiac resynchronization therapy.

More recently, the Comparison of Medical Therapy, Pacing and Defibrillation in Chronic Heart Failure (COMPANION) trial results were published |6,7|. This trial enrolled patients with moderate to severe heart failure despite maximized medical therapy. Inclusion criteria included a QRS duration >120 ms and a PR interval >150 ms. The trial had three treatment arms: one out of five patients was to receive optimal pharmacological therapy, two out of five were to receive optimal pharmacological therapy plus biventricular pacing, while the remaining two out of five were to receive biventricular pacing, plus backup ICD therapy. In contrast to all others, this study was powered to evaluate a primary end-point of combined all-cause mortality and hospitalization. Data were analysed using an intention to treat statistical approach. In total, 1520 patients were randomized (93%) and 1080 patients were implanted with a cardiac resynchronization therapy pacer (CRT group) or defibrillator (CRT-D group). Of these, 118 patients failed the initial implant (88% implant success for the CRT group and 92% for the CRT-D group). Left ventricular lead dislodgement was seen in 2 and 2.5% in the CRT and CRT-D groups, respectively. As compared with patients treated with medical therapy only, there was a statistically significant event rate reduction in the primary combined end-point of total hospitalization and total mortality at 1 year in the CRT/CRT-D group (OR 0.82; $P = 0.05$ and 0.81; $P = 0.015$, respectively), as well as in the combined end-point of hospitalization for heart failure and death (OR 0.64 and 0.60, respectively; $P = 0.05$). Mortality at 1 year decreased by 24% ($P = 0.059$, ns) in the CRT group and 36% ($P = 0.003$) in the CRT-D group. The effects of cardiac resynchronization therapy on hospitalization due to heart failure appeared to be more pronounced in patients with left bundle branch block (as opposed to intraventricular conduction defect or right bundle branch block), patients with longer QRS duration (>148 ms) and in patients receiving β blockers. Despite the findings of this trial, little can be ascertained to help guide the clinician in the selection of patients who should receive cardiac resynchronization therapy alone, or in combination with a defibrillator since the study was not powered to detect differences between these two groups.

ICDs in heart failure: preventing sudden death

Because less than 20% of patients survive an episode of sudden cardiac death, the majority who experience a life-threatening ventricular tachyarrhythmia do not

survive to benefit from an ICD. Because of this, the concept of the ICD for primary
prevention of sudden cardiac death has received considerable attention. Although
β blockers and aldosterone antagonists in patients with heart failure, particularly
in the post-myocardial infarction setting, have demonstrated benefits in reducing
sudden death, prophylactic ICDs have shown the greatest promise in this regard.

Prophylactic implantation of a defibrillator in patients with myocardial infarction and reduced ejection fraction

Moss AJ, Zareba W, Hall WJ, *et al. N Engl J Med* 2002; **346**: 877–83

BACKGROUND. This trial was designed to determine if the ICD reduces mortality in
patients with prior myocardial infarction and decreased left ventricular systolic function.
The belief was that Holter monitoring and electrophysiological testing may not be
necessary to identify patients who benefit from an ICD. In total, 1232 with prior
myocardial infarction (56% with prior surgical revascularization) and left ventricular
ejection fraction (LVEF) <0.30 were randomized to ICD or no ICD therapy. Exclusion
criteria included myocardial infarction within 1 month, coronary artery bypass graft or
percutaneous transluminal coronary angioplasty within 2 months, and any patient
already satisfying criteria for receiving an automatic implantable cardiac defibrillator
(AICD) by satisfying the entry criteria for the first Multicenter Automatic Defibrillator
Implantation Trial II (MADIT II). The primary end-point was all-cause mortality. A
30% survival benefit with ICD therapy ensued at 20 months, but a trend to increased
heart failure episodes was also seen in the device arm.

INTERPRETATION. In patients with myocardial infarction and an LVEF <0.30, strong
consideration should be given to prophylactic placement of an ICD.

Comment

This investigation was designed to follow a simple clinical algorithm based on easily
available diagnostic tests to identify the patients enrolled. Thus, unlike prior studies,
no requirement for electrophysiological studies or ambient ventricular ectopy were
required for entry into this study. Indeed, analyses of ICD discharges and electrophysiological studies performed in the subgroup of those patients who received the
device confirmed the poor predictive capacity for formal testing in this population.
Thus, whereas those patients with inducible ventricular tachycardia were more likely
to receive shocks for sustained ventricular tachycardia, those who were non-
inducible suffered as many shocks but for ventricular fibrillation. One of the most
important issues with this technology is the cost implication. Before considering
prophylactic ICD placement, patients should receive optimal medical therapy with
β blockers, ACE inhibitors and aldosterone antagonists. Left ventricular function
should be evaluated at a time remote from the time of the myocardial infarction,
allowing sufficient time to elapse to allow recovery of ventricular function. Some
have argued that we need to define subgroups within the context of the MADIT II

population who may be most likely to benefit, but a clear-cut subpopulation has been difficult to ascertain.

More recently, the Sudden Cardiac Death in Heart Failure Trial (SCD-HeFT) has been completed and presented by Dr Gust Bardy. The SCD-HeFT tested the hypothesis that either amiodarone or the automatic cardiac defibrillator improves survival compared to placebo in patients with heart failure. This study enrolled 2521 patients with New York Heart Association II or III heart failure and a LVEF <0.35 (either ischaemic or non-ischaemic aetiology) and randomly allocated them to a strategy of ICD, amiodarone or placebo. The patients were well treated with 87% on ACE inhibitors or ARBs and 78% on β blockers at last follow-up. This investigation suggested no benefit of amiodarone compared with placebo (hazard ratio [HR] 1.06; 97.5% CI 0.86–1.3; $P = 0.53$). On the other hand, ICD therapy decreased mortality by 23% compared to control, a finding consistent across ischaemic and non-ischaemic aetiology of heart failure (HR 0.77; 97.5% CI 0.62–0.96; $P = 0.007$). Interestingly, most of the benefit of the ICD strategy was confined to those with New York Heart Association II heart failure at study entry while no significant benefit was observed in the New York Heart Association III group. This study now suggests that patients with mild heart failure and left ventricular dysfunction should be strongly considered as candidates for automatic cardiac defibrillator implantation.

Dual-chamber pacing or ventricular backup pacing in patients with an implantable defibrillator: the Dual Chamber and VVI Implantable Defibrillator (DAVID) Trial

Wilkoff BL, Cook JR, Epstein AE, et al. Dual Chamber and VVI Implantable Defibrillator Trial Investigators. JAMA 2002; **288**(24): 3115–23

BACKGROUND. All of the prospective multicentre trials that support the use of implantable defibrillators have used single chamber pacemakers/ICDs. Despite the significantly increased cost of dual chamber pacemaker/ICD devices and the lack of outcome data, these devices accounted for approximately two-thirds of the ICDs implanted in the real world setting. Dual chamber pacemaker trials have not provided data that would support this trend, but the high incidence of atrial fibrillation, bradycardia, and congestive heart failure, as comorbid conditions, suggests that the situation could be different in the defibrillator patient population. The Dual Chamber and VVI Implantable Defibrillator (DAVID) Trial, a single-blind, parallel-group, randomized clinical trial, enrolled 506 patients with indications for ICD therapy. All patients had an LVEF of 40% or less, no indication for antibradycardia pacemaker therapy, and no persistent atrial arrhythmias. Patients were randomly assigned to have the ICDs programmed to ventricular backup pacing at 40/min (VVI-40; $n = 256$) or dual chamber rate-responsive pacing at 70/min (DDDR-70; $n = 250$). Maximal tolerated medical therapy for left ventricular dysfunction, including ACE inhibitors and β blockers, was prescribed to all patients and the composite end-point of time to death or first hospitalization for congestive heart failure was evaluated. One-year survival free of the

composite end-point was 83.9% for patients treated with VVI-40 compared with 73.3% for patients treated with DDDR-70 (relative hazard 1.61; 95% CI 1.06–2.44). The components of the composite end-point, mortality of 6.5% for VVI-40 vs 10.1% for DDDR-70 (relative hazard 1.61; 95% CI 0.84–3.09) and hospitalization for congestive heart failure of 13.3% for VVI-40 vs 22.6% for DDDR-70 (relative hazard 1.54; 95% CI 0.97–2.46) also trended in favour of VVI-40 programming.

INTERPRETATION. For patients with standard indications for ICD therapy, no indication for cardiac pacing, and an LVEF of 40% or less, dual chamber pacing offers no clinical advantage over ventricular backup pacing and may be detrimental by increasing the combined end-point of death or hospitalization for heart failure.

Comment

This important trial suggests that the observed worsening of heart failure noted in trials of prophylactic ICD placement may be explained not only by post-shock stunning, but more commonly by the use of backup pacing. This is most likely due to the development of right ventricular pacing-induced left bundle branch block resulting in intra- and interventricular dys-synchrony with resultant further worsening of left and right ventricular systolic and diastolic function.

Laplace therapeutics in heart failure

The management of late-stage heart failure often frustrates seasoned clinicians and is fraught with oscillating haemodynamic instability coupled with multi-organ dysfunction. Even the option of cardiac transplantation is fraught with limitations due to a scarce donor organ pool and restrictive criteria. This difficult situation has led researchers to develop mechanical alternatives to provide palliation in the form of 'destination therapy' that is fundamentally designed to enhance quality of life. The lack of viable therapeutic strategies in treating the late-stage heart failure patient have led to a flurry of activity in the surgical domain to reshape an adversely remodelled ventricle. This premise seeks to decrease wall stress by exploiting Laplace's law that describes the stress and strain relationship as a measure of cavity size and wall thickness |8| (Fig. 14.2). One of the many surgical approaches to decreasing ventricular wall stress is perhaps the notion of ventricular assistance, which provides active assistance by serving as a 'ventricular vacuum' for providing rest to the cavity. Ventricular assist devices (VADs) have ushered in the era of 'ultimate haemodynamic unloading' by the use of pumps that either replace most of the native ventricular function, or partially unload the ventricle by assistance in parallel. Another approach is to attempt reshaping of the ventricle using passive cardiac restraint devices or actively altering the stress–strain relationships within the ventricular cavity by the use of myocardial splints (Table 14.2).

CONCEPT OF LAPLACE THERAPEUTICS

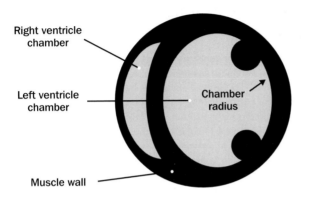

Right ventricle
chamber

Left ventricle
chamber

Chamber
radius

Muscle wall

$$\text{Stress} = \frac{P \leftrightarrow r}{h} = \frac{\text{Pressure x radius}}{\text{Wall thickness}}$$

If pressure or radius increases, stress increases

Fig. 14.2 Laplace's law defines the stress–strain relationship within a cavity. Therapeutic manoeuvres that decrease pressure or cavity size will decrease wall stress, as will thickening of the heart muscle.

Table 14.2 Laplace therapeutics: decreasing wall stress with device therapy

Target	Modality
Decrease pressure within cavity	Ventricular assist device
Decrease work of ejection	Cardiac resynchronization therapy
Decrease cavity size	Passive cardiac restraint
	Myosplint
Increase myocardial thickness	Myoblast transplantation
	Stem cell therapy

Long-term mechanical left ventricular assistance for end-stage heart failure

Rose EA, Gelijns AC, Moskowitz AJ, *et al*. Randomized Evaluation of Mechanical Assistance for the Treatment of Congestive Heart Failure (REMATCH) Study Group. *N Engl J Med* 2001; **345**(20): 1435–43

BACKGROUND. Implantable left ventricular assist devices (LVADs) have been established as an important bridge to cardiac transplantation, although some devices have been placed long term and few have recovered enough to be weaned. This trial was designed to evaluate the suitability of LVADs as long-term myocardial replacement therapy in patients ineligible for cardiac transplantation. One hundred and twenty-nine patients with end-stage heart failure who were ineligible for cardiac transplantation were randomly assigned to receive an LVAD or optimal medical therapy, with a primary end-point of all-cause mortality. To be eligible, patients had to have New York Heart Association class IV heart failure for at least 90 days despite attempted therapy with an ACE inhibitor, diuretics, and digoxin; an EF ≤25%; and an exercise peak O_2 uptake ≤12 ml/kg/min (later increased to 14 ml/kg/min). Survival was significantly improved from 25% at 1 year in the medical therapy group to 52% in the LVAD group (relative risk 0.52; 95% CI 0.34–0.78; $P = 0.001$). However, at 2 years, only 23% in the LVAD group were alive (compared with 8% in the medical group).

INTERPRETATION. The use of an LVAD resulted in improved survival and quality of life in patients with extremely severe heart failure. An LVAD may be an acceptable alternative therapy in selected patients who are not candidates for cardiac transplantation.

Comment

Whereas a superficial evaluation of these trial findings suggests a remarkable survival advantage with LVAD therapy, a closer appraisal of the evidence points to the tremendous clinical cost that has to be borne in order to achieve these salutary results. Thus, at 2 years, only 23% in the LVAD group were alive (compared with 8% in the medical group). The modes of death in the LVAD group included sepsis ($n = 17$), VAD failure ($n = 7$), cerebrovascular disease ($n = 4$), pulmonary embolus ($n = 2$), and only one categorized as pump failure. Similarly, the probability of infection with the device was 28%, bleeding 42% and device failure 35%, requiring device replacement in ten of 68 patients. In regard to hospitalizations, device-treated patients spent more days in the hospital compared with the medical therapy arm. Thus, from a clinical standpoint, one could argue that device therapy 'delayed death compared with medical therapy' but at a very high rate of unpleasant and largely iatrogenic complications. In fact, the median prolongation in life with LVADs was 8 months, of which 3 months were spent in the hospital. Although the investigators suggested that quality of life was improved, no calculation of the 'quality of death' was ascertained in the overall equation to define benefit with device therapy. It should therefore be emphasized that appropriate patient selection for destination therapy is critical, as application to less morbidly ill situations might alter the risk–benefit ratio adversely against such a therapeutic approach. More recently, proposals for care standards for destination therapy have been proposed which have led third party payers to adopt restricted coverage criteria that allow destination therapy to be performed only at centres with multidisciplinary experienced teams and demonstrated proficiency in using VAD therapy. Furthermore, coverage requirements include the transfer of centre-specific data to a central registry such that universal tracking of outcomes along with bench-marking of 'best practices' can be achieved.

Clinical experience with an implantable, intracardiac, continuous flow circulatory support device: physiologic implications and their relationship to patient selection

Frazier OH, Myers TJ, Westaby S, Gregoric ID. *Ann Thorac Surg* 2004; **77**(1): 133–42

BACKGROUND. Unlike pulsatile assist devices, continuous-flow pumps have a simplified pumping mechanism and they do not require compliance chambers or valves. In the 1980s, clinical experience with the Hemopump proved that a high-speed, intravascular, continuous-flow pump could safely augment the circulation. Subsequently, a decade of animal experiments with a larger, longer-term continuous-flow pump (the Jarvik 2000) confirmed the safety and efficacy of intraventricular placement, leading to its clinical application. In this observational study, the investigators analysed the physiological and anatomical effects of using the Jarvik 2000 pump for cardiac support in 23 patients in whom the device was applied as a bridge to transplant under the protocol approved by the Food and Drug Administration Investigational Device Exemption. The device was used as a bridge to transplantation in 20 patients and as destination therapy in three. In the bridge-to-transplant group, 14 patients underwent transplantation, five died during the circulatory support period and one is in an ongoing study. The support period lasted an average of 90 days. For the survivors, the follow-up period averaged 16 months. In the destination therapy group, one patient died unexpectedly from an accident 382 days after device implantation. The two survivors remain in New York Heart Association functional class I at 700–952 days after implantation.

INTERPRETATION. The Jarvik 2000 can offer effective long-term support for patients with chronic heart failure and New York Heart Association class IV status. However, the new physiology produced by continuous offloading of the heart throughout the cardiac cycle has introduced unique clinical problems. The understanding of the problems generated by this biotechnological interface is essential for obtaining optimal clinical outcomes.

Comment

As newer generation devices become available, the hope that the cost and morbidity associated with these devices will be lower will probably become a reality. Mechanical assist devices are increasingly evolving towards smaller devices that are associated with lesser morbidity and transcutaneous energy sources that avoid the near universal risk of infection. Continuous-flow axial impeller pumps besides the Jarvik 2000 have been introduced to clinical application offering new advantages. Wieselthaler *et al.* |9| investigated six male patients (mean age 53 ± 11 years) with end-stage left heart failure who were implanted with a DeBakey VAD axial-flow pump for bridge to transplantation. Three patients were successfully transplanted after 74, 115 and 117 days. Two other patients died after 25 and 133 days. Noon and colleagues |10| have reported more extensively on the MicroMed DeBakey VAD. A detailed evaluation of the first 32 of more than 50 patients implanted with this device has been completed. With current data, the probability of survival at 30 days after implant is 81%. This preliminary experience suggests that this long-term axial-flow circulatory assist device is capable of providing adequate haemodynamic support in patients with severe heart failure, sufficient to recover and return to normal activities while awaiting heart transplantation. The concept of destination therapy using VADs is promising and validated. Yet, gaps in translating this information to the clinical realm exist, due to the device limitations of iatrogenic complications and durability. The field of mechanical assistance is progressing rapidly with the introduction of smaller devices that are more durable and with less risk of infection or haematological aberrances. The most important advance will occur with the structured implementation and development of strategies designed to achieve the maximal potential for device removal, ushering in a more universal opportunity for destination to recovery.

Recovery from heart failure with circulatory assist: a working group of the National Heart, Lung, and Blood Institute

Reinlib L, Abraham W. *J Cardiac Fail* 2003; **9**(6): 459–63

BACKGROUND. Anecdotal evidence suggests that heart failure patients fitted with mechanical assist devices experience direct cardiac benefits manifested by reverse remodelling and some are successfully separated from their device in follow-up. To investigate this phenomenon, on 2–3 August 2001, the National Heart, Lung, and Blood Institute convened the working group, 'Recovery from Heart Failure with Circulatory Assist' in Bethesda (Maryland, USA). The team included cardiac surgeons, cardiologists, and experts in experimental research. The goal was to prioritize recommendations to guide future programmes in: (1) elucidating the mechanisms leading to reverse remodelling associated with an LVAD; (2) exploring advanced treatments, including novel pharmacologies, tissue engineering, and cell therapies, to optimize recovery with LVAD therapy; and (3) identifying target genes, proteins, and cellular pathways to focus on for the production of novel therapies for myocardial recovery and cardiovascular disease.

INTERPRETATION. The working group made research and clinical recommendations to eventually translate findings into improved therapeutic strategies and device design: (1) support collaborations among clinical and basic scientists with an emphasis on clinical/translational research that might eventually lead to clinical trials; (2) identify candidate patients most likely to benefit from LVAD as a destination therapy; (3) explore potential biomarkers indicating when patients could most successfully be weaned from devices; and (4) promote clinical and experimental study of mechanically assisted organs and the tissue derived from them.

Comment

The challenge in the notion of destination therapy is inherent in our ability to separate those likely to improve after cardiac reparation has been allowed from those who present an irreversible illness that requires ongoing mechanical support. Several recent lines of evidence suggest the potential for cardiac recovery, leading to the development of the notion that the 'destination' could in fact eventually be cardiac recovery, offering an opportunity for pump explantation. In this regard, it is useful to evaluate the cellular and biochemical effects of mechanical unloading using VAD support. It has been demonstrated that mechanically induced haemodynamic restoration is accompanied by regression of cellular hypertrophy, normalization of the neuroendocrine axis, improved expression of contractile proteins, enhanced cellular respiratory control, and decreases in markers of apoptosis and cellular stress |11|. Due to the mechanistic lines of evidence supporting the notion that device explantation is reasonable, several investigators have sought to develop algorithms whereby the VAD can be removed. The evidence in this regard is controversial, with some investigators reporting marked success along with others recommending great caution in this approach. One of the biggest dilemmas that confronts the clinician is in the optimal clinical evaluation of cardiac recovery. Because the negative pressure exerted by the mechanical device alters loading conditions unusually, investigators have yet to settle upon the best method for the determination of explant feasibility. Others have suggested active ways to facilitate cardiac recovery, a premise that is still experimental. Mancini and colleagues |12| used exercise testing and exercise haemodynamic evaluations to distinguish patients on VAD support who might be candidates for explantation due to significant recovery. These investigators reported a low rate of explant success (five of 111 implants). These researchers have recently reported two cases of successful device explantation only to suffer recrudescence of disease in late follow-up. Other groups in larger populations have reported better success. Muller *et al.* |13|, as well as Hetzer and colleagues |14|, reported on 28 explants among 96 VAD-treated patients. These investigators used routine echocardiographic parameters to assess recovery with devices turned on and then off for up to 20 min. Others have suggested that inotropic stimulation using dobutamine echocardiography might be useful in determining cardiac recovery. These same investigators also revealed variability in the clinical response and histological improvement as evidenced by inconsistency between clinical responses and collagen alteration in the myocardium. More recently, Gorcsan *et al.* |15| used on-line quantitative echocardiography alone or combined with exercise cardiopulmonary testing to assess myocardial recovery in patients receiving LVAD support and thereby identifying patients who are clinical candidates for device removal. It should be noted that the scant support for device explantation in routine late-stage heart failure is further amplified by the inconsistency and lack of agreement in the best technique to identify those likely to be successful. A tantalizing concept proposed recently seeks to actively attempt maximal reverse ventricular remodelling by the use of pharmacological stimuli. The concept revolves around the induction of physiological cardiac hypertrophy using clenbuterol, a selective β2-adrenergic receptor agonist, in carefully selected patients, followed by device explantation |16|. This interesting approach remains under systematic investigation.

Initial experience with the AbioCor implantable replacement heart system

Dowling RD, Gray LA Jr, Etoch SW, *et al. J Thorac Cardiovasc Surg* 2004; **127**(1): 131–41

BACKGROUND. This study sought to evaluate the safety and efficacy of the first available totally implantable replacement heart (AbioCor implantable replacement heart system) in the treatment of severe, irreversible biventricular heart failure in human patients. Seven male adult patients with severe, irreversible biventricular failure (>70% 30-day predicted mortality) who were not candidates for transplantation met all institutional review board study criteria and had placement of the AbioCor implantable replacement heart. All were in cardiogenic shock despite maximal medical therapy, including inotropes and intra-aortic balloon pumps. Their mean age was 66.7 + 10.4 years (range 51–79 years). Four of seven patients had prior operations. Six had ischaemic and one had idiopathic cardiomyopathy. All had three-dimensional computer-simulated implantation of the thoracic unit that predicted adequate fit. At the time of the operation, the internal transcutaneous energy transfer coil, battery, and controller were placed. Biventriculectomy was then performed, and the thoracic unit was placed in an orthotopic position and attached to the atrial cuffs and outflow conduits with quick-connects. The flow was adjusted to 4–8 l/min. Central venous and left atrial pressures were maintained at 5–15 mmHg. The device is powered through transcutaneous energy transfer. An atrial flow-balancing chamber is used to adjust left/right balance. The balance chamber and transcutaneous energy transfer eliminate the need for percutaneous lines. There was one intra-operative death caused by coagulopathic bleeding and one early death caused by an aprotinin reaction. There have been multiple morbidities primarily related to pre-existing illness severity: five patients had prolonged intubation, two had hepatic failure (resolved in one), four had renal failure (resolved in three), and one each had recurrent gastrointestinal bleeding, acute cholecystitis requiring laparotomy, respiratory failure that resolved after 3 days of extracorporeal membrane oxygenation, and malignant hyperthermia (resolved). There were three late deaths: one caused by multiple systems organ failure (post-operative day 56), one caused by a cerebrovascular accident (post-operative day 142), and one caused by retroperitoneal bleeding and resultant multiple systems organ failure (post-operative day 151). This latter patient was not able to tolerate anticoagulation (no anticoagulation or antiplatelet therapy alone for 80% of the first 60 days) and had a transient ischaemic attack on post-operative day **61** and a cerebrovascular accident on post-operative day **130**. At autopsy, blood pumps were clean. The two patients who had large cerebrovascular accidents had thrombus on the atrial cage struts. These struts have been removed for future implants. There were no significant haemolysis or device-related infections. The balance chamber allowed for left/right balance in all patients (left atrial pressure within 5 mmHg of right atrial pressure). Three patients have taken multiple (>50) trips out of the hospital, and two have been discharged from the hospital. Total days on support with the AbioCor are **759**.

INTERPRETATION. The initial clinical experience suggests that the AbioCor might be effective therapy in patients with advanced biventricular failure.

Comment

One of the most technologically advanced devices, the AbioCor totally implantable heart is designed to completely replace the human heart and not merely 'assist' it. As such, this technique is a true destination therapy with no opportunity for recovery of the native heart. Thus, this technology is best suited for those individuals who suffer from severe irreversible pulmonary hypertension and biventricular failure who have little potential for any meaningful recovery. The longest survivor with this total replacement heart lived 17 months and died due to device malfunction. In others, the results have been quite mixed with marked device-related morbidity of bleeding complications and stroke.

Myosplint implant and shape-change procedure: intra- and peri-operative safety and feasibility
Schenk S, Reichenspurner H, Boehm DH, *et al. J Heart Lung Transplant* 2002; **21**(6): 680–6.

BACKGROUND. To attempt a decrease in ventricular wall stress, transventricular tension members (Myosplint) were implanted to change the left ventricle effective radius and to reduce the left ventricle wall stress by 20%. Myosplints were implanted in seven patients, all diagnosed with dilated cardiomyopathy. New York Heart Association class ranged from III to IV, and left ventricular end-diastolic diameter ranged from 70 to 102 mm. Mitral valve regurgitation was classified as mild in three cases and moderate in four. Four patients underwent mitral valve annuloplasty. These investigators observed no significant device-related complications, such as thromboembolism, bleeding, device instability, or vascular damage, at 90 days. Early indications in a small patient population demonstrate some improvements in clinical parameters.

INTERPRETATION. From this initial experience, one may conclude that placement of the Myosplint devices can be safely performed without early, significant adverse events. In patients with significant mitral valve incompetence, concomitant mitral valve repair is indicated to realize the full benefit of the procedure. The long-term effect of each procedure on cardiac function and survival will require further evaluation.

Comment

The Myocor Myosplint is a transcavitary tensioning device designed to change left ventricular shape and reduce wall stress. Studies have shown that this technique reduces fibre stress without a decrement in the stress–strain relationship. The tension rods that are inserted within the ventricular cavity require precise estimates of location and placement in order to achieve optimal benefits in reducing wall stress. Data in humans are still quite limited and clinical trends and benefits with this device are unclear.

Global surgical experience with the Acorn cardiac support device

Oz MC, Konertz WF, Kleber FX, *et al. J Thorac Cardiovasc Surg* 2003; **126**(4): 983–91

BACKGROUND. Providing end-diastolic support with an innovative mesh-like cardiac support device reduces mechanical stress, improves function, and reverses cardiac remodelling in animal models without safety issues. The objective of this study was to review the global clinical safety and feasibility experience of this device. The Acorn CorCap cardiac support device has been implanted world-wide in more than 130 patients with dilated cardiomyopathy with or without concomitant cardiac surgery. The device is positioned around the ventricles and given a custom fit. A series of 48 patients were implanted with the device in initial safety and feasibility studies, of whom 33 also received concomitant cardiac surgery. At implantation, eleven patients were in New York Heart Association class II, 33 were in class III, and four were in class IV. The average CorCap implantation time was 27 min. The mean intra-operative reduction in left ventricular end-diastolic dimension was 4.6 ± 1%. There were no device-related intra-operative complications. Eight early and nine late deaths occurred during follow-up extending to 24 months. Actuarial survival was 73% at 12 months and 68% at 24 months. There were no device-related adverse events or evidence of constrictive disease, and coronary artery flow reserve was maintained. Ventricular chamber dimensions decreased, whereas EF and New York Heart Association class were improved in patients overall and in those patients implanted with the CorCap device without concomitant operations.

INTERPRETATION. The CorCap device appears safe for patients with dilated cardiomyopathy. Randomized clinical trials are underway in Europe, Australia, and North America.

Comment

Passive cardiac restraint devices attempt to reshape the heart over time. Concerns about the development of constrictive physiology and impediments to coronary blood flow have appeared unfounded in animal studies and initial human trials. Whether cardiac restraint devices can be beneficial in isolation or only in the context of concomitant operations such as mitral valve repair remains unproven. This concept is currently under investigation in a randomized trial that will share preliminary results in late 2004 |**17**|.

Conclusion

The device era in heart failure therapeutics has now been realized. Never before have clinicians had as diverse a repertoire of treatment options as now. However, we must be careful that we do not rush to judgement in the application of device therapy before the accumulation of an appropriate evidence base to help refine our treatment approaches. The availability of devices ushers with it responsibility to weigh factors such as device-based complications, incremental benefit potential and cost-effectiveness. The populations who are most likely to benefit require clarification. Despite these limitations, device therapy represents a fulfilment of therapeutic principles in heart failure that seek to modify the problem at the 'heart' and not simply to target the peripheral consequences of the manifest disorder.

References

1. Mehra MR, Uber PA, Potluri S. Renin angiotensin aldosterone and adrenergic modulation in chronic heart failure: contemporary concepts. *Am J Med Sci* 2002; **324**(5): 267–75.

2. Mehra MR, Uber PA, Francis GS. Heart failure therapy at a crossroad: are there limits to the neurohormonal model? *J Am Coll Cardiol* 2003; **41**: 1606–10.

3. Cohn JN, Tognoni G. Valsartan Heart Failure Trial Investigators. A randomized trial of the angiotensin-receptor blocker valsartan in chronic heart failure. *N Engl J Med* 2001; **345**(23): 1667–75.

4. McMurray JJ, Ostergren J, Swedberg K, Granger CB, Held P, Michelson EL, Olofsson B, Yusuf S, Pfeffer MA. CHARM Investigators and Committees. Effects of candesartan in patients with chronic heart failure and reduced left-ventricular systolic function taking angiotensin-converting-enzyme inhibitors: the CHARM-Added trial. *Lancet* 2003; **362**(9386): 767–71.

5. Pitt B, Remme W, Zannad F, Neaton J, Martinez F, Roniker B, Bittman R, Hurley S, Kleiman J, Gatlin M. Eplerenone Post-Acute Myocardial Infarction Heart Failure Efficacy and Survival Study Investigators. Eplerenone, a selective aldosterone blocker, in patients with left ventricular dysfunction after myocardial infarction. *N Engl J Med* 2003; **348**(14): 1309–21.

6. Mehra MR, Greenberg BH. Cardiac resynchronization therapy: caveat medicus! *J Am Coll Cardiol* 2004; **43**: 1145–8.

7. Bristow MR, Saxon LA, Boehmer J, Krueger S, Kass DA, De Marco T, Carson P, DiCarlo L, DeMets D, White BG, DeVries DW, Feldman AM; Comparison of Medical Therapy, Pacing, and Defibrillation in Heart Failure (COMPANION) Investigators. Cardiac-resynchronization therapy with or without an implantable defibrillator in advanced chronic heart failure. *N Engl J Med* 2004; **350**: 2140–50.

8. Mehra MR, Uber PA. Emergence of Laplace therapeutics: declaring an end to 'end-stage' heart failure. *Congest Heart Fail* 2002; **8**(4): 228–31.

9. Wieselthaler GM, Schima H, Lassnigg AM, Dworschak M, Pacher R, Grimm M, Wolner E. Lessons learned from the first clinical implants of the DeBakey ventricular assist device axial pump: a single center report. *Ann Thorac Surg* 2001; **71**(3 Suppl): S139–43; discussion S144–6.

10. Noon GP, Morley DL, Irwin S, Abdelsayed SV, Benkowski RJ, Lynch BE. Clinical experience with the MicroMed DeBakey ventricular assist device. *Ann Thorac Surg* 2001; **71** (3 Suppl): S133–8; discussion S144–6.

11. Van Meter Jr CH, Mehra MR. Update on left ventricular assist devices as a bridge to cardiac recovery. *Curr Opin Organ Trans* 2001; **6**: 211–15.

12. Mancini DM, Beniaminovitz A, Levin H, Catanese K, Flannery M, DiTullio M, Savin S, Cordisco ME, Rose E, Oz M. Low incidence of myocardial recovery after left ventricular assist device implantation in patients with chronic heart failure. *Circulation* 1998; **98**(22): 2383–9.

13. Muller J, Wallukat G, Weng YG, Dandel M, Spiegelsberger S, Semrau S, Brandes K, Theodoridis V, Loebe M, Meyer R, Hetzer R. Weaning from mechanical cardiac support in patients with idiopathic dilated cardiomyopathy. *Circulation* 1997; **96**(2): 542–9.

14. Hetzer R, Muller JH, Weng Y, Meyer R, Dandel M. Bridging-to-recovery. *Ann Thorac Surg* 2001; **71**(3 Suppl): S109–13.

15. Gorcsan J, Severyn D, Murali S, Kormos RL. Non-invasive assessment of myocardial recovery on chronic left ventricular assist device: results associated with successful device removal. *J Heart Lung Transplant* 2003; **22**(12): 1304–13.

16. Hon JK, Yacoub MH. Bridge to recovery with the use of left ventricular assist device and clenbuterol. *Ann Thorac Surg* 2003; **75**(6 Suppl): S36–41.

17. Mann DL, Acker MA, Jessup M, Sabbah HN, Starling RC, Kubo SH; Acorn Investigators and Study Coordinators. Rationale, design, and methods for a pivotal randomized clinical trial for the assessment of a cardiac support device in patients with New York health association class III–IV heart failure. *J Card Fail* 2004; **10**(3): 185–92.

15

Genetics of heart failure

RAY HERSHBERGER, EMILY BURKETT

Introduction

Multiple factors, both genetic and environmental, contribute to the development of heart failure. With the recent completion of the Human Genome Project, the opportunity to gain a better understanding of the genetic contributions to heart failure has generated much hope and excitement. In this chapter we review some of the recent developments in the effort to elucidate the genetic basis of heart failure.

The first section of this chapter reviews genetic risk factors: polymorphisms associated with a predisposition to heart failure. A *polymorphism* (literally 'many forms') is a DNA sequence alteration having at least two relatively common forms (frequencies of >1% in the population), or alleles, at a particular gene locus. In contrast to deleterious mutations in single genes that cause disease (which usually have frequencies of <1%), polymorphisms are widespread in the population; it has been estimated that any individual is likely to have polymorphisms at ~6% of their enzyme-encoding loci. Polymorphisms may contribute to variations in normal or abnormal physiological processes. Probably the most widely known example of a polymorphic system is the ABO blood group system, in which the varieties of ABO blood types are determined by allelic differences at the ABO locus, each allele having a frequency of >1% in the general population. The effort to elucidate and understand the multitude of polymorphisms that affect and alter the development of heart failure is currently a major area of interest to researchers.

The second section of this chapter reviews mutations in single genes that appear to cause dilated cardiomyopathy (DCM), the most common substrate for the development of heart failure. A *mutation* is any permanent, heritable change in the sequence of genomic DNA. Conditions that are caused by a mutation at a single gene locus appear in families in a defined pattern of inheritance, referred to as Mendelian. The three major Mendelian patterns of inheritance are autosomal dominant, autosomal recessive, and X-linked. Mutations in genes located on chromosomes 1–22 are transmitted in an autosomal manner, whereas genes on the X chromosome are transmitted in an X-linked pattern.

A *dominant* trait is one in which expression of the trait requires the presence of a mutation in only one of the two alleles at the trait's locus. An individual may have a dominant trait from either of two mechanisms: (1) inheriting the gene mutation from one of his or her parents who also carried the mutation, or (2) as a new mutation (that occurred in one of the parents' gametes during meiosis). Individuals who carry a mutation for a dominant trait have a 50% chance of passing on the mutation and a 50% chance of passing on the normal allele to each of their offspring.

Recessive traits require two copies of the gene mutation at the locus for obvious expression of the condition. For an individual to be affected with a recessive condition, they must have received a mutant allele from each of their parents.

X-linked traits are those caused by mutations in genes on the X chromosome. Males who carry an X-linked gene mutation will express the trait; in contrast, females, who have two copies of the X chromosome, may carry the mutant gene but not express it, or may express a much milder form of the condition. Females carrying the mutation have a 50% chance of transmitting the gene to each son or daughter.

The genetic constitution of an individual—or the specific genetic make-up at a particular gene locus—is referred to as his or her *genotype*. The expression of the individual's genotype (which includes environmental influences on the genotype) is referred to as his or her *phenotype*. The concept of *variable expression* refers to the extent to which a genotype is expressed, since even in individuals with identical genotypes the phenotype may vary from person to person. Variable expression is seen extensively with the genes known to cause DCM in families, which are reviewed later in the chapter. *Penetrance* refers to the all-or-none expression of a mutation. For example, if a phenotype is expressed in fewer than 100% of the individuals who carry the deleterious genotype, it is said to have reduced penetrance. Dilated cardiomyopathy is often said to have age-dependent penetrance; that is, as individuals who carry a deleterious gene for DCM get older, they have an increased chance of expressing the DCM phenotype.

Genetic polymorphisms associated with susceptibility to heart failure

Numerous variations in the heart failure phenotype, which may give rise to physiological and at times pathophysiological consequences, have recently been described in association with polymorphisms. The usual approach is to carefully identify and measure a phenotypic characteristic of interest in a well-defined population and assess the variation of this phenotype with differences in genotype. For example, phenotypic characteristics commonly assessed in patients with heart failure include the duration of survival, left ventricular enlargement, the degree of systolic dysfunction (usually measured by a left ventricular ejection fraction [LVEF]), exercise limitation, haemodynamic abnormalities, the level of an elevated humour (such as norepinephrine or brain natriuretic peptide), and a host of other clinical, biochemical or functional measures.

As above, genetic variations (polymorphisms) are relatively common changes in genotype found in the population, usually defined as having a frequency of >1%.

A genetic variation may be associated with no, little or substantial change in the physiological function of its cognate protein. Polymorphisms are commonly observed in most genes. However, one attractive hypothesis is that a subset of polymorphisms, especially those that significantly affect protein function, might contribute to the diversity of presentation, symptoms, progression and response to treatment in a disease process such as heart failure.

The development of the heart failure syndrome involves a vast and diverse set of proteins – and hence genes that code for protein structure – in a variety of tissues in the heart (myocytes, vascular endothelium and smooth muscle, cardiac interstitium, specialized conductive tissues, etc.), the kidney, the sympathetic nervous system and other tissues. Hence, numerous polymorphisms from scores of candidate genes could potentially be examined in patients with heart failure. Particularly tractable hypotheses can be generated for polymorphisms that affect function in proteins known to be implicated in the development of heart failure.

Reviewed below are recent reports of the effects of various polymorphisms on heart failure presentation, progression, or response to treatment, taken from the renin–angiotensin and adrenergic receptor signalling systems. Both systems have been shown to participate extensively in the onset and perpetuation of the heart failure syndrome. It is therefore predictable that variations in protein or enzyme structure that affect their function could in turn alter the phenotypic expression of selected heart failure characteristics.

Pharmacogenetic interactions between β-blocker therapy and the angiotensin-converting enzyme deletion polymorphism in patients with congestive heart failure

McNamara DM, Holubkov R, Janosko K, *et al. Circulation* 2001; **103**: 1644–8

BACKGROUND. Activation of the renin–angiotensin and sympathetic nervous systems adversely affect heart failure progression. The angiotensin-converting enzyme (ACE) deletion (ACE D) allele is associated with increased renin–angiotensin activation compared with the I allele; however, its influence on patient outcomes remains uncertain, and the pharmacogenetic interactions with β blocker therapy have not been evaluated previously. The authors prospectively followed 328 patients (age 56.1 ± 11.9 years) with systolic dysfunction (LVEF 0.24 ± 0.08) to assess the impact of the ACE D allele on transplant-free survival (median follow-up 21 months). Transplant-free survival was compared by genotype for the whole cohort and separately in patients with (*n* = 120) and those without β blocker therapy (*n* = 208) at the time of entry.

INTERPRETATION. Transplant-free survival was significantly poorer for patients with the D allele (1-year percentage survival for the genotypes II, ID and DD respectively was 94, 77 and 75; 2-year survival was 78, 65 and 60; ordered log-rank test *P* = 0.044). In patients not treated with β blockers, the adverse impact of ACE D allele was dramatically increased (1-year percentage survival for the three genotypes was 95, 75 and 67; 2-year survival was 81, 61 and 48; $P = 0.005$). In contrast, in patients receiving β blocker therapy, no influence of ACE genotype on transplant-free survival was evident (1-year percentage survival for genotypes II, ID and DD was 91, 80 and 86 respectively; 2-year survival was 70, 71 and 77; $P = 0.73$; Fig. 15.1). It was concluded that, in a cohort of patients with systolic dysfunction, the ACE D allele was associated with significantly poorer transplant-free survival. This effect was primarily evident in patients not treated with β blockers and was not seen in patients receiving therapy. These findings suggest a potential pharmacogenetic interaction between the ACE D/I polymorphism and therapy with β blockers in the determination of heart failure survival.

Comment

The well-known ACE polymorphism in this study affected the progression of the heart failure syndrome. Not all prior studies have demonstrated that ACE gene polymorphisms are associated with heart failure progression, especially ambulatory outpatients with heart failure from idiopathic DCM (IDC). The current work suggests that the ACE genotype may not affect the presence or progression of the underlying DCM, but rather may be a disease modifier of the heart failure syndrome. Additional work in larger cohorts of patients with heart failure will be required to sort out these important issues.

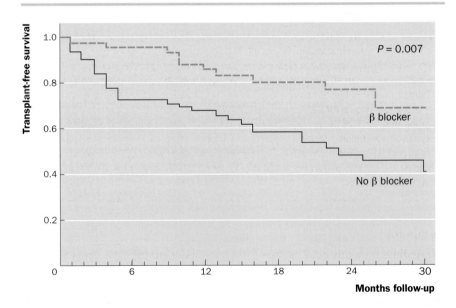

Fig. 15.1 Transplant-free survival compared by β blocker use for patients with ACE DD genotype only, $n = 1–5$. Event-free survival was significantly better for patients treated with β blockers ($n = 43$) compared with those not receiving therapy ($n = 62$) ($P = 0.0007$ by log-rank test). Source: McNamara *et al.* (2001).

Angiotensin-converting enzyme genotype modulates pulmonary function and exercise capacity in treated patients with congestive stable heart failure

Abraham MR, Olson LJ, Joyner MJ, Turner ST, Beck KC, Johnson BD.

Circulation 2002; **106**: 1794–9

BACKGROUND. The gene encoding ACE exhibits an insertion/deletion polymorphism resulting in three genotypes (DD, ID, and II), which affects serum and tissue ACE activity as well as other vasoactive substances. Pulmonary function is frequently abnormal in patients with congestive heart failure, the mechanism of which has not been completely characterized. ACE inhibition has been shown to improve diffusion across the alveolar–capillary membrane and to improve exercise capacity and gas exchange in congestive heart failure. The aim of this study was to determine if ACE genotype is associated with altered pulmonary function and exercise intolerance in patients with treated congestive heart failure. Fifty-seven patients (stratified according to ACE genotype as 17 DD, 28 ID, 12 II) with ischaemic and dilated cardiomyopathy, LVEF <35% and <10 pack-years of smoking history were studied. All patients were receiving standard therapy for left ventricular systolic dysfunction. Pulmonary function, LVEF, serum ACE, plasma angiotensin II, atrial natriuretic peptide and brain natriuretic peptide were measured at baseline. Peak VO$_2$ and gas exchange measurements were assessed with graded exercise.

INTERPRETATION. Resting LVEF was similar among the genotype groups (25–28%), and no differences were observed in diastolic function or pulmonary artery pressures (P >0.05). Mean peak VO$_2$ and forced vital capacity (% predicted) were significantly reduced (P <0.05) whereas mean serum ACE activity and plasma angiotensin II concentration were highest in DD homozygotes. Subjects homozygous for the D allele also demonstrated higher mean ventilatory equivalents for carbon dioxide (VE/VCO$_2$) during exercise (P <0.05). The authors conclude that the ACE DD genotype is associated with decreased exercise tolerance in congestive heart failure, possibly mediated by altered pulmonary function. Pharmacological strategies effecting more complete inhibition of serum and tissue ACE and/or potentiation of bradykinin may improve exercise capacity in patients with congestive heart failure and the ACE DD genotype.

Comment

The findings from this small cohort of stable, comprehensively evaluated outpatients are intriguing. Greater confidence will come with evaluation in a larger cohort. As noted by the authors, potential mechanisms for the differences observed between groups include differences in pulmonary or cardiac function, or other neurohumoral or organ effects. The authors also speculate about an ACE polymorphism dosage effect for exercise capacity. While this hypothesis is attractive, testing it will require a much larger population of patients with heart failure.

Synergistic polymorphisms of β_1- and α_{2C}-adrenergic receptors and the risk of congestive heart failure

Small KM, Wagoner LE, Levin AM, Kardia SLR, Liggett SB. *N Engl J Med* 2002; **347**: 1135–42

BACKGROUND. Sustained cardiac adrenergic stimulation has been implicated in the development and progression of heart failure. Release of norepinephrine is controlled by negative feedback from presynaptic α_{2C}-adrenergic receptors, and the targets of the released norepinephrine on myocytes are β_1-adrenergic receptors. In transfected cells, a polymorphic α_{2C}-adrenergic receptor (α_{2C}Del322–325) has decreased function, and a variant of the β_1-adrenergic receptor (β_1Arg389) has increased function. The authors hypothesized that this combination of receptor variants, which results in increased synaptic norepinephrine release and enhanced receptor function at the myocyte, would predispose persons to heart failure. Genotyping at these loci was performed in 159 patients with heart failure and 189 controls. Logistic-regression methods were used to determine the potential effect of each genotype and the interaction between them with respect to the risk of heart failure.

INTERPRETATION. Among black subjects, the adjusted odds ratio for heart failure among persons who were homozygous for α_{2C}Del322–325 compared with those with the other α_{2C}-adrenergic receptor genotypes was 5.65 (95% confidence interval [CI], 2.67 to 11.95; $P <0.001$). There was no increase in risk with β_1Arg389 alone. However, there was a marked increase in the risk of heart failure among persons who were homozygous for both variants (adjusted odds ratio 10.11; 95% CI, 2.11–48.53; $P = 0.004$) (Table 15.1). The patients with heart failure did not differ from the controls in the frequencies of nine short tandem-repeat alleles. Among white subjects, there were too few who were homozygous for both polymorphisms to allow an adequate assessment of risk. The α_{2C}Del322–325 and β_1Arg389 receptors act synergistically to increase the risk of heart failure in blacks. Genotyping at these two loci may be a useful approach for the identification of persons at risk for heart failure or its progression, who may be candidates for early preventive measures.

Comment

This important contribution connects previously demonstrated altered functions of known β_1- and α_{2C}-adrenergic receptor polymorphisms with the risk of heart failure. The β_1-adrenergic variants (Arg- or Gly-389) and their physiology have been investigated previously by this group |**1**| as summarized briefly in Fig. 15.2. The β_1-adrenergic receptor variants and their physiology in heart failure are reviewed more extensively in the review that follows. A substantial part of the interpretation of this study rests on known neurohormonal and adrenergic receptor pathway alterations in patients with heart failure—the increased norepinephrine exposure of myocardium mediated principally via β_1-adrenergic receptors. Thus, as shown in Fig. 15.2, alterations to the function of the α_{2C} receptor to augment norepinephrine release in sympathetic nerve terminals, especially when combined with altered

Table 15.1 Genotype and gene–gene interactions of α_2- and β_1-adrenergic receptor variants in relation to heart failure*

Racial group	α_{2c}-adrenergic receptor	β_1-adrenergic receptor	Controls	Patients with heart failure	Adjusted odds ratio for heart failure (95% CI)	P value
			no. of subjects			
Black subjects			84	78		
	≥1 Wild-type	≥1 Gly389	49	29	1.00	
	≥1 Wild-type	Arg389/Arg389	21	8	0.55 (0.21–1.44)	0.23
	Del322–325/Del322–325	≥1 Gly389	12	26	3.87 (1.65–9.05)	0.002
	Del322–325/Del322–325	Arg389/Arg389	2	15	10.11 (2.11–48.53)	0.004
White subjects			105	81		
	≥1 Wild-type	≥1 Gly389	42	35	1.00	
	≥1 Wild-type	Arg389/Arg389	61	40	0.85 (0.39–1.85)	0.68
	Del322–325/Del322–325	≥1 Gly389	0	3	Undefined	–
	Del322–325/Del322–325	Arg389/Arg389	2	3	2.14 (0.13–36.85)	0.60

*Subjects with at least one wild-type α_{2c}-adrenergic receptor allele and at least one β_1-Gly389 allele served as the reference group. Odds ratios are adjusted for sex and age. In the analysis of white subjects, because there were no subjects in one of the cells, the odds ratios for the other two genotypes represent single (two-by-two) comparisons with the reference group.
Source: Small et al. (2002).

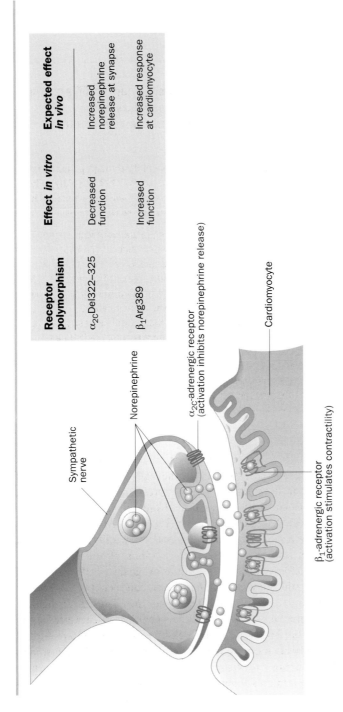

Receptor polymorphism	Effect *in vitro*	Expected effect *in vivo*
α_{2C}Del322–325	Decreased function	Increased norepinephrine release at synapse
β_1Arg389	Increased function	Increased response at cardiomyocyte

Fig. 15.2 Basis of the hypothesis that the α_{2C}Del322–325 and β_1Arg389 receptors act synergistically as risk factors for heart failure. The 2C-adrenergic receptor (along with the 2A-adrenergic receptor) inhibits norepinephrine release at cardiac presynaptic nerve endings through negative feedback. The presence of the dysfunctional 2CDel322–325 receptor would be expected to result in enhanced norepinephrine release. The 1-adrenergic receptor is the receptor for norepinephrine on the cardiomyocyte, and the presence of the hyperfunctional 1Arg389 receptor would be expected to increase contractile response at the myocyte. The combination of increased norepinephrine release and increased responsiveness of the receptor was hypothesized to be a risk factor for heart failure. Source: Small *et al.* (2002).

sensitivity of β_1-adrenergic receptors, build a plausible scenario that might affect heart failure outcomes.

β_1-Adrenergic receptor polymorphisms confer differential function and predisposition to heart failure
Mialet Perez JM, Rathz DA, Petrashevskaya NN, *et al. Nat Med* 2003; **9**: 1300–5

BACKGROUND. Catecholamines stimulate cardiac contractility through β_1-adrenergic receptors, which in humans are polymorphic at amino acid residue 389 (Arg/Gly). The authors used cardiac-targeted transgenesis in a mouse model to delineate mechanisms accounting for the association of Arg389 with human heart failure phenotypes.

INTERPRETATION. Hearts from young Arg389 mice had enhanced receptor function and contractility compared with Gly389 hearts. Older Arg389 mice displayed a phenotypic switch, with decreased β-agonist signalling to adenylyl cyclase and decreased cardiac contractility compared with Gly389 hearts. Arg389 hearts had abnormal expression of fetal and hypertrophy genes and calcium-cycling proteins, decreased adenylyl cyclase and $G\alpha_s$ expression, and fibrosis with heart failure This phenotype was recapitulated in homozygous, end-stage, failing human hearts. In addition, haemodynamic responses to β-receptor blockade were greater in Arg389 mice, and homozygosity for Arg389 was associated with improvement in ventricular function during carvedilol treatment in heart failure patients. Thus, the human Arg389 variant predisposes to heart failure by instigating hyperactive signalling programmes leading to depressed receptor coupling and ventricular dysfunction, and influences the therapeutic response to β-receptor blockade.

Comment

This important contribution from Dr Liggett and his Cincinnati colleagues now adds data from murine transgenic lines expressing either the Arg389 or Gly389 variants of the β_1-adrenergic receptor with cardiac-restricted expression using the β-myosin heavy-chain promoter. Isolated heart preparations from non-transgenic animals (NTG) or the Gly389 or Arg389 animals are shown (Fig. 15.3). At 3 months of age, the responses of the Gly389 variant show elevated basal contractility and heart rate, and contractility is greater with increasing concentrations of the β-adrenergic agonist dobutamine (Fig. 15.3). However, by 6 months of age the Gly389 β-receptor signalling pathway, while still showing elevated basal contractility, has lost all responsiveness to dobutamine. To further elucidate the mechanisms of this loss of contractility in the murine hearts, adenylyl cyclase activity was measured using the β_1-adrenergic agonist GW805415, the non-selective agent isoproterenol and forskolin, which stimulates adenylyl cyclase directly (Fig. 15.4). These studies demonstrated that the reduction in contractility could be explained by receptor uncoupling. The similar experiments shown in panel B used preparations from failing human left ventricular myocardium selected by β_1-adrenergic receptor variant.

Greater dysfunction was observed in the Arg389 variant in preparations from these end-stage failing hearts with advanced disease, congruent with the experimental findings in murine hearts at the later time point (6 months). The summary of these experiments suggests that the Arg389 variant provides greater β_1-adrenergic receptor signalling in early life, but with time, particularly with a chronic myocardial disease

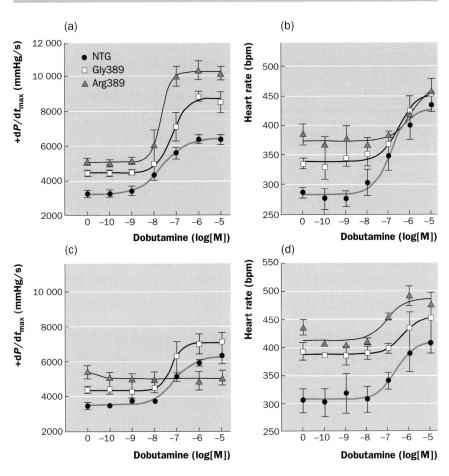

Fig. 15.3 Functional consequences of polymorphic 1-AR expression in transgenic mouse hearts. (a,b) Work-performing heart studies at 3 months of age reveal enhanced contractility (+dP/dtmax) a) and heart rates (b) at baseline, and an enhanced contractile response to the 1-AR agonist dobutamine ($n = 5$; $P < 0.01$ for Arg389 compared with Gly389 1-AR transgenic mice). (c,d) Studies at 6 months of age of contractile (c) and heart rate (d) responses reveal a loss of contractile responses to agonist in Arg389, but not Gly389, 1-AR transgenic mice ($P < 0.01$; $n = 5$). NTG, non-transgenic. Symbols in b–d are same as in a. Source: Mialet Perez *et al.* (2003).

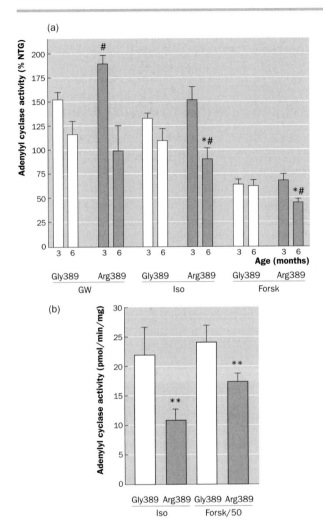

Fig. 15.4 Phenotypic switching of Arg389 and Gly389 1-AR signalling in mouse and human ventricles. (a) -AR stimulation of adenylyl cyclase activity by the agonists GW805415 (GW) and isoproterenol (Iso) undergoes a marked decrease between the ages of 3 and 6 months, in Arg389 ventricular membranes of mice. Similarly, forskolin (Forsk)-stimulated activities are reduced in an age-dependent fashion in Arg389, but not Gly389, mice. * $P < 0.02$ for 3 months compared with 6 months, within genotype; # $P < 0.02$ between genotypes of the same age ($n = 5$–9). (b) Membranes from homozygous 1-AR variant human end-stage failing hearts show depressed function of the Arg389 variant. Stimulation of Arg389 membranes with isoproterenol and forskolin (Forsk/50, values divided by 50) show decreased signalling compared with Gly389 membranes. ** $P < 0.01$ for Arg389 versus Gly389. ($n = 6$ in each group). Source: Mialet Perez *et al.* (2003).

such as heart failure, signalling progressively diminishes. This 'phenotype switching' with progression of disease is a novel observation. It implies that different therapeutic emphases may be tailored for receptor variants, depending upon the stage of disease.

Mutations of single genes associated with dilated cardiomyopathy

The link between DCM and heart failure is intuitively obvious to most clinicians. Yet it is important to clearly define the interrelationships of DCM and heart failure.

Heart failure is a multisystem neurohormonal disease characterized by a clinical syndrome with manifold signs, symptoms and presentations. The key features of heart failure are symptoms: the recent American Heart Association/American College of Cardiology (AHA/ACC) guidelines define heart failure as 'a complex clinical syndrome that can result from any structural or functional cardiac disorder that impairs the ability of the ventricle to fill with or eject blood' |2|. This definition includes heart failure that results from a variety of myocardial disorders (excluding pericardial and other diseases of the great vessels, as well as aetiologies from thyroid and anaemias), but the most common final cause of heart failure is from the systolic dysfunction that is usually associated with left ventricular enlargement (LVE). This duo, systolic dysfunction and LVE, forms the basis of the diagnosis of DCM, an anatomical description of the most common cause of heart failure. Of note, it is common that some patients are discovered to have DCM but have no symptoms, and thus do not have heart failure. This may be particularly prevalent in patients with early DCM and relatively preserved ventricular function.

To understand the genetic causes of heart failure, it is necessary to investigate the specific disorders that underlie its development. The most common cause of heart failure is DCM. DCM is a specific disease of the myocardium defined by LVE and reduced systolic function. Idiopathic dilated cardiomyopathy (IDC) is defined as DCM without an identifiable aetiology following a comprehensive evaluation; the term indicates that an aetiological search has been completed, and common aetiologies, such as coronary artery disease (associated with 'ischaemic cardiomyopathy'), have been excluded.

We now know that one-quarter to one-half of patients diagnosed with IDC have family members similarly involved |3–5|. Prior to 1985, scattered case reports suggested that approximately 1–2% of patients with IDC had family members with a similar condition, termed familial DCM (FDC). FDC was therefore thought to be infrequent and genetic factors were considered an unusual cause of IDC. However, systematic studies in the mid-1980s to the early 1990s, usually using the family history, suggested rates from 2 to 10%. When first-degree relatives of individuals with IDC were systematically examined by echocardiography, FDC rates were observed to be 10–33% |3,6,7|. A keynote clinical study that used echocardiography to screen first-degree relatives in 1992 |3| provided the most compelling evidence that

FDC was present in 20% of patients with IDC and suggested that a genetic basis was likely. Using less stringent criteria, such as isolated LVE to identify familial disease, the two largest and most recent studies have suggested that 35–48% of all patients with IDC have relatives with a similar condition |4,5|.

FDC has been reported most commonly (70–90%) with autosomal dominant inheritance |8|, and to date mutations in 14 autosomal genes have been suggested to be causative, including: lamin A/C |9,10–13|, desmin |14|, actin |15|, δ-sarcoglycan |16|, β-myosin heavy chain |17|, cardiac troponin T |17–19|, α-tropomyosin |20|, titin |21|, metavinculin |22|, myosin-binding protein C |23|, muscle LIM protein |24,25|, α-actinin-2 |25|, phospholamban |26| and Cypher |27|. While mutations in the lamin A/C and β-myosin heavy chain genes may together be responsible for 10–20% of FDC, the other putative genes appear to be rare causes of IDC and FDC, accounting for only a handful of cases each. Collectively, these reports may explain approximately 20–25% of the observed familial DCM.

Two X-linked genes, dystrophin |28| and G4.5 |29|, have also been shown to cause IDC and FDC. Autosomal recessive and mitochondrial inheritance has also been reported, though less commonly.

One of the most challenging issues in the investigation of genetic causes of heart failure is the establishment of genotype–phenotype relationships. This is especially important in order to establish the causation of DCM from a mutation, which in the case of autosomal dominant inheritance is usually a single-base missense or nonsense mutation. The difficulty stems from proving that the DCM phenotype – LVE and systolic dysfunction – have resulted from a single base mutation. How does the researcher convince the scientific community that the identified mutation may cause DCM? The disease phenotype should segregate with the mutation in a large family containing members that have both normal and affected phenotypes. Ideally, these associations can be identified in multiple families. Other evidence that builds the case includes a plausible pathophysiological role of the putative disease gene in DCM. Further evidence of DCM in an animal model harbouring the same mutation also strengthens the case.

A number of other major scientific issues remain in this rapidly evolving field. How many additional genes will be implicated in FDC? Are there one or two disease genes that may account for a substantial fraction of FDC? The answers to these questions remain to be elucidated in the years to come.

Expanding the phenotype of *LMNA* mutations in dilated cardiomyopathy and functional consequences of these mutations

Sébillon P, Bouchier C, Bidot LD, *et al. J Med Genet* 2003; **40**: 560–7

BACKGROUND. Mutations in the lamin A/C gene (*LMNA*) were first implicated in DCM associated with conduction system disease and/or skeletal myopathy in 1999. Since then, other groups have identified *LMNA* mutations in families with similar phenotypes. The aim of this study was to perform a mutational analysis of *LMNA* in a large white population of patients affected by DCM with or without associated symptoms. The authors performed screening of the coding sequence of *LMNA* on DNA samples from 66 index cases, and carried out cell transfection experiments to examine the functional consequences of the mutations identified.

INTERPRETATION. Three mutations were identified: (1) a new missense mutation was identified in a family with early atrial fibrillation; (2) a previously described mutation was identified in a family with a quadriceps myopathy associated with DCM; and (3) a new mutation leading to a premature stop codon was identified in a family affected by DCM with conduction defects. All three index patients had affected family members who also carried the mutation; no mutation in *LMNA* was found in cases with isolated DCM. The authors also performed functional analyses, and proposed potential physiopathological mechanisms for the identified mutations, including haploinsufficiency and intermediate filament disorganization.

Comment

Mutations in *LMNA* are a rare but important cause of DCM. The 4.5% incidence observed in this study is at the low end of the 5–15% frequency range reported by other groups. Although each of the mutations identified in this paper was in an individual who had affected family members, *LMNA* mutations have also been reported in individuals with IDC and have been demonstrated to be *de novo* in these individuals. As these authors propose, the variable phenotypes observed in *LMNA*-associated DCM might be explained by the variability of functional consequences of *LMNA* mutations.

Natural history of dilated cardiomyopathy due to lamin A/C gene mutations
Taylor MRG, Fain PR, Sinagra G, *et al. J Am Coll Cardiol* 2003; **41**: 771–80

BACKGROUND. Mutations in *LMNA* have been found in patients with DCM with familial conduction defects and muscular dystrophy, but the clinical spectrum, prognosis and clinical relevance of laminopathies in DCM are largely unknown. The authors examined the prevalence, genotype–phenotype correlation and natural history of *LMNA* gene mutations in subjects with DCM. A cohort of 49 nuclear families, 40 with familial DCM and nine with sporadic DCM (269 subjects, 105 affected), was screened for mutations in *LMNA* using denaturing high-performance liquid chromatography and sequence analysis. Bivariate analysis of clinical predictors of *LMNA* mutation carrier status and Kaplan–Meier survival analysis were performed.

INTERPRETATION. Mutations in *LMNA* were detected in 4/49 individuals (8%); three with familial DCM and one with sporadic DCM. There was significant phenotypic variability, but the presence of skeletal muscle involvement (*P* <0.001), supraventricular arrhythmia (*P* = 0.003), conduction defects (*P* = 0.01) and 'mildly' dilated cardiomyopathy (*P* = 0.006) were predictors of *LMNA* mutations. The *LMNA* mutation carriers had a significantly poorer cumulative survival compared with non-carrier DCM patients: event-free survival at the age of 45 years was 31% versus 75% in non-carriers. Mutations in *LMNA* cause severe and progressive DCM in a relevant proportion of patients. Mutation screening should be considered in patients with DCM, in particular when clinical predictors of *LMNA* mutation are present, regardless of the family history.

Comment

The authors suggest a role for *LMNA* mutation screening in patients with DCM, whether or not they have a positive family history of DCM. DNA testing of patients with DCM is not currently part of routine cardiovascular assessment, but the authors suggest that it could play a meaningful role.

Dilated cardiomyopathy and heart failure caused by a mutation in phospholamban

Schmitt JP, Kamisago M, Asahi M, *et al. Science* 2003; **299**: 1410–13

BACKGROUND. Phospholamban (PLN) is an abundant, 52-amino acid transmembrane sarcoplasmic reticulum phosphoprotein that regulates the Ca^{2+} adenosine triphosphatase SERCA2a pump. Studies in mice had suggested that PLN plays a fundamental role in heart failure: PLN protein levels were shown to correlate with cardiac contractile parameters; superinhibitory PLN molecules were known to impair heart function; and PLN ablation was demonstrated to rescue a mouse heart failure model. The authors therefore speculated that PLN has a role in human heart failure.

INTERPRETATION. The PLN gene was sequenced in 20 unrelated individuals with inherited DCM and heart failure. An Arg→Cys missense mutation was identified at residue 9 in one individual. The mutation was demonstrated to cosegregate with other affected individuals in the proband's family (Fig. 15.5). The authors then created transgenic PLN^R9C mice, which recapitulated human heart failure with premature death (Fig. 15.6). They also performed cellular and biochemical studies that revealed that, unlike wild-type PLN, PLN^R9C did not directly inhibit SERCA2a. Rather, PLN^R9C trapped protein kinase A (PKA), which blocked PKA-mediated phosphorylation of wild-type PLN and in turn delayed the decay of calcium transients in myocytes. The authors concluded that myocellular calcium dysregulation can initiate human heart failure.

Comment

This important contribution expands our understanding of the pathophysiological basis of DCM, as all of the mutations implicated in DCM prior to this paper were in genes encoding proteins of the sarcomere or cytoskeleton, thought to cause DCM through impairment of force production or transmission. In contrast, the mechanism behind PLN-associated DCM is proposed to involve direct disturbance of myocellular Ca^{2+} metabolism due to constitutive SERCA2a inhibition.

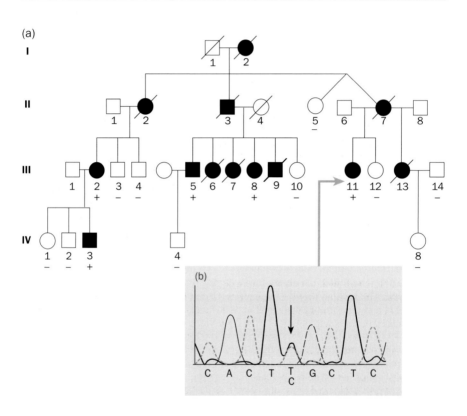

Fig. 15.5 Cosegregation of PLNR9C and dilated cardiomyopathy in a large family. (a) Pedigree showing clinical status (circle, female; square, male; solid symbol, affected; clear symbol, unaffected; slashed symbol, death) and genetic status (+, PLNR9C/+; –, PLNwt). Clinical status was assessed without knowledge of genotype. Subjects III-2, III-5, III-8, and III-13 underwent heart transplantation. Individual III-11 (arrow) was the proband, (b) DNA sequence analysis of the PLN gene in the proband revealing a cytosine-to-thymidine substitution at nucleotide 25. The line of the trace reflects the presence of a specific nucleotide residue: C, thick; A, thin; T, short dash; and G, long dash. Source: Schmitt *et al.* (2003).

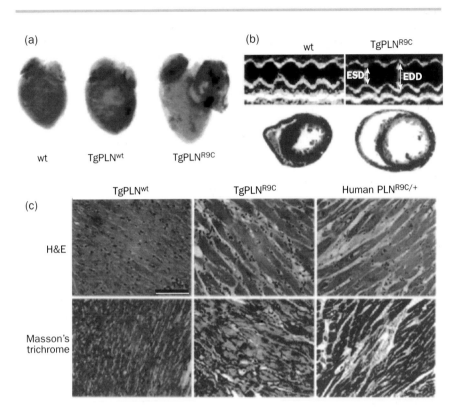

Fig. 15.6 Characterization of hearts expressing PLNR9C. (a) Hearts of strain-matched wild-type (wt), TgPLNwt, and TgPLNR9C mice at 4 months of age, showing enlargement of TgPLNR9C hearts only. (b) Upper panels: *in vivo* assessment of left ventricular diameters and function by echocardiography (M-mode). End-systolic diameters (ESD) and end-diastolic diameters (EDD) were increased in the TgPLNR9C mice. Lower panels: *ex vivo* cross sections show biventricular dilatation of the TgPLNR9C heart (right). (c) Histopathology of left ventricular heart tissue from 12-week-old, strain-matched TgPLNwt and TgPLNR9C mice and a human heterozygous for PLNR9C. Upper panels: haematoxylin and eosin (H&E) staining reveals normal tissue in TgPLNwt mice and enlarged myocytes and nuclei in the TgPLNR9C mouse and human PLNR9C/+ tissue. Lower panels: collagen staining (Masson's trichrome) shows massive interstitial fibrosis in PLNR9C mouse and human hearts. All images are shown at equal magnification. Scale bar, 100 μm. Source: Schmitt *et al.* (2003).

Idiopathic restrictive cardiomyopathy is part of the clinical expression of cardiac troponin I mutations

Mogensen J, Kubo T, Duque M, *et al. J Clin Invest* 2003; **111**: 209–16

BACKGROUND. Restrictive cardiomyopathy (RCM) is an uncommon heart muscle disorder characterized by impaired filling of the ventricles with reduced volume in the presence of normal or near-normal wall thickness and systolic function. The disease may be associated with systemic disease but is most often idiopathic. The authors recognized a large family in which individuals were affected by either idiopathic RCM or hypertrophic cardiomyopathy (HCM).

INTERPRETATION. Linkage analysis to selected sarcomeric contractile protein genes identified cardiac troponin I (*TNNI3*) as the likely disease gene in the family. Subsequent mutation analysis revealed a novel missense mutation, which cosegregated with the disease in the family. To determine if idiopathic RCM is part of the clinical expression of *TNNI3* mutations, genetic investigations of the gene were performed in an additional nine unrelated RCM patients with restrictive filling patterns, biatrial dilatation, normal systolic function and normal wall thickness. *TNNI3* mutations were identified in six of these nine RCM patients. Two of the mutations identified in young individuals were *de novo* mutations. All mutations appeared in conserved and functionally important domains of the gene.

Comment

Mutations in genes encoding sarcomeric proteins had previously been reported to be associated with HCM and DCM, and mutations in *TNNI3* specifically had been reported in a small number of HCM families |**30**|. However, this is the first report of any disease gene associated with RCM, and, interestingly, it was found in a family having some individuals with RCM and others with HCM. These findings indicate that idiopathic RCM is part of the clinical expression of sarcomeric contractile protein disease and of HCM. The fact that *TNNI3* mutations were identified in two *de novo* RCM cases (in which the parents were negative for the gene mutation) indicates that, as with HCM and DCM, not all patients with a genetic basis for their disease will have a positive family history. Clinical screening is often recommended for family members of individuals with idiopathic RCM and HCM (and DCM) in an effort to detect early signs of disease. The discovery of a gene mutation which appears to cause both idiopathic RCM and HCM in the same family suggests that clinical screening of family members should include a vigilant search for evidence of either phenotype. *TNNI3* mutations appear to be a very common cause of idiopathic restrictive cardiomyopathy, and further studies of the gene may provide insight into the pathophysiology of other forms of cardiomyopathy as well.

Mutations in *Cypher/ZASP* in patients with dilated cardiomyopathy and left ventricular non-compaction

Vatta M, Mohapatra B, Jimenez S, *et al. J Am Coll Cardiol* 2003; **42**: 2014–27

BACKGROUND. *Cypher/ZASP* is a recently identified gene encoding a protein that is a component of the Z-line in both skeletal and cardiac muscle. A *Cypher/ZASP* knockout mouse had been shown to develop a severe congenital myopathy and DCM; therefore the authors evaluated the role of this gene in the pathogenesis of human DCM with or without isolated non-compaction of the left ventricular myocardium (INLVM). INLVM is characterized by a hypertrophic dilated left ventricle, ventricular dysfunction and deep trabeculations. Like DCM, it is often inherited, although the causative genes identified to date differ from those causing DCM. The authors screened (by echocardiogram, electrocardiogram, physical examination and creatine kinase measurement) and performed mutation analysis (by denaturing high-performance liquid chromatography and direct deoxyribonucleic acid sequencing) on 100 probands with left ventricular dysfunction (DCM or INLVM). Five mutations in six probands (6% of cases) were identified in patients with familial or sporadic DCM or INLVM. *In vitro* studies showed cytoskeleton disarray in cells transfected with mutated *Cypher/ZASP*. The authors suggest that mutated *Cypher/ZASP* can cause DCM and INLVM and identify a mechanistic basis.

INTERPRETATION. *Cypher/ZASP* is the most recent in a now long list of genes shown to be associated with DCM and, in this case, other forms of left ventricular dysfunction. No definitive genotype–phenotype correlations can be generated.

Comment

This work suggests that disruption of the *Cypher/ZASP* gene is responsible for approximately 6% of cases of left ventricular dysfunction (DCM or INLVM). This gene encodes a specific Z-line PDZ-domain protein that plays a potentially important role in bridging the sarcomere to the cytoskeletal network. This supports the concept that disruption of the cytoarchitecture, comprising the cytoskeleton, sarcolemma and interacting components, is pivotal to the development of LV dysfunction.

Conclusion

The identification and investigation of genes contributing to and/or causing the development of heart failure is proceeding rapidly. Despite these advances, however, DNA testing is not currently widely available as a part of routine cardiovascular risk assessment and management. The development of clinically useful, comprehensive genetic tests for heart failure is currently complicated by (1) the number of different putative genes, most of which could have mutations at many different locations throughout the gene (locus and allelic heterogeneity); (2) the knowledge that a significant proportion of heart failure cases are not attributable to any of the known genes; and (3), perhaps most importantly, the difficulty of establishing meaningful genotype–phenotype correlations. Additional genes that cause or contribute to the development of heart failure are likely to be identified. However, sensitive, comprehensive and affordable DNA tests may not be widely available for years.

Once we have the ability to identify specific putative gene mutations in individual patients, DNA diagnostics will add an important component to the comprehensive evaluation of the heart failure patient. As reliable genotype–phenotype correlations are elucidated, they may provide useful knowledge about the likely disease course and severity as well as the effectiveness of various medications and other therapies.

DNA diagnostics will also allow family members of patients with known mutations to consider presymptomatic genetic testing. Individuals identified as having the at-risk genotype could plan aggressive surveillance for early signs of disease at appropriate intervals, as well as prophylactic treatment. Those found to be negative could be provided with some degree of reassurance, and could avoid years of unnecessary and costly screening tests.

A greater understanding of the genes that play a role in the development of heart failure will eventually enhance cardiovascular patient evaluation. The identification of the specific molecular bases of heart failure may also allow the use of genotype-specific therapies. However, it will be imperative for those providing genetic counselling to understand the implications and limitations of DNA testing and genotype–phenotype correlations |31|.

References

1. Beta-Blocker Evaluation of Survival Trial Investigators. A trial of the beta-blocker bucindolol in patients with advanced chronic heart failure. *N Engl J Med* 2001; **344**: 1659–67.

2. Hunt S, Baker D, Chin M, Cinquegrani M, Feldman A, Francis G, Ganiats T, Goldstein S, Gregoratos G, Jessup M, Noble R, Packer M, Silver M, Stevenson L. ACC/AHA guidelines for the evaluation and management of chronic heart failure in the adult: a report of the American College of Cardiology/American Heart Association Task Force on Practice Guidelines. http://www.acc.org/clinical/guidelines/failure/hf_index.htm. 2001.

3. Michels VV, Moll PP, Miller FA, Tajik J, Chu JS, Driscoll DJ, Burnett JC, Rodeheffer RJ, Chesebro JH, Tazelaar HD. The frequency of familial dilated cardiomyopathy in a series of patients with idiopathic dilated cardiomyopathy. *New Engl J Med* 1992; **326**: 77–82.

4. Baig MK, Goldman JH, Caforio AP, Coonar AS, Keeling PJ, McKenna WJ. Familial dilated cardiomyopathy: cardiac abnormalities are common in asymptomatic relatives and may represent early disease. *J Am Coll Cardiol* 1998; **31**: 195–201.

5. Grünig E, Tasman JA, Kücherer H, Franz W, Kubler W, Katus HA. Frequency and pheno-types of familial dilated cardiomyopathy. *J Am Coll Cardiol* 1998; **31**: 186–94.

6. Fragola PV, Autore C, Picelli A, Sommariva L, Cannata D, Sangiorgi M. Familial idio-pathic dilated cardiomyopathy. *Am Heart J* 1988; **115**: 912–14.

7. Keeling P, Gang Y, Smith G, Seo H, Bent SE, Murday V, Caforio A, McKenna W. Familial dilated cardiomyopathy in the United Kingdom. *Br Heart J* 1995; **73**: 417–21.

8. Mestroni L, Rocco C, Gregori D, Sinagra G, DiLenarda A, Miocic S, Vatta M, Pinamonti B, Muntoni F, Caforio L, McKenna W, Falaschi A, Giacca M, Camerini F. Familial dilated cardiomyopathy: evidence for genetic and phenotypic heterogeneity. *J Am Coll Cardiol* 1999; **34**: 181–90.

9. Fatkin D, MacRae C, Sasaki T, Wolff M, Porcu M, Frenneaux M, Atherton J, Vidaillet H, Spudich S, Girolami U, Seidman J, Seidman C. Missense mutations in the rod domain of the lamin A/C gene as causes of dilated cardiomyopathy and conduction-system disease. *N Engl J Med* 1999; **341**: 1715–24.

10. Becane HM, Bonne G, Varnous S, Muchir A, Ortega V, Hammouda EH, Urtizberea JA, Lavergne T, Fardeau M, Eymard B, Weber S, Schwartz K, Duboc D. High incidence of sudden death with conduction system and myocardial disease due to lamins A and C gene mutation. *Pacing Clin Electrophysiol* 2000; **23**(11 Pt 1): 1661–6.

11. Brodsky G, Muntoni F, Miocic S, Sinagra G, Sewry C, Mestroni L. Lamin A/C gene muta-tion associated with dilated cardiomyopathy with variable skeletal muscle involvement. *Circulation* 2000; **101**: 473–6.

12. Jakobs PM, Hanson E, Crispell KA, Toy W, Keegan H, Schilling K, Icenogle T, Litt M, Hershberger RE. Novel lamin A/C mutations in two families with dilated cardiomyopathy and conduction system disease. *J Card Fail* 2001; **7**: 249–56.

13. Hershberger RE, Hanson E, Jakobs PM, Keegan H, Coates K, Bousman S, Litt M. A novel lamin A/C mutation in a family with dilated cardiomyopathy, prominent conduction system disease, and need for permanent pacemaker implantation. *Am Heart J* 2002; **144**: 1081–6.

14. Li D, Tapscoft T, Gonzalez O, Burch P, Quinones M, Zoghbi W, Hill R, Bachinski L, Mann D, Roberts R. Desmin mutation responsible for idiopathic dilated cardiomyopathy. *Circulation* 1999; **100**: 461–4.

15. Olson TM, Michels VV, Thibodeau SN, Tai YS, Keating MT. Actin mutations in dilated cardiomyopathy, a heritable form of heart failure. *Science* 1998; **280**: 750–2.

16. Tsubata S, Bowles KR, Vatta M, Zintz C, Titus J, Muhonen L, Bowles NE, Towbin JA. Mutations in the human delta-sarcoglycan gene in familial and sporadic dilated cardio-myopathy. *J Clin Invest* 2000; **106**: 655–62.

17. Kamisago M, Sharma SD, DePalma SR, Solomon S, Sharma P, McDonough B, Smoot L, Mullen MP, Woolf PK, Wigle ED, Seidman JG, Seidman CE. Mutations in sarcomere protein genes as a cause of dilated cardiomyopathy. *N Engl J Med* 2000; **343**: 1688–96.

18. Li D, Czernuszewicz GZ, Gonzalez O, Tapscott T, Karibe A, Durand JB, Brugada R, Hill R, Gregoritch JM, Anderson JL, Quinones M, Bachinski LL, Roberts R. Novel cardiac troponin T mutation as a cause of familial dilated cardiomyopathy. *Circulation* 2001; **104**: 2188–93.

19. Hanson E, Jakobs P, Keegan H, Coates K, Bousman S, Dienel N, Litt M, Hershberger R. Cardiac troponin T lysine-210 deletion in a family with dilated cardiomyopathy. *J Card Fail* 2002; **8**: 28–32.

20. Olson TM, Kishimoto NY, Whitby FG, Michels VV. Mutations that alter the surface charge of alpha-tropomyosin are associated with dilated cardiomyopathy. *J Mol Cell Cardiol* 2001; **33**: 723–32.

21. Gerull B, Gramlich M, Atherton J, McNabb M, Trombitas K, Sasse-Klaassen S, Seidman JG, Seidman C, Granzier H, Labeit S, Frenneaux M, Thierfelder L. Mutations of TTN, encoding the giant muscle filament titin, cause familial dilated cardiomyopathy. *Nat Genet* 2002; **14**: 14.

22. Olson TM, Illenberger S, Kishimoto NY, Huttelmaier S, Keating MT, Jockusch BM. Metavinculin mutations alter actin interaction in dilated cardiomyopathy. *Circulation* 2002; **105**: 431–7.

23. Daehmlow S, Erdmann J, Knueppel T, Gille C, Froemmel C, Hummel M, Hetzer R, Regitz-Zagrosek V. Novel mutations in sarcomeric protein genes in dilated cardio-myopathy. *Biochem Biophys Res Commun* 2002; **298**: 116–20.

24. Knoll R, Hoshijima M, Hoffman HM, Person V, Lorenzen-Schmidt I, Bang ML, Hayashi T, Shiga N, Yasukawa H, Schaper W, McKenna W, Yokoyama M, Schork NJ, Omens JH, McCulloch AD, Kimura A, Gregorio CC, Poller W, Schaper J, Schultheiss HP, Chien KR. The cardiac mechanical stretch sensor machinery involves a Z disc complex that is defective in a subset of human dilated cardiomyopathy. *Cell* 2002; **111**: 943–55.

25. Mohapatra B, Jimenez S, Lin JH, Bowles KR, Coveler KJ, Marx JG, Chrisco MA, Murphy RT, Lurie PR, Schwartz RJ, Elliott PM, Vatta M, McKenna W, Towbin JA, Bowles NE. Mutations in the muscle LIM protein and alpha-actinin-2 genes in dilated cardio-myopathy and endocardial fibroelastosis. *Mol Genet Metab* 2003; **80**: 207–15.

26. Schmitt JP, Kamisago M, Asahi M, Li GH, Ahmad F, Mende U, Kranias EG, MacLennan DH, Seidman JG, Seidman CE. Dilated cardiomyopathy and heart failure caused by a mutation in phospholamban. *Science* 2003; **299**: 1410–13.

27. Vatta M, Mohapatra B, Jimenez S, Sanchez X, Faulkner G, Perles Z, Sinagra G, Lin JH, Vu TM, Zhou Q, Bowles KR, Di Lenarda A, Schimmenti L, Fox M, Chrisco MA, Murphy RT, McKenna W, Elliott P, Bowles NE, Chen J, Valle G, Towbin JA. Mutations in Cypher/ZASP in patients with dilated cardiomyopathy and left ventricular non-compaction. *J Am Coll Cardiol* 2003; **42**: 2014–27.

28. Towbin JA, Hejtmancik JF, Brink P, Gelb B, Zhu XM, Chamberlain JS, McCabe ER, Swift M. X-linked dilated cardiomyopathy. Molecular genetic evidence of linkage to the Duchenne muscular dystrophy (dystrophin) gene at the Xp21 locus. *Circulation* 1993; **87**: 1854–65.

29. Bione S, D'Adamo P, Maestrini E, Gedeon A, Bolhuis P, Toniolo D. A novel X-linked gene, G4.5, is responsible for Barth syndrome. *Nat Genet* 1996; **12**: 385–9.

30. Kimura A, Harada H, Park J, Nishi H, Satoh M, Takahashi M, Hiroi S, Sasaoka T, Ohbuchi N, Nakamura T, Koyanagi T, Hwang T, Choo J, Chung K, Hasegawa A, Nagai R, Okazaki O, Nakamura H, Matsuzaki M, Sakamoto T, Toshima H, Koga Y, Imaizumi T, Sasazuki T. Mutations in the cardiac troponin I gene associated with hypertrophic cardiomyopathy. *Nat Genet* 1997; **16**: 379–82.

31. Hanson E, Hershberger RE. Genetic counseling and screening issues in familial dilated cardiomyopathy. *J Genet Couns* 2001; **10**: 397–415.

Abbreviations

ACE	angiotensin-coverting enzyme	
ACED	ACE deletion	
AHA/ACC	American Heart Association/American College of Cardiology	
AHI	apnoea–hypopnoea index	
AICD	automatic implantable cardiac defibrillator	
ALVD	asymptomatic left ventricular systolic dysfunction	
ARB	angiotensin receptor blocker	
ATLAS	Assessment of Treatment with Lisinopril and Survival	
ATTACH	Anti-TNFα Therapy Against CHF	
BEST	Beta-blocker Evaluation of Survival Trial	
biw	twice a week	
BNP	brain natriuretic peptide	
BUN	blood urea nitrogen	
CABG	coronary artery bypass grafting	
CAD	coronary artery disease	
CHARM	Candesartan in Heart Failure—Assessment of Reduction in Mortality and Morbidity	
CHF	congestive heart failure	
CI	confidence interval	
CIBIS	Cardiac Insufficiency Bisoprolol Study	
CM	cardiomyopathy	
COMET	Carvedilol Or Metoprolol European Trial	
COMPANION	Comparison of Medical Therapy, Pacing and Defibrillation in Chronic Heart Failure	
CONSENSUS	Cooperative North	

	Scandinavian Enalapril Survival Study
COPERNICUS	Carvedilol Prospective Randomized Cumulative Survival
CPAP	continuous positive airway pressure
CRT	cardiac resynchronization therapy
CSA	central sleep apnoea
CSD	cardiac support device
DAVID	Dual Chamber And VVI Implantable Defibrillator trial
DATASUS	DATA Sistema Unificado de Saúde
DCM	dilated cardiomyopathy
DHF	diastolic heart failure
DIG	Digitalis Investigation Group
Ea	arterial elastance
EARTH	Endothelin A Receptor Antagonist Trial in Heart Failure
EDP	end-diastolic pressure
Ees	end-systolic elastance
EF	ejection fraction
ELITE	Evaluation of Losartan in the Elderly
ENABLE	Endothelin Antagonist Bosentan for Lowering Cardiac Events in Heart Failure
EPHESUS	Eplerenone Post-acute Myocardial Infarction Heart Failure Efficacy and Survival Study
ET	endothelin
FDC	familial dilated cardiomyopathy
FIAU	fluoroiodoarabinouracil

GCSF	granulocyte colony stimulating factor	MONICA	Monitoring Trends and determinants in Cardiovascular Disease
GUSTO	Global Utilization of Streptokinase and t-PA for Occluded Coronary Arteries	MOXCON	Moxonidine in Congestive Heart Failure
		mRNA	messenger RNA
HCM	hypertrophic cardiomyopathy	MSNA	muscle sympathetic nerve activity
HF	heart failure	MUSTIC	multisite stimulation in cardiomyopathy
HF-ACTION	Heart Failure–A Controlled Trial Investigating Outcomes of Exercise Training	NTG	non-transgenic
		NYHA	New York Heart Association
HF-nIEF	heart failure and preserved ejection fraction	OPTIME-CHF	Outcomes of the Prospective Trial of Intravenous Milrinone for Exacerbations of Chronic Heart Failure
HR	hazard ratio		
HSV1-tk	herpesviral thymidine kinase reporter gene	OR	odds ratio
ICD	implantable cardioverter defibrillator	OSA	obstructive sleep apnoea
		OVERTURE	Omapatrilat Versus Enalapril Randomized Trial of Utility in Reducing Events
IDC	idiopathic dilated cardiomyopathy		
IL	interleukin		
INLVM	isolated non-compaction of the left ventricular myocardium	PKA	protein kinase A
		PLN	phospholamban
		pRER	peak respiratory exchange ratio
IRC	idiopathic restrictive cardiomyopathy	PROVED	Prospective Randomized Study of Ventricular Failure and Efficacy of Digoxin
LVAD	left ventricular assist device		
LVE	left ventricular enlargement	PTCA	percutaneous coronary angioplasty
LVEF	left ventricular ejection fraction	PVR	pulmonary vascular resistance
MADIT	Multicenter Automatic Defibrillator Implantation Trial	qw	once a week
		RADIANCE	Randomized Assessment of Digoxin on Inhibitors of the Angiotensin-Converting Enzyme
MERIT	Metoprolol CR/XL Randomized Intervention Trial		
MERIT-HF	Metoprolol Extended-Release Randomized Intervention Trial in Heart Failure	RALES	Randomized Aldactone Evaluation Study
		RCM	restrictive cardiomyopathy
MIRACLE	Multicentre In Sync Randomized Clinical Evaluation	REACH-1	Research on Endothelin Antagonism in Chronic Heart Failure

RECOVER	Research into Etanercept Cytokine Antagonism in Ventricular Dysfunction	SOLVD-P	Studies of Left Ventricular Dysfunction Prevention trial
REMATCH	Randomized Evaluation of Mechanical Assistance for the Treatment of Congestive Heart Failure	SOLVD-T	Studies of Left Ventricular Dysfunction Treatment trial
RENAISSANCE	Randomized Etanercept North American Strategy to Study Antagonism of Cytokines	SPECT	simple photon emission computed tomography
		STICH	Surgical Treatment for Ischaemic Cardiomyopathy trial
RENEWAL	Randomized Etanercept Worldwide Evaluation	SUS	Sistema Unificado de Saúde (Brazil's government medical care)
RESTORE	Reconstructive Endoventricular Surgery, Returning Torsion Original Radius Elliptical Shape to the Left Ventricle	SVT	supraventricular tachycardia
		tiw	three times a week
		TNF	tumour necrosis factor
RITZ	Randomized Intravenous Tezosentan Study	TRACE	Trandolapril Cardiac Evaluation
RR	relative risk	TUNEL	terminal deoxynucleotidyl transferase-mediated deoxyuridine triphosphate nick end labelling
SAVE	Survival and Ventricular Enlargement		
SAVER	surgical anterior ventricular endocardial restoration		
		UNE	urinary norepinephrine
		VAD	ventricular assist device
SCD	sudden cardiac death	Val-HeFT	Valsartan Heart Failure Trial
SCDF-1	stromal cell-derived factor-1		
SCD HeFT	Sudden Cardiac Death Heart Failure Trial	VALIANT	Valsartan in Acute Myocardial Infarction
SCF	stem cell factor	VEGF	vascular endothelial growth factor
SERCA	sarcoplasmic reticulum calcium ATPase	VF	ventricular fibrillation
		V-HeFT	Vasodilator Heart Failure Trial
SHF	systolic heart failure		
SNS	sympathetic nervous system	VT	ventricular tachycardia

Index of papers reviewed

Abraham MR, Olson LJ, Joyner MJ, Turner ST, Beck KC, Johnson BD. Angiotensin-converting enzyme genotype modulates pulmonary function and exercise capacity in treated patients with congestive stable heart failure. *Circulation* 2002; **106**: 1794–9. **241**

Abraham WT, Fisher WG, Smith AL, Delurgio DB, Leon AR, Loh E, Kocovic DZ, Packer M, Clavell AL, Hayes DL, Ellestad M, Trupp RJ, Underwood J, Pickering F, Truex C, McAtee P, Messenger J; Multicenter InSync Randomized Clinical Evaluation (MIRACLE) Study Group. Cardiac resynchronization in chronic heart failure. *N Engl J Med* 2002; **346**(24): 1845–53. **221**

Allman KC, Shaw LJ, Hachamovitch R, Udelson JE. Myocardial viability testing and impact of revascularization on prognosis in patients with coronary artery disease and left ventricular dysfunction: a meta-analysis. *J Am Coll Cardiol* 2002; **39**(7): 1151–8. **106**

Ancoli-Israel S, DuHamel ER, Stepnowsky C, Engler R, Cohen-Zion M, Marler M. The relationship between congestive heart failure, sleep apnea, and mortality in older men. *Chest* 2003; **124**(4): 1400–5. **142**

Aronson E, Burger AJ. Relation between pulse pressure and survival in patients with decompensated heart failure. *Am J Cardiol* 2004; **93**: 785–8. **32**

Arzt M, Harth M, Luchner A, Muders F, Holmer SR, Blumberg FC, Riegger GA, Pfeifer M. Enhanced ventilatory response to exercise in patients with chronic heart failure and central sleep apnea. *Circulation* 2003; **107**(15): 1998–2003. **146**

Ascione R, Narayan P, Rogers CA, Lim KH, Capoun R, Angelini GD. Early and midterm clinical outcome in patients with severe left ventricular dysfunction undergoing coronary artery surgery. *Ann Thorac Surg* 2003; **76**: 793–9. **109**

Baker DW, Einstadter D, Thomas C, Cebul RD. Mortality trends for 23 505 Medicare patients hospitalized with heart failure in Northeast Ohio, 1991 to 1997. *Am Heart J* 2003; **146**(2): 258–64. **5**

Beanlands RS, Ruddy TD, deKemp RA, Iwanochko RM, Coates G, Freeman M, Nahmias C, Hendry P, Burns RJ, Lamy A, Mickleborough L, Kostuk W, Fallen E, Nichol G; PARR Investigators. Positron emission tomography and recovery following revascularization (PARR-1): the importance of scar and the development of a prediction rule for the degree of recovery of left ventricular function. *J Am Coll Cardiol* 2002; **40**(10): 1735–43. **108**

Bengel FM, Anton M, Richter T, Simoes MV, Haubner R, Henke J, Erhardt W, Reder S, Lehner T, Brandau W, Boekstegers P, Nekolla SG, Gansbacher B, Schwaiger M. Non-invasive imaging of transgene expression by use of positron emission tomography in a pig model of myocardial gene transfer. *Circulation* 2003; **108**(17): 2127–33. **29**

Blanchet M, Ducharme A, Racine N, Rouleau JL, Tardif JC, Juneau M, Marquis J, Larivee L, Nigam A, Fortier A, White M. Effects of cold exposure on submaximal exercise performance and adrenergic activation in patients with congestive heart failure and the effects of beta-adrenergic blockade (carvedilol or metoprolol). *Am J Cardiol* 2003; **92**: 548–53. **175**

Bradley DJ, Bradley EA, Baughman KL, Berger RD, Calkins H, Goodman SN, Kass DA, Powe NR. Cardiac resynchronization and death from progressive heart failure: a meta-analysis of randomized controlled trials. *JAMA* 2003; 289(6): 730–40. **222**

Bradley TD, Tkacova R, Hall MJ, Ando S, Floras JS. Augmented sympathetic neural response to simulated obstructive apnoea in human heart failure. *Clin Sci (Lond)* 2003; 104(3): 231–8. **150**

Braunstein JB, Anderson GF, Gerstenblith G, Weller W, Niefield M, Herbert R, Wu AW. Non-cardiac comorbidity increases preventable hospitalizations and mortality among Medicare beneficiaries with chronic heart failure. *J Am Coll Cardiol* 2003; 42(7): 1226–33. **20**

Burger AJ, Horton DP, LeJemtel T, Ghali JK, Torre G, Dennish G, Koren M, Dinerman J, Silver M, Cheng ML, Elkayam U. Effect of nesiritide (B-type natriuretic peptide) and dobutamine on ventricular arrhythmias in the treatment of patients with acutely decompensated congestive heart failure: the Prospective Randomized Evaluation of Cardiac Ectopy with Dobutamine or Natrecor Therapy (PRECEDENT) study. *Am Heart J* 2002; 144: 1102–8. **82**

Chung ES, Packer M, Lo KH, Fasanmade AA, Willerson JT; Anti-TNF Therapy Against Congestive Heart Failure Investigators. Randomized, double-blind, placebo-controlled, pilot trial of infliximab, a chimeric monoclonal antibody to tumor necrosis factor-alpha, in patients with moderate-to-severe heart failure: results of the anti-TNF Therapy Against Congestive Heart Failure (ATTACH) trial. *Circulation* 2003; 107: 3133–40. **84**

Curtis JP, Sokol SI, Wang Y, Rathore SS, Ko DT, Jadbabaie F, Portnay E, Marshalko SJ, Radford MJ, Krumholz HM. The association of left ventricular ejection fraction, mortality, and cause of death in stable outpatients with heart failure. *J Am Coll Cardiol* 2003; 42(4): 736–42. **21 52**

Delagardelle C, Feiereisen P, Autier P, Shita R, Krecke R, Beissel J. Strength/endurance training versus endurance training in congestive heart failure. *Med Sci Sports Ex* 2002; 34 (12): 1868–72. **167**

de Lissovoy G, Stier DM, Ciesla G, Munger M and Burger AJ. Economic implications of nesiritide versus dobutamine in the treatment of patients with acutely decompensated congestive heart failure. *Am J Cardiol* 2003; 92: 631–3. **83**

Di Napoli P, Taccardi AA, Grilli A, Felaco M, Balbone A, Angelucci D, Gallina S, Calafiore AM, De Caterina R, Barsotti A. Left ventricular wall stress as a direct correlate of cardiomyocyte apoptosis in patients with severe dilated cardiomyopathy. *Am Heart J* 2003; 146: 1105–11. **35**

Domanski M, Norman J, Pitt B, Haigney M, Hanlon S, Peyster E. Diuretic use, progressive heart failure, and death in patients in the Studies Of Left Ventricular Dysfunction (SOLVD). *J Am Coll Cardiol* 2003; 42: 705–8. **86**

Dowling RD, Gray LA Jr, Etoch SW, Laks H, Marelli D, Samuels L, Entwistle J, Couper G, Vlahakes GJ, Frazier OH. Initial experience with the AbioCor implantable replacement heart system. *J Thorac Cardiovasc Surg* 2004; 127(1): 131–41. **232**

Fischer M, Baessler A, Hense HW, Hengstenberg C, Muscholl M, Holmer S, Doring A, Broeckel U, Riegger G, Schunkert H. Prevalence of left ventricular diastolic dysfunction in the community: results from a Doppler echocardiographic-based survey of a population sample. *Eur Heart J* 2003; 24(4): 320–8. **50**

Frazier OH, Myers TJ, Westaby S, Gregoric ID. Clinical experience with an implantable, intracardiac, continuous flow circulatory support device: physiologic implications and their relationship to patient selection. *Ann Thorac Surg* 2004; 77(1): 133–42. **229**

Gattis WA, O'Connor CM, Leimberger JD, Felker GM, Adams KF, Gheorghiade M. Clinical outcomes in patients on beta-blocker therapy admitted with worsening chronic heart failure. *Am J Cardiol* 2003; 91: 169–74. **76**

Ghali JK, Krause-Steinrauf HJ, Adams KF, Khan SS, Rosenberg YD, Yancy CW, Young JB, Goldman S, Peberdy MA, Lindenfeld J. Gender differences in advanced heart failure: insights from the BEST study. *J Am Coll Cardiol* 2003; 42(12): 2128–34. **33**

Gheorghiade M, Niazi I, Ouyang J, Czerwiec F, Kambayashi J, Zampino M, Orlandi C, for the Tolvaptan Investigators. Vasopressin V2-receptor blockade with tolvaptan in patients with chronic heart failure. *Circulation* 2003; 107: 2690–6. **85**

Giannuzzi P, Temporelli PL, Corra U Tavazzi L, for the ELVD-CHF Study Group. Antiremodeling effect of long-term exercise training in patients with stable chronic heart failure. *Circulation* 2003; 108: 554–9. **159**

Gielen S, Adams V, Mobius-Winkler S, Linke A, Erbs S, Yu J, Kempf W, Schubert A, Schuler G, Hambrecht R. Anti-inflammatory effects of exercise training in the skeletal muscle of patients with chronic heart failure. *J Am Coll Cardiol* 2003; 42 (5): 861–8. **164**

Granger CB, McMurray JJ, Yusuf S, Held P, Michelson EL, Olofsson B, Ostergren J, Pfeffer MA, Swedberg K; CHARM Investigators and Committees. Effects of candesartan in patients with chronic heart failure and reduced left-ventricular systolic function intolerant to angiotensin-converting-enzyme inhibitors: the CHARM-Alternative trial. CHARM Investigators and Committees. *Lancet* 2003; 362: 772–6. **72**

Gummert JF, Rahmel A, Bucerius J, Onnasch J, Doll N, Walther T, Falk V, Mohr FW. Mitral valve repair in patients with end-stage cardiomyopathy: who benefits? *Eur J Cardiothorac Surg* 2003; 23: 1017–22. **115**

Haider AW, Larson MG, Franklin SS, Levy D. Systolic blood pressure, diastolic blood pressure, and pulse pressure as predictors of risk for congestive heart failure in the Framingham Heart Study. *Ann Intern Med* 2003; 138(1): 10–16. **19**

Hayakawa Y, Chandra M, Miao W, Shirani J, Brown JH, Dorn GW 2nd, Armstrong RC, Kitsis RN. Inhibition of cardiac myocyte apoptosis improves cardiac function and abolishes mortality in the peripartum cardiomyopathy of $G\alpha(q)$ transgenic mice. *Circulation* 2003; 108: 3036–41. **28**

Hryniewicz K. Androne AS, Hudaihed A, Katz SD. Partial reversal of cachexia by β-adrenergic receptor blocker therapy in patients with chronic heart failure. *J Card Fail* 2003; 9: 464–8. **36**

Hu K, Li Q, Yang J, Hu S, Chen X. The effect of theophylline on sleep-disordered breathing in patients with stable chronic congestive heart failure. *Chin Med J (Engl)* 2003; 116(11): 1711–16. **152**

Kaneko Y, Floras JS, Usui K, Plante J, Tkacova R, Kubo T, Ando S, Bradley TD. Cardiovascular effects of continuous positive airway pressure in patients with heart failure and obstructive sleep apnea. *N Engl J Med* 2003; 348(13): 1233–41. **153**

Kawaguchi M, Hay I, Fetics B, Kass DA. Combined ventricular systolic and arterial stiffening in patients with heart failure and preserved ejection fraction: implications for systolic and diastolic reserve limitations. *Circulation* 2003; 107: 714–20. **42**

Peterson LR, Schechtman KB, Ewald GA, Geltman EM, Meyer T, Krekeler P, Rogers JG. The effect of β-adrenergic blockers on the prognostic value of peak exercise oxygen uptake in patients with heart failure. *J Heart Lung Transplant* 2003; 22: 70–7. **173**

Pfeffer MA, McMurray JJ, Velazquez EJ, Rouleau JL, Køber L, Maggioni AP, Solomon SD, Swedberg K, Van de Werf F, White H, Leimberger JD, Henis M, Edwards S, Zelenkofske S, Sellers MA, Califf RM, for the Valsartan in Acute Myocardial Infarction Trial Investigators. Valsartan, captopril, or both in myocardial infarction complicated by heart failure, left ventricular dysfunction, or both. *N Engl J Med* 2003; 349: 1893–906. **74**

Pitt B, Remme W, Zannad F, Neaton J, Martinez F, Roniker B, Bittman R, Hurley S, Kleiman J, Gatlin M; Eplerenone Post-Acute Myocardial Infarction Heart Failure Efficacy and Survival Study Investigators. Eplerenone, a selective aldosterone blocker, in patients with left ventricular dysfunction after myocardial infarction. *N Engl J Med* 2003; 348: 1309–21. **68**

Poole-Wilson PA, Swedberg K, Cleland JG F, Di Lenarda A, Hanrath P, Komajda M, Lubsen J, LutigerB, Metra M, Remme WJ, Torp-Pedersen C, Scherhag A, Skene A, and COMET investigators. Comparison of carvedilol and metoprolol on clinical outcomes in patients with chronic heart failure in the Carvedilol Or Metoprolol European Trial (COMET): randomized controlled trial. *Lancet* 2003; 362: 7–13. **75**

Rathore SS, Curtis JP, Wang Y, Bristow MR, Krumholz HM. Association of serum digoxin concentration and outcomes in patients with heart failure. *JAMA* 2003; 289: 871–8. **79**

Rathore SS, Foody JM, Wang Y, Smith GL, Herrin J, Masoudi FA, Wolfe P,

Havranek EP, Ordin DL, Krumholz HM. Race, quality of care, and outcomes of elderly patients hospitalized with heart failure. *JAMA* 2003; 289(19): 2517–24. **23**

Redfield MM, Jacobsen SJ, Burnett JC Jr, Mahoney DW, Bailey KR, Rodeheffer RJ. Burden of systolic and diastolic ventricular dysfunction in the community: appreciating the scope of the heart failure epidemic. *JAMA* 2003; 289: 194–202. **10 48**

Reinlib L, Abraham W. Recovery from heart failure with circulatory assist: a Working Group of the National Heart, Lung, and Blood Institute. *J Card Fail* 2003; 9(6): 459–63. **230**

Rickli H, Kiowski W, Brehm M, Weilenmann D, Schalcher C, Bernheim A, Oechslin E, Brunner-La Rocca HP. Combining low-intensity and maximal exercise test results improves prognostic prediction in chronic heart failure. *J Am Coll Cardiol* 2003; 42: 116–22. **169**

Rose EA, Gelijns AC, Moskowitz AJ, Heitjan DF, Stevenson LW, Dembitsky W, Long JW, Ascheim DD, Tierney AR, Levitan RG, Watson JT, Meier P, Ronan NS, Shapiro PA, Lazar RM, Miller LW, Gupta L, Frazier OH, Desvigne-Nickens P, Oz MC, Poirier VL; Randomized Evaluation Of Mechanical Assistance for the Treatment of Congestive Heart Failure (REMATCH) Study Group. Long-term mechanical left ventricular assistance for end-stage heart failure. *N Engl J Med* 2001; 345(20): 1435–43. **228**

Roveda F, Middlekauff HR, Rondon MU, Reis SF, Souza M, Nastari L, Barretto AC, Krieger EM, Negrao CE. The effects of exercise training on sympathetic neural activation in advanced heart failure. *J Am Coll Cardiol* 2003; 42(5): 854–60. **161**

Sabbah HN, Sharov VG, Gupta RC, Mishra S, Rastogi S, Undrovinas AI, Chaudhry PA, Todor A, Mishima T, Tanhehco EJ, Suzuki G. Reversal of chronic molecular and cellular abnormalities due to

Vasan RS, Sullivan LM, Roubenoff R, Dinarello CA, Harris T, Benjamin EJ, Sawyer DB, Levy D, Wilson PW, D'Agostino RB. Inflammatory markers and risk of heart failure in the elderly subjects without prior myocardial infarction: the Framingham Heart Study. *Circulation* 2003; 107(11): 1486–91. **16**

Vatta M, Mohapatra B, Jimenez S, Sanchez X, Faulkner G, Perles Z, Sinagra G, Lin JH, Vu TM, Zhou Q, Bowles KR, Di Lenarda A, Schimmenti L, Fox M, Chrisco MA, Murphy RT, McKenna W, Elliott P, Bowles NE, Chen J, Valle G, Towbin JA. Mutations in *Cypher/ZASP* in patients with dilated cardiomyopathy and left ventricular non-compaction. *J Am Coll Cardiol* 2003; 42(11): 2014–27. **255**

Wang TJ, Evans JC, Benjamin EJ, Levy D, LeRoy EC, Vasan RS. Natural history of asymptomatic left ventricular systolic dysfunction in the community. *Circulation* 2003; 108(8); 977–82. **7**

Wang TJ, Larson MG, Levy D, Vasan RS, Leip EP, Wolf PA, D'Agostino PB, Murabito JM, Kannel WB, Benjamin AJ. Temporal relations of atrial fibrillation and congestive heart failure and their joint influence on mortality: the Framingham Heart Study. *Circulation* 2003; 107(23): 2920–5. **14**

Wilkoff BL, Cook JR, Epstein AE, Greene HL, Hallstrom AP, Hsia H, Kutalek SP, Sharma A; Dual Chamber and VVI Implantable Defibrillator Trial Investigators. Dual-chamber pacing or ventricular backup pacing in patients with an implantable defibrillator: the Dual Chamber And VVI Implantable Defibrillator (DAVID) Trial. *JAMA* 2002; 288(24): 3115–23. **225**

Yamaguchi H, Yoshida J, Yamamoto K, Sakata Y, Mano T, Akehi N, Hori M, Lim YJ, Mishima M, Masuyama T. Elevation of plasma brain natriuretic peptide is a hallmark of diastolic heart failure independent of ventricular hypertrophy. *J Am Coll Cardiol* 2004; 43: 55–60. **46**

Yasumura Y, Takemura K, Sakamoto A, Kitakaze M, Miyatake K MD. Changes in myocardial gene expression associated with β blocker therapy in patients with chronic heart failure. *J Card Fail* 2003; 9: 469–74. **31**

Yusuf S, Pfeffer MA, Swedberg K, Granger CB, Held P, McMurray JJ, Michelson EL, Olofsson B, Ostergren J; CHARM Investigators and Committees. Effects of candesartan in patients with chronic heart failure and preserved left-ventricular ejection fraction: the CHARM-Preserved Trial. *Lancet* 2003; 362(9386): 777–81. **56** **73**

General index

KEEPING UP TO DATE IN ONE SERIES

"The Year in ..."

EXISTING AND FUTURE VOLUMES

The Year in Allergy 2003	ISBN 1 904392 05 9
The Year in Allergy 2004	ISBN 1 904392 25 3
The Year in Diabetes 2003	ISBN 1 904392 02 4
The Year in Diabetes 2004	ISBN 1 904392 20 2
The Year in Dyslipidaemia 2003	ISBN 1 904392 07 5
The Year in Dyslipidaemia 2004	ISBN 1 904392 21 0
The Year in Gynaecology 2001	ISBN 0 9537339 2 0
The Year in Gynaecology 2002	ISBN 1 904392 01 6
The Year in Gynaecology 2003	ISBN 1 904392 10 5
The Year in Hypertension 2003	ISBN 1 904392 13 X
The Year in Hypertension 2004	ISBN 1 904392 28 8
The Year in Infection 2003	ISBN 1 904392 12 1
The Year in Interventional Cardiology 2002	ISBN 0 9537339 7 1
The Year in Interventional Cardiology 2003	ISBN 1 904392 14 8
The Year in Neurology 2003	ISBN 1 904392 03 2
The Year in Neurology 2004	ISBN 1 904392 22 9
The Year in Osteoporosis 2004	ISBN 1 904392 27 X
The Year in Post-Menopausal Health 2004	ISBN 1 904392 23 7
The Year in Respiratory Medicine 2003	ISBN 0 9537339 8 X
The Year in Respiratory Medicine 2004	ISBN 1 904392 31 8
The Year in Rheumatic Disorders 2002	ISBN 0 9537339 9 8
The Year in Rheumatic Disorders 2003	ISBN 1 904392 09 1
The Year in Rheumatic Disorders Volume 4	ISBN 1 904392 29 6
The Year in Urology 2003	ISBN 1 904392 06 7

To receive more information about these books and future volumes,
or to order copies, please contact us at the address below:

Atlas Medical Publishing Ltd
Oxford Centre for Innovation
Mill Street
Oxford OX2 0JX, UK

T: +44 1865 811116
F: +44 1865 251550
E: info@clinicalpublishing.co.uk
W: www.clinicalpublishing.co.uk